Early Detection and Treatment of Head & Neck Cancers
Theoretical Background and Newly Emerging Research

头颈肿瘤的早期诊断与治疗

理论背景与前沿研究

主编

［美］Rami El Assal

［美］Dyani Gaudilliere

［美］Stephen Thaddeus Connelly

主译

田 皞　阮 敏

安常明　单小峰

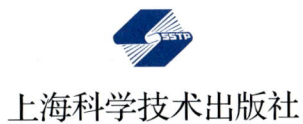

上海科学技术出版社

图书在版编目（CIP）数据

头颈肿瘤的早期诊断与治疗：理论背景与前沿研究 / （美）拉米·阿萨勒等主编；田皞等主译. -- 上海：上海科学技术出版社，2025.8. -- ISBN 978-7-5478-7281-9

Ⅰ. R739.91

中国国家版本馆CIP数据核字第2025485MX6号

First published in English under the title
Early Detection and Treatment of Head & Neck Cancers
by Stephen Thaddeus Connelly, Rami El Assal and Dyani Gaudilliere
Copyright © Springer Nature Switzerland AG 2021
This edition has been translated and published under licence from Springer Nature Switzerland AG.

上海市版权局著作权合同登记号 图字：09-2025-0478号

封面图片由译者提供

头颈肿瘤的早期诊断与治疗：理论背景与前沿研究
主编 ［美］Rami El Assal
　　　［美］Dyani Gaudilliere
　　　［美］Stephen Thaddeus Connelly
主译　田　皞　阮　敏　安常明　单小峰

上海世纪出版(集团)有限公司
上海科学技术出版社　　出版、发行
(上海市闵行区号景路159弄A座9F-10F)
邮政编码201101　www.sstp.cn
山东京沪印刷科技有限公司印刷
开本 889×1194　1/16　印张 10.5
字数 275千字
2025年8月第1版　2025年8月第1次印刷
ISBN 978-7-5478-7281-9/R·3329
定价：168.00元

本书如有缺页、错装或坏损等严重质量问题，请向印刷厂联系调换

内容提要

本书针对头颈肿瘤早期检测与处理，从早癌发生的机制到相关最新临床应用技术做了全面梳理与论述。本书主要内容包括：头颈肿瘤的流行病学、病因学、症状、分期和诊断的综述，口腔早期恶性病变相关研究进展，头颈癌的基因组学、促炎信号通路、循环肿瘤标志物等一些新兴研究领域的情况，头颈癌相关慢性疼痛的机制和处理策略，口腔黏膜给药系统在头颈癌领域的研究现状等。本书内容前沿，反映了当下头颈肿瘤领域的发展趋势，适合头颈外科、口腔颌面外科、放疗科、肿瘤科医生和相关研究人员阅读与参考。

献　词

谨以本专著献给斯坦福大学已故 Sam Gambhir 教授。

作为癌症早期检测领域的奠基人，Gambhir 教授毕生致力于疾病早期诊断方法的研发。他开创性地将分子影像学与纳米技术相结合，引领了在疾病萌芽阶段捕获生物信号的新纪元。Gambhir 教授生前担任斯坦福大学医学院 Virginia and D.K. Ludwig 癌症研究讲席教授、放射学系主任，同时创立并领导斯坦福大学 Canary 癌症早期检测中心、精准健康与整合诊断中心，兼任分子影像研究项目负责人。

主编 Rami El Assal 博士深切缅怀这位仁厚谦逊的学者："在我即将离开斯坦福的告别会谈中，Gambhir 教授展现出多层次的人文关怀，并特别承诺'若您希望重返斯坦福，请随时告知'。"

Assal 博士追忆道："2015 年放射学系会议上，Gambhir 教授曾立誓'愿毕生致力于人类健康事业，纵使成就不获当世认可'。而今观之，其志已成。"

译者名单

主　译
田　皞　阮　敏　安常明　单小峰

主　审
张陈平　刘绍严　蔡志刚　喻建军

副主译
陈　超·浙江省肿瘤医院头颈外科
姚志红·云南省癌症防治中心
颜仕鹏·湖南省癌症防治中心
蒋灿华·中南大学湘雅医院口腔医学中心
周　旋·天津医科大学肿瘤医院颌面耳鼻咽喉肿瘤科
黄志权·中山大学孙逸仙纪念医院口腔颌面外科

译　者（按姓氏拼音排序）
蔡　旭·湖南省肿瘤医院头颈外科
蔡永聪·四川省肿瘤医院头颈外科
陈佳铭·湖南省肿瘤医院头颈外科
陈　健·湖北省肿瘤医院头颈外科
谌　星·湖南省肿瘤医院头颈外科
戴　捷·湖南省肿瘤医院头颈外科
冯芝恩·首都医科大学附属北京口腔医院口腔颌面头颈肿瘤外科
高水超·湖南省肿瘤医院头颈外科
葛姝云·上海交通大学医学院附属第九人民医院口腔黏膜病科
韩亚骞·湖南省肿瘤医院头颈/口腔颌面肿瘤诊疗中心

黄文孝·湖南省肿瘤医院头颈/口腔颌面肿瘤诊疗中心
金和坤·湖南省肿瘤医院头颈/口腔颌面肿瘤诊疗中心
李和清·中南大学湘雅三医院耳鼻咽喉头颈外科
李晋芸·湖南省肿瘤医院头颈外科
李仕晟·中南大学湘雅二医院耳鼻咽喉头颈外科
李　赞·湖南省肿瘤医院头颈/口腔颌面肿瘤诊疗中心
林劲冠·湖南省肿瘤医院头颈/口腔颌面肿瘤诊疗中心
刘法昱·中国医科大学附属口腔医院口腔颌面外科
刘　峰·湖南省肿瘤医院头颈/口腔颌面肿瘤诊疗中心
刘　彦·湖南省肿瘤医院头颈外科
刘　勇·中南大学湘雅医院耳鼻咽喉头颈外科
苗素生·哈尔滨医科大学附属肿瘤医院头颈外科
彭小伟·湖南省肿瘤医院头颈/口腔颌面肿瘤诊疗中心
钱　永·海南省肿瘤医院头颈外科
任　玉·天津医科大学
邵　喆·武汉大学口腔医院口腔颌面－头颈肿瘤外科
盛健峰·绵阳市第三人民医院耳鼻咽喉科
宋达疆·湖南省肿瘤医院头颈/口腔颌面肿瘤诊疗中心
苏　彤·中南大学湘雅医院口腔颌面外科
孙传政·云南省肿瘤医院头颈外科
王　成·中山大学附属口腔医院口腔颌面外科
王鸿涵·湖南省肿瘤医院头颈外科
王　健·中国医学科学院肿瘤医院头颈外科
王　宇·天津医科大学肿瘤医院颌面耳鼻咽喉肿瘤科
魏　攀·北京大学口腔医院口腔黏膜科
闫　冰·四川大学华西口腔医院头颈肿瘤外科
张海林·湖南省肿瘤医院头颈外科
张　胜·中南大学湘雅二医院口腔颌面外科
张松涛·河南省肿瘤医院甲状腺头颈外科
张　泽·天津医科大学肿瘤医院颌面耳鼻咽喉肿瘤科
章文博·北京大学口腔医院口腔颌面外科
朱小峰·福建医科大学附属第一医院口腔颌面外科
左　良·湖南省肿瘤医院头颈外科

主编简介

Rami El Assal

Canary Center at Stanford for Cancer Early Detection

Stanford University School of Medicine

Palo Alto, CA

USA

Dyani Gaudilliere

Division of Plastic & Reconstructive Surgery, Department of Surgery

Stanford University School of Medicine

Palo Alto, CA

USA

Stephen Thaddeus Connelly

Department of Oral and Maxillofacial Surgery

University of California, San Francisco

San Francisco, CA

USA

编者名单

Hamzah Alkofahi Division of Plastic & Reconstructive Surgery, Department of Surgery, Stanford University School of Medicine, Stanford, CA, USA
Department of Oral and Maxillofacial Surgery, Jordanian Royal Medical Services, Irbid, Jordan

Zhong Chen Tumor Biology Section, Head and Neck Surgery Branch, National Institute on Deafness and Other Communication Disorders, National Institutes of Health, Bethesda, MD, USA

Stephen Thaddeus Connelly Department of Oral and Maxillofacial Surgery, University of California San Francisco (UCSF) School of Dentistry, San Francisco, CA, USA
San Francisco VA Health Care System, San Francisco, CA, USA

Mehdi Ebrahimi Prince Philip Dental Hospital, The University of Hong Kong, Pok Fu Lam, Hong Kong, China

Lisa M. Evangelista Department of Otolaryngology/Head & Neck Surgery, University of California at Davis Medical Center, Sacramento, CA, USA

Ayman Fouad Department of Otolaryngology, Head & Neck Surgery, Stanford University, Stanford, CA, USA
Department of Otolaryngology, Head & Neck Surgery, Tanta University, Tanta, Egypt

Jennifer R. Grandis Department of Otolaryngology–Head and Neck Surgery, University of California at San Francisco, San Francisco, CA, USA

Jun Jeon Tumor Biology Section, Head and Neck Surgery Branch, National Institute on Deafness and Other Communication Disorders, National Institutes of Health, Bethesda, MD, USA

Daniel E. Johnson Department of Otolaryngology–Head and Neck Surgery, University of California at San Francisco, San Francisco, CA, USA

Nagarjun Konduru Department of Cellular and Molecular Biology, University of Texas Health Science Center at Tyler, Tyler, TX, USA

Shilpa Kusampudi Department of Cellular and Molecular Biology, University of Texas Health Science Center at Tyler, Tyler, TX, USA

Peter Luke Santa Maria Department of Oral Rehabilitation, Prince Philip Dental Hospital, The University of Hong Kong, Pok Fu Lam, Hong Kong, China

Solange Massa Department of Otolaryngology, Head & Neck Surgery, Stanford University, Stanford, CA, USA

Ethan L. Morgan Tumor Biology Section, Head and Neck Surgery Branch, National Institute on Deafness and Other Communication Disorders, National Institutes of Health, Bethesda, MD, USA

Taichiro Nonaka Center for Oral/Head and Neck Oncology Research, School of Dentistry, University of California, Los Angeles, Los Angeles, CA, USA
Division of Oral Biology and Medicine, School of Dentistry, University of California, Los Angeles, Los Angeles, CA, USA

Kelechi Nwachuku School of Medicine, University of California at San Francisco, San Francisco, CA, USA

M. Anthony Pogrel Department of Oral and Maxillofacial Surgery, University of California, San Francisco, San Francisco, CA, USA

Carter Van Waes Tumor Biology Section, Head and Neck Surgery Branch, National Institute on Deafness and Other Communication Disorders, National Institutes of Health, Bethesda, MD, USA

Ramya Viswanathan Tumor Biology Section, Head and Neck Surgery Branch, National Institute on Deafness and Other Communication Disorders, National Institutes of Health, Bethesda, MD, USA

David T. W. Wong Center for Oral/Head and Neck Oncology Research, School of Dentistry, University of California, Los Angeles, Los Angeles, CA, USA
Division of Oral Biology and Medicine, School of Dentistry, University of California, Los Angeles, Los Angeles, CA, USA

Justin M. Young Private Practice, San Francisco, CA, USA
Department of Oral & Maxillofacial Surgery, University of the Pacific, Arthur A. Dugoni School of Dentistry, San Francisco, CA, USA

中文版序

早诊早治——破解头颈癌生存困局的金钥匙

头颈部这片结构精密的狭小疆域,承载着人类最复杂的生理功能与社会属性。当癌症盘踞于此——一位喉癌患者失去发声能力,一位舌癌患者无法品尝食物滋味,一位上颌窦癌患者因面容改变而闭门不出——我们面对的不仅是肿瘤细胞的肆虐,更是人之为人的尊严崩塌。然而,临床实践与循证医学反复验证着一个真理:早期检测与诊断是扭转这场悲剧的最有力杠杆。数据显示,早期(Ⅰ~Ⅱ期)头颈鳞癌患者的 5 年生存率达到甚至超过 90%,而晚期(Ⅲ~Ⅳ期)患者骤降至 30%~40%。这悬殊的数字背后,是成千上万家庭截然不同的命运轨迹。

早期检测:在沉默中聆听癌变的"第一声啼哭"

头颈部解剖结构的特殊性,使得早期病灶往往隐匿于生理性不适的"伪装"之下。慢性咽炎与下咽癌早期均可表现为咽部异物感,口腔溃疡与舌癌初期均可引起局部疼痛——这种症状的重叠性导致头颈癌初诊误诊率接近一半患者。突破这一困局需要以下革新。

- 技术赋能:从肉眼观察到分子探针
  - 光学增强内镜:窄带成像(NBI)技术可使早期喉癌的检出率从传统白光镜的 58% 提升至 89%。
  - 液体活检突破:唾液外泌体 miRNA 检测在口腔癌前病变中已实现 84.7% 的敏感度。
  - 人工智能(AI)辅助诊断:深度学习模型对口腔白斑恶变预测的 AUC 值达 0.91,较专家肉眼判断提高 27%。
- 高危人群精准锚定
  - 风险分层模型:EPIC-HN 评分系统整合 HPV 感染、吸烟包年、EB 病毒抗体等多项指标,可筛出需重点监测的 5% 高危人群。
  - 癌前病变管理:口腔黏膜下纤维性变患者每年 3 次活检的监测方案,使癌变检出时间提前。

诊断革新：多维解码肿瘤的"生命密码"

当前，早期诊断的精准化正经历从形态学到功能学的范式转移。
- 空间维度：显微与宏观的融合
  - 共聚焦激光显微内镜：在体显示喉黏膜基底层的细胞异型性，实现"光学活检"（敏感度 92.3%，特异度 88.6%）。
  - 多模态影像导航：PET-MRI 融合技术将鼻咽癌 T 分期准确率提升至 93%，较传统 MRI 提高 19 个百分点。
- 时间维度：捕捉恶变的"临界瞬间"
  - 表观遗传时钟：通过检测抑癌基因甲基化程度，可预测口腔白斑在 18 个月内的恶变风险。
  - 动态荧光追踪：肿瘤特异性探针 MMP-2-ICG 能在术中发现 0.5 mm 的卫星病灶。

治疗策略：微创与功能保留的平衡艺术

早期诊断的价值，最终要转化为治疗策略的优化。
- 外科的"毫米级革命"
  - 经口机器人手术（TORS）对早期口咽癌的 3 年无病生存率达 91%，且 83% 患者术后无需气管切开。
  - 声带癌的激光显微手术可使 92% 患者保留接近正常的发声功能。
- 精准放疗的进化
  - 质子治疗对早期鼻咽癌的腮腺剂量降低 56%，显著减少口干症。
  - 自适应放疗通过每周 CT 重塑形，将局部控制率提升至 97%。
- 免疫预防的前沿探索
  - HPV 疫苗在男性中的推广使口咽癌发病率下降 21%。
  - 治疗性疫苗 EBV-LMP2 在鼻咽癌前病变中的有效率突破 67%。

未来展望：构建早诊早治的生态系统

当我们在实验室研发纳米探针、在手术室操作机械臂、在数据中心训练 AI 模型时，必须清醒认识到：技术突破必须与公共卫生策略同频共振。建议构建三级防控网络。

- 社区级：口腔科/耳鼻喉科医生主导的"3 分钟快速筛查"（白光检查＋风险问卷）。
- 区域级：配备 NBI 内镜的癌症早诊中心，实现"可疑病例 48 小时转诊"。
- 国家级：建立头颈部癌前病变注册系统，动态追踪百万级高危人群。

这本专著的每个章节，都凝聚着广大学者在头颈癌早诊早治道路上的智慧结晶。在中国抗癌协会口腔癌整合防筛专业委员会支持下，我们汇聚了耳鼻咽喉头颈外科、口腔颌面外科、放疗科、肿瘤科等领域专家来翻译本专著。从分子探针的实验室研发到乡村医生的筛查培训，从手术机器人的精度优化到患者发音重建的心理干预——我们期待这些知识能转化为临床实践的具体行动。因为每一个被早期发现的患者，不仅意味着统计学上的生存率提升，更是让一个家庭免于破碎——让一个孩子继续拥有说话发音的权利，让一位艺术家保住传递情感、塑造角色和表达艺术理念的能力……这正是医学最崇高的使命。

湖南省肿瘤医院　周　晓
2025 年 5 月

中文版前言

头颈癌作为全球范围内严重威胁人类健康的恶性肿瘤之一，其发病率近年来呈上升趋势。据统计，头颈癌位居全球常见癌症第六位，每年新增病例逾 70 万例，其中约 2/3 患者在确诊时已处于中晚期，导致治疗难度大、预后不佳。这一严峻现状凸显了早期检测与精准治疗在头颈癌管理中的核心地位。

近年来，随着分子生物学、影像学及基因组学技术的飞速发展，头颈癌的诊疗模式正经历革命性变革。传统依赖临床症状和病理活检的诊断方式逐步向多模态整合迈进。液体活检技术（如循环肿瘤 DNA、外泌体 miRNA）的兴起，为非侵入性早期筛查提供了新路径。研究表明，唾液与血浆中的肿瘤特异性标志物可灵敏反映口腔癌、鼻咽癌等病变，为高危人群筛查及治疗后监测开辟了广阔前景。与此同时，癌症基因组图谱（TCGA）计划的推进，揭示了头颈癌的突变谱系差异——HPV 阳性与阴性肿瘤在驱动基因（如 *TP53*、*PIK3CA*）和表观遗传特征上的分化，为个体化靶向治疗奠定了分子基础。

在治疗领域，微创手术［如经口机器人手术（TORS）］与精准放疗［如调强放疗（IMRT）］的应用显著提升了功能保留率；免疫治疗（如 PD-1/PD-L1 抑制剂）和靶向药物（如 EGFR 单抗）的突破，则为晚期患者带来了生存希望。然而，挑战依然存在：早期病变的隐匿性、治疗耐药性的频发、吞咽功能与生活质量的长期管理，仍需多学科协作与技术创新。

在中国抗癌协会口腔癌整合防筛专业委员会的支持下，我们组织国内头颈外科、口腔颌面外科、肿瘤科等多个领域的专家翻译了这本专著。本书立足于全球头颈癌研究前沿，系统梳理了从流行病学、病因机制到临床诊疗的全链条知识体系。书中不仅详述了传统诊疗技术的优化路径，更聚焦于新兴技术转化——纳米技术、基因治疗、ctDNA 动态监测等，勾勒出未来"早筛-早诊-精准干预"的一体化蓝图。

展望未来，头颈癌的防控必将迈向更高维度的整合医学时代。通过跨学科协作、大数据驱动的风险预测模型，以及患者全程管理体系的完善，我们有望在降低发病率的同时，实现"治愈"与"生存质量"的双重突破。谨以此书献给奋战在头颈癌领域的同仁，愿我们携手共进，为终结这一疾病的威胁而不懈努力。

湖南省肿瘤医院　田 皞
2025 年 4 月

英文版序

谨为本书作序，幸甚至哉。随着理论体系日臻完善与临床实践持续深化，癌症生物学领域早期检测与治疗技术正经历跨越式发展。

2015年，Nature杂志发布了迄今最全面的头颈癌基因组数据，该研究源自美国国立卫生研究院资助的癌症基因组图谱（The Cancer Genome Atlas, TCGA）计划。此项突破使科研人员得以优化现有头颈癌生物标志物目录，并发现新型早期诊断标志物。鉴于约2/3头颈癌确诊时已届晚期且预后不良，知识体系的持续拓展尤为重要。当前亟需创新早期检测手段以改善治疗效果，其中循环DNA作为非侵入性生物标志物在多项头颈癌队列研究中展现显著优势。通过分析体液中头颈癌特征性突变谱识别肿瘤DNA的技术，在早期肿瘤筛查、复发监测及疗效评估方面凸显出临床应用潜力。

精准医疗时代背景下，基于个体化数据制订最优治疗方案已成为可能。整合多模态医学数据（包括液体活检、唾液生物标志物、影像学检查等），并应用经严格验证的创新疗法（涵盖基因治疗、免疫治疗、手术、放疗等），可显著提升头颈癌诊疗效能。

尽管早期检测领域已取得长足进步，其学科发展仍处于初级阶段。我们在基础理论层面成果丰硕，但在检测技术转化、诊断标准优化及治疗体系完善等方面仍需持续探索，以期最终实现包括头颈癌在内的肿瘤的有效预防。

诚邀读者深入研读本书作者团队精心编写的学术内容，这些成果既植根于坚实的科学证据，又凝聚了多年临床实践积累的宝贵经验。

R. Bruce Donoff, DMD, MD
Dean of Harvard School of Dental Medicine (1991–2019)
Boston, MA, USA

荣休院长 R. Bruce Donoff 简介

R. Bruce Donoff 博士于 1991—2019 年间担任哈佛大学牙医学院（HSDM）院长。生于纽约布鲁克林，本科就读于布鲁克林学院，1967 年获哈佛大学牙医学院牙科博士学位（DMD），1973 年获哈佛医学院医学博士学位（MD）。其职业生涯始终扎根于哈佛大学医学部及麻省总医院口腔颌面外科：1967 年以实习医师身份开启职业生涯，1982—1993 年间担任科室主任兼首席医师，至今仍坚持临床诊疗工作。

除担任院长外，Donoff 博士在口腔颌面外科领域的研究贡献卓著，尤专注于口腔及头颈癌诊疗。已发表学术论文逾百篇，主编多部教科书并在全球开展学术讲座。近期主导推动"HSDM 口腔医学整合计划"，该跨学科项目系其学术理念的重要实践载体。

Donoff 博士曾任口腔颌面外科基金会理事（任期 12 年）、美国国立牙科与颅面研究院之友协会主席，现任《麻省总医院口腔颌面外科诊疗规范》主编，兼任《口腔颌面外科杂志》及《麻省牙科学会期刊》编委。

其学术生涯荣膺多项殊荣：美国口腔颌面外科医师协会研究成就奖、William J. Gies 口腔颌面外科学基金会奖、美国科学促进会会士、Alpha Omege 杰出成就奖、哈佛大学牙医学院杰出校友及教师奖等。2014 年获颁 Shils-Meskin 牙科领袖奖，以表彰其对牙科专业的卓越领导力。

英文版前言

本书系统梳理了头颈肿瘤领域的理论基础与前沿研究进展，旨在为读者呈现当前医学界对该疾病的深入认知与创新探索。

本书开篇全面综述了头颈癌的流行病学特征、病因学机制、临床表现、诊断标准及临床分期体系，并着重探讨口腔潜在恶性疾病的诊疗要点——此类疾病是头颈癌的重要亚型之一。

随后，本书聚焦头颈癌研究领域的新兴方向。例如，近数十年来基因组学技术的突破性进展，助力研究者更精准地解析头颈癌的基因突变谱；对促炎信号通路的系统性研究，为早期生物标志物的发现及新型治疗策略的开发提供了科学依据。此外，越来越多的研究表明，循环肿瘤 DNA（ctDNA）、循环肿瘤细胞（CTC）及外泌体 miRNA 等液体活检标志物，为头颈癌的全程监测、早期筛查与精准干预开辟了新路径。这些研究的终极目标在于推动精准医学的临床应用，从而为患者提供个体化诊疗方案。

本书末章深入探讨了头颈癌相关慢性疼痛的病理机制与综合管理策略，并介绍了新兴的口腔黏膜黏附给药技术。无论是临床医师、科研人员、医学生，抑或是深受疾病影响的患者及家属，皆能从中理解疼痛对患者生存质量与康复进程的深远影响。

本书编写团队秉承学术严谨性，力求通过翔实的数据支持、典型的案例剖析及相关领域专家评述，为读者构建多维知识体系。我们希望本书能为头颈癌的基础研究与临床实践提供有价值的参考，助力学界与医疗工作者提升诊疗水平，最终惠及广大患者。

Rami El Assal
Palo Alto, CA, USA

Dyani Gaudilliere
Palo Alto, CA, USA

Stephen Thaddeus Connelly
San Francisco, CA, USA

致 谢

历 史 回 眸

未来岁月里某个时刻，我必将叹息着诉说：
林中有双径歧分，我择罕行之途，
而这抉择改变了一切。

——罗伯特·弗罗斯特《未择之路》（1916）

首先谨以至诚感恩我的家人。

致母亲：您以非凡坚忍伴我走过漫漫长路，步履间尽显优雅，明眸中蕴含星辰，举手投足皆展露慈爱尊严。我之所有与所求，皆承恩于您——我的天使母亲。

致爱妻 Somayeh 与爱子 Adam：你们是我的世界与存在的意义。感谢你们理解我从事医疗服务的职业常需夙夜匪懈，感恩你们的耐心与包容。

致胞妹 Lina：您始终如一的支持与指引伴我前行；挚诚的妹夫 Ghiath；以及四位淑媛侄女：Sana、Maria、Naya、Zeina。

致手足 Shadi：您永远是我坚实的后盾。

永志先父：您集刚毅与仁厚于一身（愿您安息）。

致堂兄 Hussein：珍视与您肝胆相照的友谊。

致岳家双亲、内弟 Wahid，以及四位贤淑妻姐：Susan、Samira、Sudaba、Saeeda。

致视若家人的挚友们：你们塑造了我的学术根基，始终支持我在专业领域的不断求索。

特别鸣谢联合主编 Dyani 与 Thaddeus：本书付梓仰赖二位鼎力相助。我以你们为荣，这份情谊铭感五内。期待未来继续携手并进，共筑学术理想。

衷心感谢全体撰稿学者：本书之成，端赖诸君学术精粹。

承蒙哈佛大学荣休院长 R. Bruce Donoff 教授赐序，谨致谢忱。

致授业恩师、学术引路人与同窗益友：冀本书不负诸位昔日之厚赐。

致全球同仁：感谢你们持续的专业支持。

最后，谨向头颈癌患者致以崇高敬意。为践行服务承诺，近期我与 Thaddeus 联合创立"早期疾病检测与治疗基金"（Early Disease Detection & Treatment Fund），致力推动实验室创新成果临床转化。幸得远见卓识的企业家携手投资，以期共克头颈癌诊疗难题。

Rami El Assal
Palo Alto, CA, USA

目　录

第 1 章 头颈癌概述：病因、症状、诊断、分期、预防和治疗 ………………………… 001
General Introduction to Head and Neck Cancer: Etiology, Symptoms, Diagnosis, Staging, Prevention, and Treatment
Shilpa Kusampudi and Nagarjun Konduru

第 2 章 口腔潜在恶性病变 ……………………………………………………………… 035
Potentially Malignant Disorders of the Oral Cavity
Hamzah Alkofahi and Mehdi Ebrahimi

第 3 章 口内上皮异常增生的诊断和治疗 ……………………………………………… 050
Diagnosis and Management of Intraoral Epithelial Dysplasia
M. Anthony Pogrel

第 4 章 头颈肿瘤中的吞咽困难 ………………………………………………………… 059
Dysphagia in Head and Neck Cancers
Lisa M. Evangelista

第 5 章 头颈鳞癌的突变景观：通过分析循环肿瘤 DNA 进行检测和监测 …………… 069
The Mutational Landscape of Head and Neck Squamous Cell Carcinoma: Opportunities for Detection and Monitoring Via Analysis of Circulating Tumor DNA
Kelechi Nwachuku, Daniel E. Johnson, and Jennifer R. Grandis

第 6 章　头颈癌循环生物标志物 ······ 080
Circulating Biomarkers in Head and Neck Cancer
Taichiro Nonaka and David T. W. Wong

第 7 章　头颈癌中的促炎信号通路和基因组特征 ······ 094
Proinflammatory Signaling Pathways and Genomic Signatures in Head and Neck Cancers
Zhong Chen, Ramya Viswanathan, Ethan L. Morgan, Jun Jeon, and Carter Van Waes

第 8 章　头颈癌相关疼痛 ······ 122
Pain Associated with Head and Neck Cancers
Justin M. Young and Stephen Thaddeus Connelly

第 9 章　口腔黏膜黏附给药治疗头颈癌的发展趋势 ······ 131
Emerging Trends in Oral Mucoadhesive Drug Delivery for Head and Neck Cancer
Solange Massa, Ayman Fouad, Mehdi Ebrahimi, and Peter Luke Santa Maria

第 1 章

Shilpa Kusampudi and Nagarjun Konduru

头颈癌概述：病因、症状、诊断、分期、预防和治疗

General Introduction to Head and Neck Cancer: Etiology, Symptoms, Diagnosis, Staging, Prevention, and Treatment

引 言

头颈癌是一组起源于嘴唇、口腔、口咽、唾液腺、喉、咽、下咽、鼻咽和鼻窦的癌症（图1-1）。这些癌症最常累及鳞状细胞，约占所有头颈癌的90%[1-4]。在20世纪50年代，颜面骨肿瘤、颈部原发及转移性肿瘤和甲状腺肿瘤也被称为头颈肿瘤[5]。但当前已将这些恶性肿瘤归属为不同的类别，如甲状腺和甲状旁腺恶性肿瘤被归类为内分泌肿瘤，淋巴结肿瘤被归类为血液系统恶性肿瘤等。

人体各部位的肿瘤有特定的编码，其中C00～C14、C30和C32是头颈癌的编码（表1-1）。

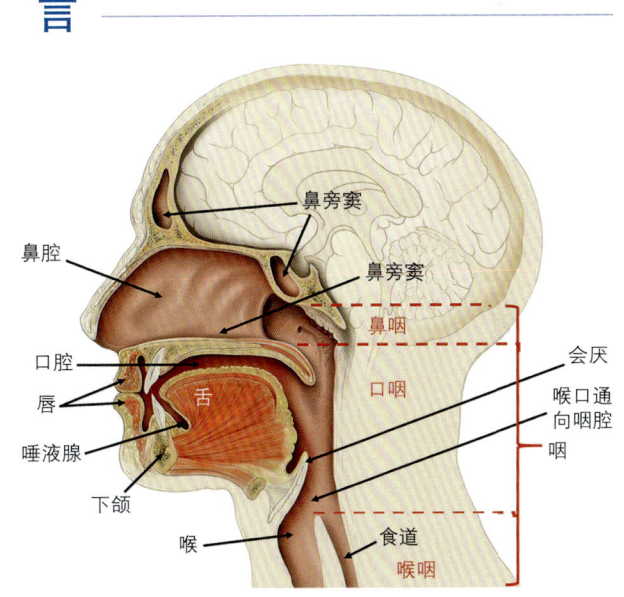

图1-1 头颈癌区域[6]

表1-1 头颈癌编码

癌症编码	癌	癌症编码	癌
C00～C06	唇、口腔	C002	部位未特指的唇外侧面恶性肿瘤
C000	上唇外侧面恶性肿瘤	C003	上唇内侧面恶性肿瘤
C001	下唇外侧面恶性肿瘤	C004	下唇内侧面恶性肿瘤

S. Kusampudi · N. Konduru (✉)
Department of Cellular and Molecular Biology, University of Texas Health Science Center at Tyler, Tyler, TX, USA
e-mail: nagarjun.konduruvenkata@uthct.edu

续　表

癌症编码	癌	癌症编码	癌
C005	部位未特指的唇内侧恶性肿瘤	C07～C08	唾液腺
C006	部位未特指的唇接合部恶性肿瘤	C07	腮腺恶性肿瘤
C008	唇交界部恶性肿瘤	C080	颌下腺恶性肿瘤
C009	部位未特指的唇部恶性肿瘤	C081	舌下腺恶性肿瘤
C010	舌根恶性肿瘤	C089	部位未特指的大唾液腺恶性肿瘤
C020	舌背恶性肿瘤	C09～C10	口咽
C021	舌缘恶性肿瘤	C090	扁桃体窝恶性肿瘤
C022	舌腹恶性肿瘤	C091	（前后）扁桃体柱恶性肿瘤
C023	部位未特指的舌前2/3的恶性肿瘤	C098	扁桃体交界部位的恶性肿瘤
C024	舌扁桃体恶性肿瘤	C099	部位未特指的扁桃体恶性肿瘤
C028	舌交界部位的恶性肿瘤	C100	舌根凹陷处恶性肿瘤
C029	部位未特指的舌恶性肿瘤	C101	会厌前部恶性肿瘤
C030	上牙龈恶性肿瘤	C102	口咽侧壁恶性肿瘤
C031	下牙龈恶性肿瘤	C103	口咽后壁恶性肿瘤
C039	部位未特指的牙龈恶性肿瘤	C104	鳃裂恶性肿瘤
C040	口底前部恶性肿瘤	C108	口咽交界部位的恶性肿瘤
C041	口底外侧恶性肿瘤	C109	部位未特指的口咽部恶性肿瘤
C048	口底交界部位的恶性肿瘤	C11	鼻咽
C049	部位未特指的口底恶性肿瘤	C110	鼻咽上壁恶性肿瘤
C050	硬腭恶性肿瘤	C111	鼻咽后壁恶性肿瘤
C051	软腭恶性肿瘤	C112	鼻咽侧壁恶性肿瘤
C052	悬雍垂恶性肿瘤	C113	鼻咽前壁恶性肿瘤
C058	腭交界部位的恶性肿瘤	C118	鼻咽交界部位的恶性肿瘤
C059	部位未特指的腭恶性肿瘤	C119	部位未特指的鼻咽部恶性肿瘤
C060	颊黏膜恶性肿瘤	C12～C13	下咽部
C061	口腔前庭恶性肿瘤	C12	梨状窝恶性肿瘤
C062	磨牙后区恶性肿瘤	C130	环后区恶性肿瘤
C0680	部位未特指的口腔重叠部位的恶性肿瘤	C131	下咽侧构会厌襞恶性肿瘤
C0689	口腔其他部位交界的恶性肿瘤	C132	下咽后壁恶性肿瘤
C069	部位未特指的口腔恶性肿瘤	C138	下咽交界部位的恶性肿瘤

续 表

癌症编码	癌	癌症编码	癌
C139	部位未特指的下咽恶性肿瘤	C312	额窦恶性肿瘤
C14	部位未特指	C313	蝶窦恶性肿瘤
C140	部位未特指的咽恶性肿瘤	C318	鼻窦交界部位恶性肿瘤
C142	咽淋巴环恶性肿瘤	C319	部位未特指的鼻窦恶性肿瘤
C148	唇部、口腔和咽部交界部位的恶性肿瘤	C32	声门
C30～C31	鼻腔、鼻窦	C321	声门上恶性肿瘤
C30	鼻腔恶性肿瘤	C322	声门下恶性肿瘤
C301	中耳恶性肿瘤	C323	喉软骨恶性肿瘤
C310	上颌窦恶性肿瘤	C328	喉交界部位的恶性肿瘤
C311	筛窦恶性肿瘤	C329	部位未特指的喉部恶性肿瘤

流 行 病 学

据估计，头颈癌发病位居所有恶性肿瘤第六位（图1-2）。2018年，全球新增1 800万癌症病例中有710 237例为头颈癌。

根据2018年Globocan全球癌症数据，全球头颈癌的发病数占所有癌症的4.9%（图1-3）。在各种头颈癌中，唇和口腔癌占全球头颈癌病例

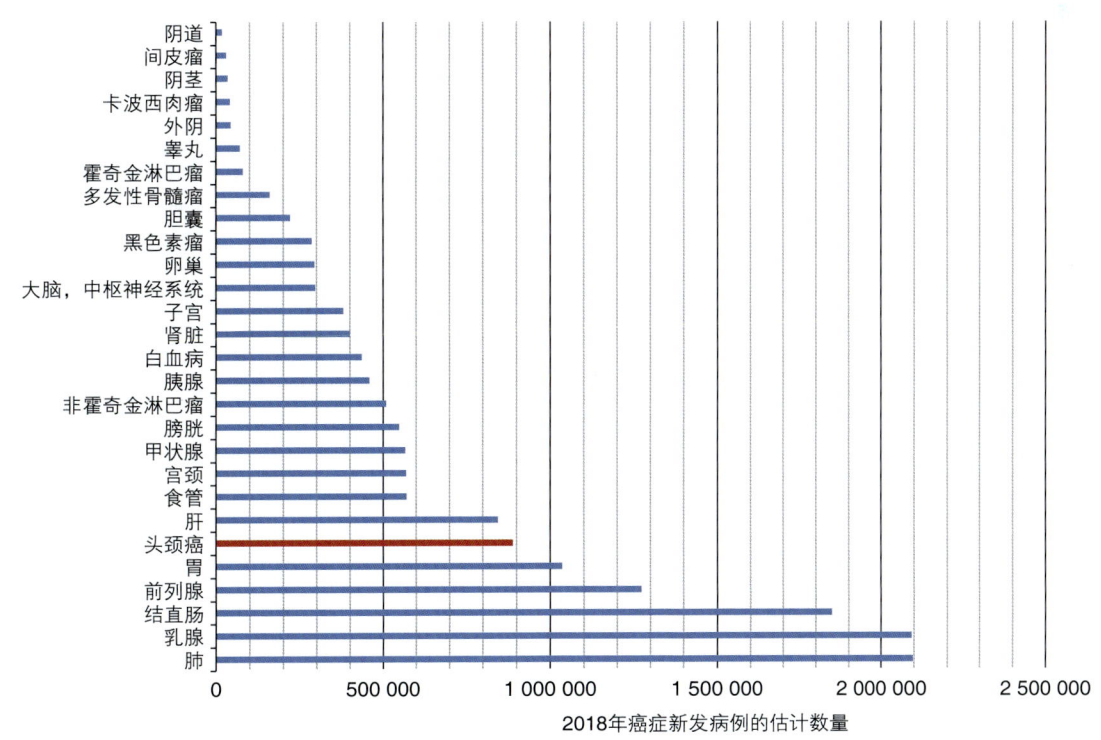

图1-2 2018年全球癌症新发病例数估计

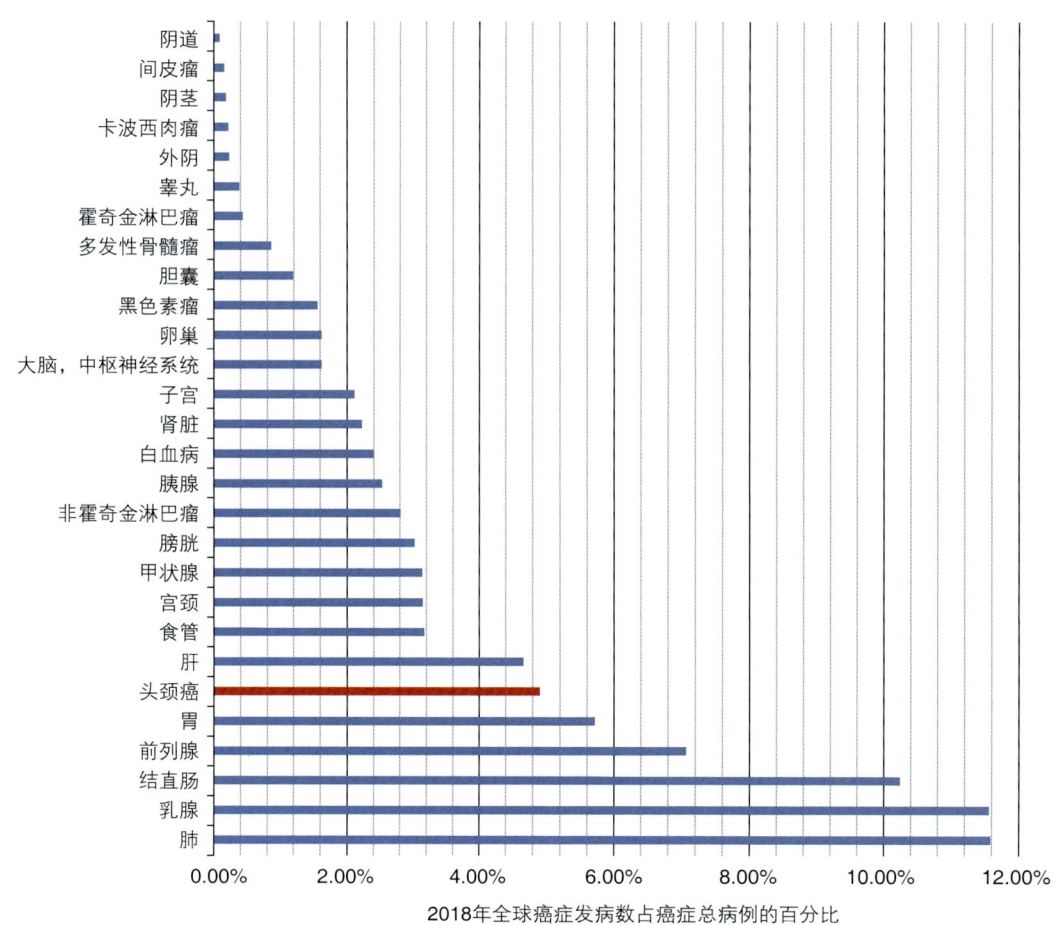

图1-3 不同癌症的发病数占全球估计癌症病例总数的百分比

的比例最高（40%），其次是喉癌（20%）、鼻咽癌（15%）、口咽癌（10%）、下咽癌（9%）和唾液腺癌（6%）（图1-4）。

根据2018年Globocan数据，头颈癌新发病例数量最高的是亚洲，其次是欧洲、北美洲、拉丁美洲及加勒比地区、非洲和大洋洲。在东南亚，头颈癌的发病率实际上在所有癌症中排名第一，而在美国则排名第六。在各大洲中，头颈癌占其他癌症的比例最高的是亚洲（6.3%），其次是非洲、拉丁美洲及加勒比地区、欧洲、大洋洲和北美洲（图1-5）。在亚洲地区，唇和口腔癌占头颈癌的发病占比最高（41%），其次是鼻咽癌、喉癌、下咽癌、口咽癌和唾液腺癌。

亚洲地区头颈癌发病率高于其他大洲，引起亚洲各国的重点关注。根据2018年癌症统计数据，头颈癌新发病例增加最多的前10个国家是印度、中国、孟加拉国、印度尼西亚、巴基斯

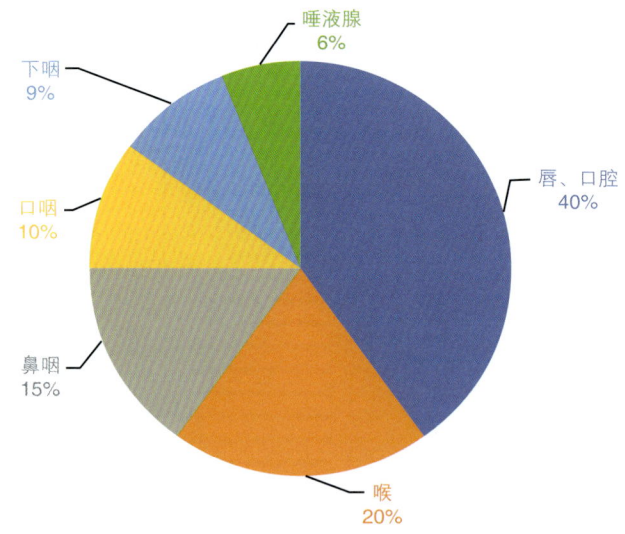

图1-4 全球不同类型头颈癌（C00～C14，C32）的发病占比

坦、日本、泰国、缅甸、土耳其和菲律宾。在印度，唇和口腔癌占头颈癌的58%，其次是喉癌（14%）、下咽癌（13%）、口咽癌（9%）、唾液腺

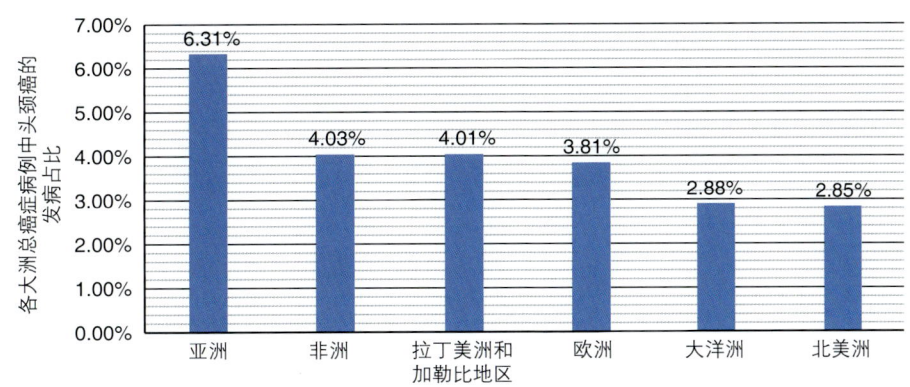

图 1-5　各大洲头颈癌（C00~C14，C32）发病占比

癌（4%）和鼻咽癌（2%）。

印度和中国的新发头颈癌病例数最高，原因可能是这两个国家的人口基数较大，均超过10亿。而孟加拉国头颈癌发病占比最高，达20.5%；亚美尼亚头颈癌的发病占比最低，仅为1%。各国头颈癌发病占比最高的前10个国家依次为：孟加拉国、印度、巴基斯坦、斯里兰卡、不丹、缅甸、阿富汗、尼泊尔、印度尼西亚和马来西亚。

孟加拉国的头颈癌中，唇和口腔癌的发病占比为43%，其次是下咽癌（23%）、喉癌（16%）、口咽癌（12%）、唾液腺癌（3%）和鼻咽癌（3%）。

各大洲不同部位头颈癌的发病占比存在差异，见图1-6。根据2018年Globocan全球癌症数据显示，头颈癌位居北美洲恶性肿瘤发病的第九顺位，总占比约2.9%（图1-7）。在不同部位头颈癌中，唇和口腔癌占全球头颈癌病例的比例最高（40%），其次是喉癌（24%）、口咽癌（20%）、唾液腺癌（8%）、下咽癌（5%）和鼻咽癌（3%）。

美国2013—2017年头颈癌年龄调整统计数据见表1-2。癌症相关死亡率在1991年前呈上升态势，此后在2017年开始下降。因此，与持续增长的死亡率相比，预计癌症死亡人数将减少290万例[8]。2018年，北美洲头颈癌的新发病

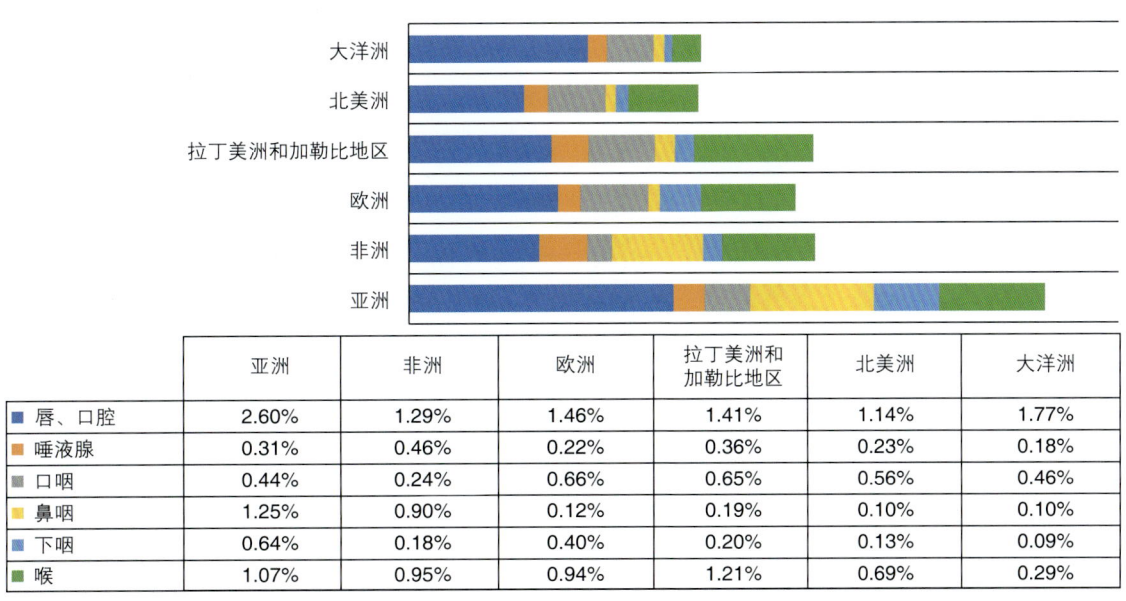

图 1-6　各大洲不同部位头颈癌（C00~C14，C32）在所有癌症中的发病占比

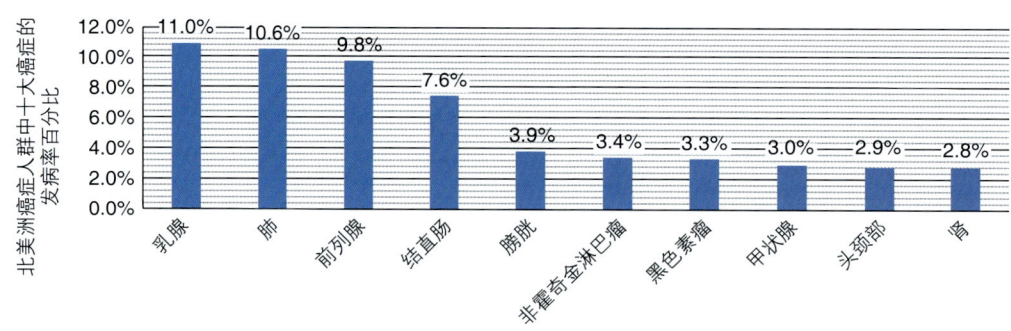

图1-7 2018年北美洲癌症人群中十大癌症的发病占比

表1-2 2013—2017年美国头颈癌监测、流行病学和最终结果统计（SEER 21）[9]

	口腔和咽喉癌	唇癌	舌癌	喉癌
2020年预计新发病例数	53 260	—	17 660	12 370
在所有新发癌症的占比	2.9%	—	1.0%	0.7%
2020年预计死亡病例数	10 750	—	2 830	3 750
在所有死亡癌症的占比	1.8%	—	0.5%	0.6%
5年相对生存率（2010—2016年）	66.2%	92.0%	67.1%	60.6%
2013—2017年男性和女性年发病率	11.4/100 000	0.6/100 000	3.5/100 000	2.9/100 000
2013—2017年男性和女性的年死亡率	2.5/100 000	0.02/100 000	0.7/100 000	1/100 000
男性和女性一生患癌风险	1.2%	0.1%	0.4%	0.3%
在美国所有新发癌症中占比	2.9%	—	1.0%	0.7%
2017年美国该癌症的发病数	383 415	—	—	96 231
发病最常见的年龄组	55～64	65～74	55～64	55～64
死亡最常见的年龄组	65～74	85+	65～74	65～74
新发病例数增加的种族和性别	非西班牙裔男性	白人男性	白人男性	黑人男性
死亡病例数增加的种族和性别	黑人男性	非西班牙裔男性和白人男性	非西班牙裔和白人	黑人男性
2008—2017年年均按年龄调整的死亡率	上涨0.5%	稳定	平均上涨1.2%	下降2.3%

例数位居全球第三，而其在所有癌症的发病占比排名第六（Globocan 2018）。据此，美国癌症协会预测，到2020年，美国的癌症新发病例数为1 806 590例，死亡病例数为606 520例[8]。

根据Globocan 2018年的数据，全球男性人群中头颈部癌新发病例数量以及不同部位头颈癌的发病占比高于女性人群（图1-8和图1-9）。男性和女性头颈癌发病率的差异通常与吸烟或咀嚼香烟、咀嚼槟榔、饮酒等有关[10]。Addala等

人（2012）的回顾性研究证实了这一点，该研究只关注头颈癌患者的组织学确诊病例，结果表明，男性比女性更容易患头颈癌，这是由于男性更常沉迷于增加头颈癌风险的习惯（吸烟和咀嚼香烟、饮酒以及两者皆有）[11]。长期暴露于这些危险因素以及特定饮食和职业会增加头颈癌的发病率[11]。然而，唇癌、口腔癌、唾液腺癌和鼻咽癌的发病率在女性中高于男性。而口咽癌、下咽癌和喉癌的男性发病率高于女性（图1-10）。

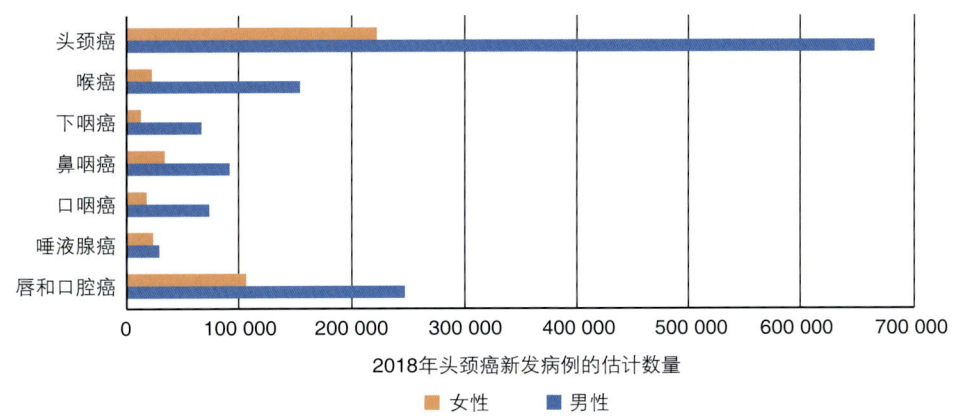

图 1-8　2018 年估计全球男性和女性人群头颈癌（C00～C14，C32）新发病例数

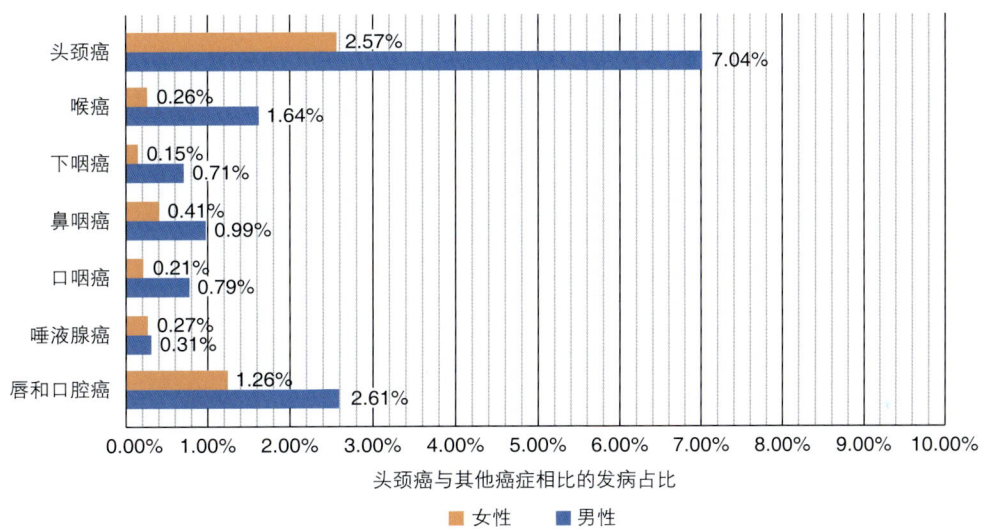

图 1-9　全球范围内头颈癌（C00～C14，C32）的发病数占所有癌症发病数的比例

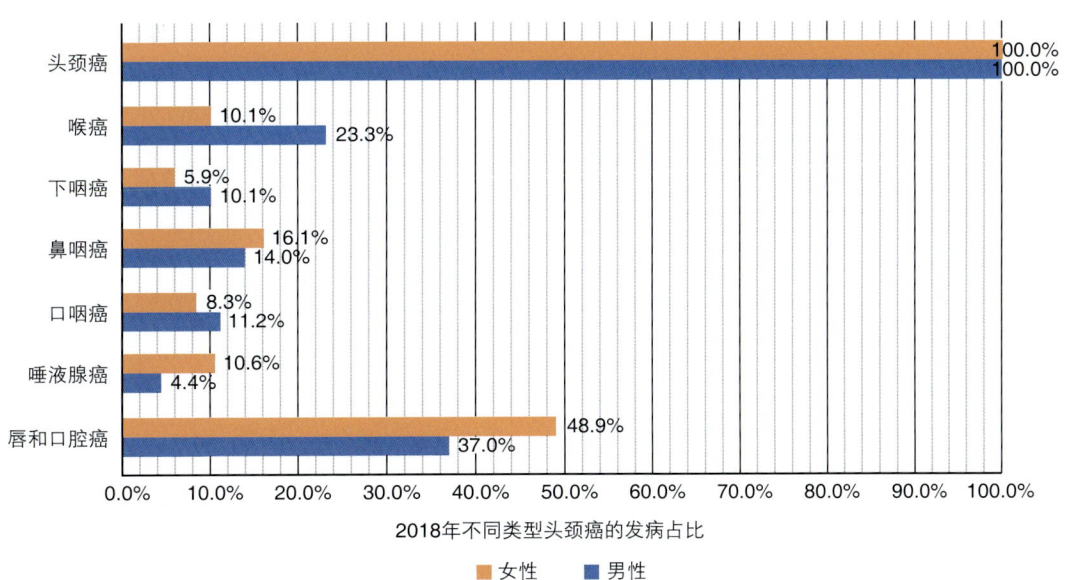

图 1-10　男性和女性人群中不同类型头颈癌的发病数（C00～C14，C32）占头颈癌总发病数的比例

病　因

"暴露"是一个术语，它指的是一个人一生中接触到的所有内部和外部暴露因素及其对健康影响的度量[12]。人们在出生前及整个生命过程中都会接触到各种环境和职业来源的暴露因素。理解暴露与个体基因学和表观遗传学之间的关系，对我们认识健康的影响因素至关重要。内部暴露体的评估发生在基因、蛋白质、脂质和代谢物的水平上[12]。外部暴露评估依赖于测量环境应激源，而环境应激源影响头颈癌的发生。我们将详细讨论引起头颈癌的各种外部因素（表1-3）。

烟草

烟草可通过多种方式使用，包括吸香烟、雪茄、烟斗、咀嚼和鼻吸，被认为是头颈癌的首要风险因素[4,10]。接触烟草及相关产品属于外部暴露的一部分，会增加罹患口腔癌、咽癌、口咽癌、下咽癌、喉上癌和鼻咽癌的风险。

在阿拉伯半岛，一种名为"沙玛"的传统无烟烟草使用与白斑病发病率呈剂量依赖性关系[13]。在东南亚、南太平洋岛屿和印度，人们使用烟草制品，如槟榔、槟榔果、查利亚、古塔卡、纳斯瓦和槟榔子，也会增加罹患口腔癌的风险[13]。无烟烟草含有亚硝胺等致癌物质，被认为是口腔癌的重要风险因素。南亚是全球无烟烟草使用的中心[14]。Khan等人（2014）报告称，咀嚼含烟草的槟榔果会增加罹患口腔癌的风险[14]。亚太地区有很大一部分人经常咀嚼槟榔[15,16]。槟榔子本身就是一种历史悠久的致癌物，会导致口腔癌[17,18]。

酒精

饮酒量增加会提高罹患口腔癌、咽癌和喉癌的风险。Elwood等人（1984）报告称，与吸烟相比，饮酒会使这些癌症的风险增加[19]。

酒精与烟草的共同作用

同时摄入酒精和烟草会显著提高罹患头颈癌的风险[4,10]。Horn-Ross等人（1997）报告称，吸烟和大量饮酒会增加男性罹患涎腺癌的风险，但这些因素与女性罹患涎腺癌的关联性并不强[31]。

无论以何种形式，如吸食比迪烟和（或）咀嚼潘烟草，酒精与烟草的共同摄入都会增加罹患口腔癌的风险[18,108]。

病毒

人乳头瘤病毒（HPV）是头颈癌的一个公认的风险因素[39]。HPV与头颈鳞状细胞癌有关，并且与口咽癌的关联性极强[40]。HPV所致头颈癌的比例在不同国家之间存在显著差异。Gheit等人（2017）在印度次大陆进行了一项研究，并报告称口咽部的HPV DNA/RNA双阳性比例最高（9.4%），其次是喉部（1.7%）和口腔（1.6%）。不同分型的HPV与某些类型癌症的发展有关。HPV16是与头颈癌相关的主要分型[109]。Smith等人（2012）报告称，与对照组相比，HPV阳性/高烟草和高酒精使用水平的个体罹患口腔癌的风险增加。然而，他们的研究还报告称，HPV阴性/高烟草和高酒精使用水平的个体罹患口咽癌的风险高于HPV阳性/高烟草和高酒精使用水平的个体[39]。

人们普遍认为，Epstein-Barr病毒（EBV）会导致鼻咽癌。在EBV感染引发的多种癌症中，已确定在部分地区（如中国南方人群）中，未分化鼻咽癌与该感染密切相关[110]。已确定EBV抗原向宿主免疫细胞呈递与鼻咽癌风险之间存在关系，并且鼻咽癌风险与6p染色体上的人类白细胞抗原（HLA）位点之间存在强烈关联[110]。

表 1-3 引起头颈癌的各种因素

暴露	暴露亚型	头颈癌的类型/部位	参考文献
烟草	吸香烟 雪茄 烟斗 倒抽 水烟壶 奇勒姆烟斗 嚼烟 鼻烟 槟榔 槟榔果包裹物 查利亚 古斯塔 纳斯瓦 槟榔果 无烟烟草 比迪烟/基尤烟［一种由日晒、未发酵的烟草卷在特姆伯尼叶（学名：*Diospyros melanoxylon*，黑檀）或香蕉叶中制成的廉价香烟］ 含亚硝胺的无烟烟草 加烟草的槟榔果 吸食烟草 "纳斯"形式的嚼烟（由槟榔叶、灰烬、石灰、棉花、芝麻油、烟草和熟石灰等成分混合而成）	硬腭癌 咽癌 口咽癌 下咽癌 声门上癌 舌根癌 口腔癌	［4，10，13，14，18，20-30］
酒精	饮酒	口腔癌 咽癌 喉癌	［18-21，24，31-33］
酒精和烟草	—	口咽癌 下咽癌 唾液腺癌 口腔癌 咽癌	［19，24，31-37］
病毒	人乳头瘤病毒（HPV）	口咽癌 口咽鳞状细胞癌 口腔癌	［18，38-45］
	Epstein-Barr 病毒（EBV）	鼻咽癌 恶性唾液腺肿瘤	［46，47］
饮食	营养不良 蔬菜和水果摄入量低 饮食中维生素 A、B、C、E，铁、硒、叶酸及其他微量元素含量低 由蔬菜和水果摄入减少导致的 β-胡萝卜素摄入量低，且饮食富含胆固醇	口腔癌 咽癌 唾液腺恶性肿瘤	［13，21，47-51］
	饮用马黛茶	口腔癌	［38，52］
	咀嚼可乐果	口腔癌	［53，54］
	食用咸鱼	鼻咽癌	［29，30，55-58］
	广式咸鱼	鼻咽癌	［59］

续 表

暴露	暴露亚型	头颈癌的类型/部位	参考文献
饮食	腌制蔬菜	鼻咽癌	[59]
	熏制/腌制肉类	鼻咽癌	[59]
	盐渍食品，包括咸蛋、叶类蔬菜和根茎类蔬菜	鼻咽癌	[57，58]
	食用其他腌制食品	鼻咽癌	[46]
	中国南方传统食品中的亚硝胺	鼻咽癌	[29，60，61]
	亚洲人群中的传统中草药	鼻咽癌	[29，30，62]
口腔卫生	多菌种龈上牙菌斑	口腔癌	[13，19]
	牙周病	口腔癌	[18，63，64]
	佩戴不合适或存在缺陷的全口义齿；修复体不良；牙齿尖锐及义齿适配性差	口腔癌	[18，38，65，66]
疾病	多发性内分泌腺病-念珠菌病-外胚层发育不良综合征 糖尿病 胃食管反流病（GERD） 喉咽反流病（LPRD）	口腔癌	[13]
	糖尿病	头颈癌	[18，67]
	Plummer-Vinson 综合征	口腔癌 口咽癌	[18]
免疫抑制剂	肾移植 硫唑嘌呤和环孢菌素	口腔癌	[18，38，68，69]
	艾滋病相关口腔癌	唇癌	[18]
	免疫抑制	恶性唾液腺肿瘤	[47]
口腔微生物	梭杆菌属、双歧杆菌属、消化链球菌属、纤毛菌属、消化链球菌属、卡氏菌属和微小消化链球菌属	口腔癌	[70]
社会经济地位低下	—	口腔癌 头颈癌	[4，38，71-74]
自由基	活性氧自由基（ROS），活性氮自由基（RNS）	口腔癌	[13]
大气气体	二氧化硫	喉癌 咽癌	[75]
	大气烟尘	喉癌 咽癌	[75]
	烟雾	鼻咽癌	[29，30，46]
	酸雾	喉癌	[75]
	由油、煤、木柴等固体燃料引起的室内空气污染	口腔癌 头颈癌	[38，76，77]

续 表

暴露	暴露亚型	头颈癌的类型/部位	参考文献
职业暴露	农业/耕作	喉癌 唾液腺癌 头颈癌	[75, 78-81]
	纺织业	喉癌 咽癌 鼻腔鼻窦癌	[75, 82, 83]
	染料	喉癌 声门癌	[75, 84]
	从事涂料和清漆工作的人员（使用含六价铬化合物的涂料）	喉癌	[85]
	手工艺劳动者	喉癌	[78, 79]
	煤矿开采	喉癌	[75]
	铁路行业	喉癌	[79]
	木材行业	喉癌	[79]
	金属板工人/铸造工人/结构金属准备和安装工人	喉癌 鼻咽癌 头颈癌	[79, 81, 82]
	物料搬运设备操作人员	头颈癌	[81]
	焊接工	头颈癌	[81]
	钎焊烟尘（电气工作）	口腔癌 咽癌	[86]
	焊接烟尘（电气工作）	咽癌 喉癌	[87]
	研磨轮操作人员	喉癌	[79]
	汽车修理工/汽车行业从业者	喉癌 唾液腺癌	[79, 80]
	木工/林业/木匠行业工作者	恶性唾液腺癌 鼻腔鼻窦癌	[75, 88-90]
	橡胶行业工作者	恶性唾液腺癌 头颈癌	[30, 80, 81, 88]
	建筑/建设行业	咽癌 头颈癌 鼻腔鼻窦癌	[75, 81, 83]
	消防员	头颈癌	[81]
	洗衣工	头颈癌	[81]
	清洁工人	头颈癌	[81]
粉尘	建筑粉尘	喉癌	[85, 89]

续　表

暴露	暴露亚型	头颈癌的类型/部位	参考文献
粉尘	水泥粉尘	喉癌 声门上癌 咽癌 头颈鳞状细胞癌	[75, 84, 85, 89, 91]
	石棉	喉癌 咽癌	[18, 87, 89, 91-93]
	硅尘/二氧化硅粉尘	唾液腺癌	[47, 51, 80]
	金属粉尘	喉癌 头颈鳞状细胞癌	[82, 89]
	木尘	鼻腔鼻窦癌 鼻癌 喉癌 咽癌 鼻咽癌	[18, 29, 75, 82, 83, 89, 90]
	煤尘	下咽癌	[36]
	木屑	喉癌 头颈鳞状细胞癌	[89]
	皮革粉尘	头颈鳞状细胞癌 鼻腔鼻窦癌 喉咽癌	[18, 75, 82, 83, 89, 90]
	烟囱烟灰	头颈鳞状细胞癌	[89]
溶剂和化学品	乙醇	喉癌	[75]
	食用油 油脂	喉癌 声门上癌	[75, 84]
	煤油（作为烹饪燃料）	唾液腺癌	[80]
	四氯乙烯和三氯乙烯	头颈癌	[94]
	石油	鼻腔鼻窦癌	[75]
	甲醛	下咽癌 鼻腔鼻窦癌 鼻咽癌	[29, 36, 83]
辐射	头部X线检查	唾液腺癌	[80]
	电离辐射	唾液腺癌	[88, 95, 96]
	高剂量或长时间辐射	唾液腺恶性肿瘤	[47, 51]
	紫外线辐射	恶性唾液腺肿瘤 唇癌	[18, 47, 97-100]
	头部或颈部的紫外线光疗	头颈癌	[31]
	太阳辐射	唇癌	[13]
	原子弹（高强度电离辐射）	头颈癌	[101]

续 表

暴露	暴露亚型	头颈癌的类型 / 部位	参考文献
辐射	辐射 / 放射性物质	头颈癌	[31]
	头部或颈部放疗（放射治疗）	头颈癌	[31，102]
	多次医疗及全口牙齿 X 线检查	头颈癌	[31]
金属	镍化合物 / 合金	恶性唾液腺癌 鼻腔鼻窦癌 头颈癌	[31，75，83，88，95，103]
	镉	头颈癌 鼻腔鼻窦癌	[103]
	铬	鼻腔鼻窦癌	[83]
其他	年龄（＜ 45 岁）	头颈癌	[104，105]
	性别	头颈癌	[40]
	黑人种族	唾液腺癌	[106]
	从不吸烟且从不饮酒者（NSND）	头颈癌	[107]
	家族史	鼻咽癌	[46]

免疫抑制剂

肾移植后，使用免疫抑制剂，如硫唑嘌呤和环孢菌素，会增加罹患唇癌的风险[68, 111]。在炎症性肠病（如克罗恩病）中，长期使用免疫抑制剂，如硫唑嘌呤，会增加罹患舌癌的风险[38, 69]。

饮食

研究表明，饮食质量不佳与头颈癌的发生有关。新鲜蔬菜和水果摄入量低，以及饮食中维生素 A、B、C、E、铁、硒、叶酸和其他微量元素含量低，会增加罹患口腔癌的风险[13, 38, 104, 112-114]。肉类和加工肉制品摄入过多会增加多种头颈癌发病风险[18, 38, 48, 115]。据报道，食用咸鱼、腌制蔬菜、食物中的亚硝胺和传统草药会增加鼻咽癌发病风险[29, 59]。在南美洲的阿根廷、乌拉圭、巴拉圭和巴西南部，人们常用金属吸管饮用非常热的马黛茶。马黛茶是由南美洲广泛种植的巴拉圭冬青制成的茶饮。饮用马黛茶会增加罹患口腔癌的风险[38, 52]。

口腔卫生

不良的口腔卫生会增加罹患口腔癌的风险[19]。不良的口腔卫生和不良的牙齿状况，包括修复不良、牙齿尖锐以及假牙不合适等，都会增加口腔癌的发病率[38, 66, 116]。菌斑是牙齿表面上的多种微生物聚集体，它与唾液发生相关的致突变相互作用，是口腔癌的一个独立风险因素[13]。Divaris 等人（2010）报告称，牙周炎与罹患头颈鳞状细胞癌的风险有关联[63]。

疾病

■ 多发性内分泌腺病-念珠菌病-外胚层发育不良综合征

这是一种在芬兰较为常见的常染色体隐性遗传病，称为多发性内分泌腺病-念珠菌病-外胚层发育不良综合征。该病与 T 淋巴细胞缺陷有关，这种缺陷似乎有利于白假丝酵母菌的生长，并使个体易于罹患慢性黏膜炎和口腔癌[13]。

■ 糖尿病

基于流行病学研究，糖尿病被认为与口腔鳞状细胞癌（OSCC）有关，涉及胰岛素受体底物-1 和局部黏着斑激酶等分子靶点[13]。

■ 胃食管反流病和喉咽反流病

胃食管反流病（GERD）和喉咽反流病（LPRD）

会导致胃酸反流至上呼吸道和喉部，从而增加罹患头颈癌的风险[13]。

口腔微生物

对于长期饮酒者而言，口腔微生物及其生物膜可能会促进乙醇在口腔内代谢为乙醛（一种强致癌物）。乙醛会增加长期饮酒者口腔细胞癌变的风险[38]。Zhao 等人（2017）在口腔鳞状细胞癌（OSCC）表面病变样本中报告了菌群失调现象，与对照组相比，细菌组成和细菌基因功能发生了显著变化[70]。他们团队观察到，包括梭杆菌属（*Fusobacterium*）、戴氏菌属（*Dialister*）、消化链球菌属（*Peptostreptococcus*）、纤毛菌属（*Filifactor*）、消化球菌属（*Peptococcus*）、卡氏菌属（*Catonella*）和微小单胞菌属（*Parvimonas*）在内的一组与牙周炎相关的菌群在 OSCC 样本中显著富集。此外，几种梭杆菌属的操作分类单元（OTU）与 OSCC 有关，并且具有良好的诊断能力。菌群失调会改变细菌栖息地的局部微环境，从而驱动致癌过程，使得适应肿瘤微环境的细菌得以繁殖，进而导致细菌群落发生变化[70]。

社会经济地位

低社会经济地位与头颈癌风险增加有关[71]。据报道，发展中国家人群因吸烟、饮酒量上升[4]及不良饮食习惯[38]，导致头颈癌的发病率较高。然而，从职业、收入或教育等方面衡量的较低社会经济地位是口腔癌的重要风险因素，且这一风险独立于生活行为方式之外[38]。

自由基

在致癌过程中，活性氧（ROS）和活性氮（RNS）等自由基起着引发和促进的作用。ROS 与 RNS 增多会消耗并降低唾液抗氧化系统，进而引发 DNA 与蛋白质氧化损伤，可能促进口腔癌的发生[13]。

大气气体

1993 年，Wake 将大气中的二氧化硫或其产物及影响与喉癌和咽癌风险增加联系起来。他还报告了大气烟雾会增加喉癌的风险[75]。

职业暴露

尽管 Elwood 等人（1984）[19]和 Purdue 等人（2006）[91]在对建筑工人进行的独立研究中，没有发现头颈癌与特定职业暴露的显著关联，而其他研究表明环境或职业性吸入物增加了头颈癌的发生风险。1994 年，Pukkala 等人报告了电工因暴露于焊接烟雾中，口腔癌和咽喉癌的风险增加[86]。1998 年，Gustavsson 等人（1998）将长期暴露于焊接烟雾与咽喉癌和喉癌的风险增加相关联[87]。

可能接触橡胶的职业与唾液腺癌风险增加相关[80]。Horn-Ross 等人（1997）也报告了在橡胶工业工作的人群中头颈癌风险增加[31]。

Williams 等人（1977）报告了某些职业的喉癌发病率不同的比率，操作工、工匠、劳动者和农民的比率分别为 1.3、1、0.9 和 0.4[78]。类似地，Flanders 和 Rothman（1982）在 1982 年估算了相同职业的发病率比率分别为 1.4、1.2、1.6 和 0.5[79]。他们还报告了铁路行业、木材行业、钣金工、砂轮操作工和汽车机械师的喉癌发病率增加[79]。

可能接触汽车工业和农业的职业与唾液腺癌的高风险相关[80]。Comba 等人（1992）报告称，鼻癌的高风险与在木材、皮革和纺织工业中工作的个体相关[82]。Paget-Bailly 等人（2013）报告，在法国人群中，清洁、洗衣、消防、农业、焊接、结构金属准备、建筑、橡胶加工、若干建筑行业以及物料处理设备操作等职业的工作时间越长，头颈癌的风险越高[81]。

- **粉尘**

粉尘是暂时悬浮在空气中的小固体颗粒，直径范围为 1~100 μm。它包含多种异质的有机物（如木屑或皮革粉尘）或无机物（如金属粉尘）。粉尘可通过其固有的化学性质而引起慢性炎症，或作为其他致癌物质的载体，进而产生致癌效应。木屑和皮革粉尘是与鼻腔和鼻旁窦癌相关的两种职业性粉尘。这两种粉尘被国际癌症研究机构（IARC）列为 1 类致癌物[89]。Langevin 等人报告，接触木屑和金属粉尘会增加喉癌的风险，而皮革粉尘暴露会增加头颈鳞状细胞癌（HNSCC）的风险[89]。

- **建筑粉尘**

据报道，建筑和施工工人的喉癌风险增加，因为建筑粉尘由多种物质组成，例如石棉、矿物纤维、砂子、金属粉末、沥青、柏油和水泥粉尘[85]。

- **水泥粉尘**

1990年，Cauvin等人报告了与暴露于水泥与声门上癌风险增加相关[84]。Dietz等人（2004）的研究得出结论，建筑工人和施工工人接触水泥粉尘会增加喉癌的风险[85]。Purdue等人（2006）也报告了暴露于水泥粉尘的工人咽癌风险增加[91]。

- **石棉**

1998年，Gustavsson等人报告了石棉暴露与喉癌之间的关联[87]。Purdue等人（2006）的研究结果与此相似，显示石棉暴露与喉癌发病率增加相关[91]。Straif等人（2009）指出，IARC将石棉暴露认定为喉癌的致因[92]。Menvielle等人（2016）在法国进行的一项研究建议避免接触含有石棉的材料，因为他们的研究显示，石棉与烟草和酒精的联合暴露会显著增加喉癌的发病率[93]。

- **硅粉尘**

Zheng等人（1996）的一项研究报告，暴露于硅粉尘会使唾液腺癌的风险增加2.5倍[80]。

- **金属粉尘**

Comba等人（1992）报告了在铸造厂工作的人群中风险增加，金属粉尘与鼻癌的风险增加相关[82]。

- **木屑粉尘**

Elwood（1981）的一项研究表明，鼻腔和鼻旁窦肿瘤的职业风险可能不仅限于家具制造商，还包括从事木材加工的初级产业工人，如林业和木工工人[90]。

- **溶剂**

Cauvin等人（1990）的一项研究显示，声门上癌与暴露于油和润滑脂有关[84]。Zheng等人（1996）报告了使用煤油作为烹饪燃料的人群中唾液腺癌风险增加[80]。Gustavsson等人（1998）报告，增加的多环芳烃（PAH）暴露与食管癌有关[87]。Carton等人（2017）研究了职业暴露于溶剂对女性头颈癌的影响[94]。研究中使用的溶剂包括5种氯化溶剂（四氯化碳、氯仿、二氯甲烷、四氯乙烯、三氯乙烯）、5种石油溶剂（苯、特种石油产品、汽油、白电油及其他轻芳烃混合物、柴油、燃料和煤油），以及5种氧化溶剂（醇类、酮类和酯类、乙二醇、二乙醚、四氢呋喃）。研究发现，暴露于四氯乙烯和三氯乙烯的女性风险增加，且随暴露时间延长而增加。Carton等人（2017）报告，其他氯化溶剂、石油或氧化溶剂的职业暴露与头颈鳞状细胞癌（HNSCC）之间没有显著关联[94]。

- **辐射**

来自广岛和长崎原子弹的高水平电离辐射[101]、放射治疗[102]以及反复的医学和牙科放射检查[117]都会增加癌症风险。Zheng等人（1996）报告了头部放射检查与唾液腺癌风险增加之间的关联[80]。Horn-Ross等人（1997）报告了头颈部接受较高剂量的医疗放射治疗、全口牙科X线、头颈部紫外线治疗以及辐射或放射性材料暴露的风险增加[31]。

长期暴露于太阳辐射是唇癌的主要风险因素。通常，唇癌发生在下唇，许多患者从事户外职业，导致日晒时间增加。唇癌在男性中的发病率是女性的3倍，这可能与职业、吸烟和日晒有关[13]。

- **金属**

Horn-Ross等人（1997）报告，接触镍化合物/合金会增加头颈癌的风险[31]。Khlif和Hamza-Chaffai（2010）指出，吸烟会增加金属工人的重金属总负荷[103]。普遍认为，镍[31,103]、铬和镉等重金属是致癌物，增加了人类患头颈癌的风险[103]。

1990年，Cauvin等人报告了声门癌与染料暴露相关[84]。油漆工和上漆工可能更容易患喉癌，因为油漆中含有致癌物质，如六价铬化合物[85]。

其他风险因素

- **年龄**

头颈癌的风险在40岁以上人群中更高，确诊的平均年龄为62岁[118]。头颈鳞状细胞癌（HNSCC）通常被认为是老年人的疾病。然而，近年来，全球报告了越来越多45岁以下患者患HNSCC的病例[105]。

▪ 性别

在中美洲和南美洲，男性患头颈癌的发生率约为女性的4倍[40]。根据2018年的Globocan数据，类似的观察显示，头颈癌在男性中是第五大常见癌症，仅次于肺癌、前列腺癌、结直肠癌和胃癌；而在女性中，头颈癌是第十一大常见癌症，排在乳腺癌、结直肠癌、肺癌、宫颈癌、甲状腺癌、子宫体癌、胃癌、卵巢癌、肝癌和非霍奇金淋巴瘤之后。

▪ 种族

研究表明，南亚人的口腔癌发病率比大多数其他国家的人群更高。在美国，黑人男性患咽喉癌的风险高于白人男性[38]。

▪ 从不吸烟且从不饮酒者（NSND）

Dahlstrom等人（2008）报告，极端年龄段的非吸烟非饮酒（NSND）女性更容易患头颈癌，并且她们的年龄显著低于曾经吸烟和（或）饮酒（ESED）的患者[107]。NSND患口腔癌和咽癌的比例高于ESED患者。在头颈癌病例中，45%的NSND女性和41%的男性有定期接触环境烟草烟雾的历史。职业中的致癌物或毒素暴露也使24%的NSND女性和36%的NSND男性头颈癌风险增加。患有胃食管反流病（GERD）的NSND患者占发病率的30%。超过一半的血清HPV16型阳性的NSND患者的原发部位为口咽部。观察到没有特定的单一已知因素是NSND罹患HNSCC的主要诱因[107]。

Diz等人（2017）报道了在口腔癌和咽癌的发病率和死亡率方面存在地区差异，这些差异归因于生活方式的不同以及某些危险因素（如吸烟、饮酒等），例如，丹麦女性的高吸烟率导致发病率较高，立陶宛男性的饮酒导致发病率上升，而比利时和葡萄牙则因吸烟和饮酒共同作用导致较高发病率。其他传统因素如日光辐射，导致唇癌发病率增加（如在西班牙），而HPV的致癌潜力解释了某些国家和地区口咽癌发病率上升的现象（如丹麦和苏格兰）[119]。

症　状

在头颈癌的早期阶段，肿瘤通常是无症状的，导致患者或医生可能忽视头颈癌的症状[120]。然而，最常见的症状是持续性的口腔肿胀或溃疡。口腔中的红斑或白斑，以及头颈部区域的肿块或肿块，可能伴有或不伴有疼痛，以上都是头颈癌的临床表现[121]。

其他症状包括：即使在保持适当口腔卫生后，仍然会出现口臭；持续鼻塞；频繁鼻出血；异常鼻分泌物；咀嚼、吞咽或移动下颌或舌头时出现疼痛或困难；下颌疼痛；唾液或痰中带血；牙齿松动；假牙不再合适；声音嘶哑或改变；呼吸困难；复视；头颈部某个部位的麻木或无力；不明原因体重下降；疲劳；耳痛或感染。面部疼痛、轻度张口受限、耳痛和头痛是鼻咽癌的细微迹象，通常会被误认为良性疾病。咽癌大多数是在晚期被发现的，并且由于症状出现较晚而导致预后较差[121,122]。

诊　断

临床检查

除了进行内镜检查外，还需通过触诊肿瘤和颈部区域淋巴结来进行临床检查，以确定疾病的分期。由于几乎所有头颈癌病例中都可以通过自然腔道进行简单的内镜检查和诊断活检，因此临床上可以通过临床检查进行诊断和分期[4,123-125]。在诊断过程中，会评估患者的病史，并进行全面的头颈部体检和活检[4, 126]。然而，在体检过程中，建议对口腔进行双合诊，并检查颈部淋巴结[4]。使用镜子或电子纤维喉镜进行检查对于诊断和分期涉及喉部和咽部的病变至关重要[126]。耳鼻喉科医生使用鼻咽镜对于头颈癌的诊断和分期是必不可少的。在检查颈部肿块时，细针穿刺抽吸是一种有用的诊断工具。

影像学检查

■ 超声检查

超声可以与细针穿刺活检（FNA）结合使用，以评估颈部淋巴结中的肿瘤存在情况或测量口腔癌的浸润深度[127, 128]。有研究表明，通过超声引导下的 FNA 进行临床检查，对评估颈部淋巴结肿大时的准确性有所提高[129, 130]，并且在这个目的上被认为优于其他影像学检查方式。由于其固有位置，超声无法评估咽后淋巴结区域，而对小淋巴结进行抽吸在技术上比较困难。超声引导的 FNA 可能会检测到在 CT 扫描中看似正常的淋巴结中的恶性肿瘤，因此可能成为颈部评估的重要辅助诊断工具[127, 128, 131]。然而，其在头颈癌患者管理中的具体作用尚待确定[132]。

■ 计算机断层（CT）扫描

CT 扫描用于可视化肿瘤和颈部淋巴结的位置及大小，就头颈癌而言，它主要有助于检测副鼻窦和鼻腔中的癌症[133]。CT 扫描通常会生成多个图像，所产生的横断面图像可以帮助重建三维图像。它用于测量肿瘤体积或确定放射治疗区域的范围[127, 128, 132]。

对于晚期肿瘤，尤其是鼻咽癌和下咽癌，发生远处转移的风险增加，可能扩散到肺部、骨骼、肝脏和纵隔淋巴结。具有较大远处转移风险的患者通常会接受胸部 CT 扫描，包括上腹部，并可能进行骨扫描评估，后者的诊断价值可能较低[132]。

颈部的 CT 和 MRI 提供有关淋巴结受累及邻近结构侵犯的信息。CT 扫描比 MRI 更快速且更经济，常用于评估颈部淋巴结肿大。CT 扫描在评估骨质侵蚀（例如，下颌骨或颅底的侵袭）和喉部病变方面准确性更高，因为这些区域在 MRI 扫描中可能产生运动伪影[131, 132]。

■ 磁共振成像（MRI）

MRI 扫描提供多平面成像，常用于可视化和描绘头颈肿瘤，并能更好地呈现软组织对比度，因为它能够检测软组织中的微妙差异。此外，可以使用不同的扫描协议来更清晰地成像不同结构或研究不同的组织特征，如扩散或灌注[127, 128]。在评估鼻咽、鼻窦、唾液腺、咽后及椎前间隙以及口咽方面，MRI 优于 CT 扫描[131]。在 MRI 扫描过程中，多平面成像可以检测软组织中的细微差异[132]。

■ 正电子发射断层（PET）扫描

这是一种使用标记有正电子发射体的不同分子（如氟代脱氧葡萄糖，FDG）来产生功能性图像的方法。注射后，这些标记分子会分布到全身并提供实时生物信息。PET 示踪剂（如 FDG）可用于通过研究不同组织的葡萄糖摄取来检测代谢活跃的肿瘤细胞。PET 扫描的优势在于可以根据研究的过程使用多种分子作为 PET 示踪剂[134]。除了 FDG 外，在放射肿瘤学中使用的其他示踪剂包括用碳-11 标记的胸苷用于测量增殖，FMISO[(^{18}F）氟咪唑]和 Cu-ATSM 用于缺氧成像，以及 ^{99m}Tc 标记的 Annexin 用于测量细胞凋亡[127, 128, 131, 132, 135]。

淋巴结转移在扁桃体、舌根和鼻咽的原发癌中常见。通过 PET 扫描、超声、CT 扫描和 MRI，OCSCC 的淋巴结组织学受累评估并不理想。隐匿性颈部淋巴结肿大会改变治疗方案，因为临床检查无法检测到。解剖学影像在诊断恶性淋巴结病变方面不够精确，通常依赖于淋巴结大小标准。因此，PET 扫描和超声引导的细针穿刺活检可用于颈部分期。FDG-PET 扫描可评估远处转移和颈部淋巴结肿大。多项研究表明，在检测癌症淋巴结受累方面，PET 扫描优于 CT 扫描和 MRI。PET 扫描的灵敏度和特异性高于 CT 扫描和 MRI，能够区分活跃肿瘤与纤维变化，因此对于治疗后复发的头颈癌有重要的诊断价值[131, 132]。

在常规断层成像未能识别原发病灶的情况

下，建议使用 PET 和 CT 的联合成像技术。这种联合应用还被推荐用于非手术治疗 12 周后检测残留病灶[136]。

探测技术

探测是一种侵入性技术。用于在肿瘤内部进行测量的探头提供肿瘤的实时信息。例如，Eppendorf pO$_2$ 的氧敏感针探头可以插入肿瘤中，从而获得实时测量数据，并在治疗过程中提供重复测量的可能性[137,138]。

肿瘤活检

对于诊断性活检，取出肿瘤的一部分用于研究肿瘤的各个方面，包括 HPV 的存在。取出的肿瘤细胞可以在体外培养，用甲苯胺蓝染色肿瘤组织切片被认为有助于在显微镜下检测局部复发或新发病灶[132]。通过对鼻咽、扁桃体、窦腔和舌根等头颈癌部位进行随机活检的全内镜检查，可以发现未知的原发恶性肿瘤。所有患者在口腔检查中明显可见的肿瘤均需进行组织学诊断，咽喉腔也需进行活检。肿瘤细胞或组织可用于研究肿瘤特定蛋白质、RNA 或 DNA 的水平[139]。然而，建议避免对颈部淋巴结进行针吸或切除活检，因为这可能会改变淋巴管结构，并影响后续淋巴结清扫的效果。

病理学/免疫组化

肿瘤组织被切成薄片并固定在玻璃载玻片上，以便在显微镜下进行观察。使用荧光染料标记的抗体的不同染色方案有助于可视化肿瘤细胞内外的各种标志物。来自不同患者的多个小肿瘤切片可以在同一载玻片上进行染色，以执行组织微阵列（TMA）分析。

结合 PCR 和 p16 免疫组化（IHC）可用于检测 HPV。p16-IHC 具有优良的特异性、可接受的敏感性以及良好的预测价值，适用于 HPV 引起的头颈癌的诊断[7]。最常见的诊断测试总结见图 1-11。

- **可能的诊断延迟**

早期诊断和治疗可以提高任何恶性肿瘤的生存概率。尽管头颈癌的位置和可见性较好，许多患者仍在晚期才被诊断。缺乏对症状的教育和意识会导致诊断延迟，这些因素共同造成了疾病的进展及更高的发病率和死亡率[24,74,114,151-153]。

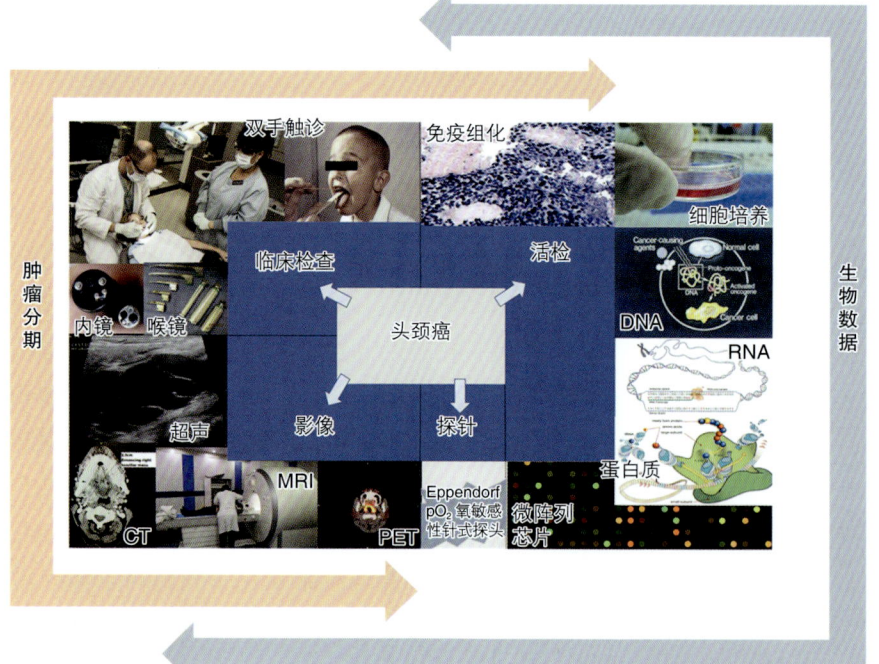

图 1-11 头颈肿瘤的诊断方法[140-150]

Agarwal 等人（2018）研究了与诊断延迟相关的各种原因，包括年龄较大、农村背景、文盲、大家庭、经济状况差、与医院的距离较远、咀嚼烟草、知识缺乏和对疾病的恐惧。提高医疗覆盖率和对可用医疗卫生服务的意识可能有助于防止诊断和治疗的延迟[152]。

分期系统

美国癌症联合委员会（AJCC）建立了一种分期系统，涵盖肿瘤生长的三个方面，包括原发肿瘤的扩展程度（T）、区域淋巴结的受累情况（N）和转移（M）。TNM 分期系统（表1-4）指导初步治疗决策，并主要基于临床检查定义肿瘤的解剖范围。此外，TNM 分期系统结合了影像学技术（例如，皮质受累将分期升级为T4）。病理分期的数据源于手术发现和组织病理学评估，并单独记录。根据肿瘤的大小及其从起始位置的扩散划分癌症的不同阶段。癌症分期因癌症类型而异，但常见的分期系统见表1-5[154]。此外，根据在显微镜下观察到的癌细胞外观进行分级，如表1-6所述。一般而言，T 分期在头颈癌的每个子类型肿瘤中相对相似，然后基于解剖学考虑而有所差异；N 分期表示肿瘤扩散到附近淋巴结；M 分期表示远处转移，这在各类型肿瘤里面是一致的。头颈癌分期、其TNM 分期及其分组见表1-7～表1-9[155, 156]。根据1997年 AJCC 系统，大约2/3的头颈癌患者被诊断为Ⅲ期或Ⅳ期的晚期疾病（局部区域晚期头颈癌），而1/3为Ⅰ期或Ⅱ期的早期阶段[132]。

表 1-4 分 期 系 统

TNM 分期	描 述
T：肿瘤	肿瘤的特征，例如其大小、在起始部位的生长情况，以及是否存在或向邻近组织的生长
T0	无原发肿瘤的证据
TX	无法测量肿瘤
Tis	原位癌或癌前病变，即癌细胞在最表层组织中生长，而未侵入更深的组织
Tn（例如T1、T2、T3和T4）	肿瘤的大小及其向邻近结构的扩散程度。T 数值越高，表示肿瘤越大且在邻近组织中的生长越明显
N：淋巴结	肿瘤扩散至附近淋巴结
NX	区域淋巴结无法评估
N0	区域淋巴结未发现癌细胞
Nn（例如N1、N2和N3）	表示区域淋巴结的大小、位置和（或）数量。N 数值越高，表示癌症向区域淋巴结的扩散程度越大
M：远处转移	癌症是否扩散至身体远处部位
M0	无远处癌症扩散的证据
M1	癌症扩散至远处器官或组织

表 1-5 癌症分期

癌症分期	描述
0 期	癌前病变（原位癌）未扩散的发生部位
Ⅰ 期	小肿瘤，未扩散
Ⅱ 期	肿瘤增大，尚未扩散
Ⅲ 期	大型癌症，可能已扩散至邻近组织和（或）淋巴结
Ⅳ 期	转移性癌症，从其发生部位扩散至身体其他远处位置

表 1-6 癌症分级

癌症分级	描述
1 级	肿瘤细胞和组织与健康细胞和组织相似。这些被称为分化良好的肿瘤，属于低级别
2 级	细胞和组织稍显异常，称为中度分化。这些是中级别肿瘤
3 级	癌细胞和组织的外观非常异常。这些癌症不再具有结构或模式，属于分化差的肿瘤。此类肿瘤被视为高级别
4 级	未分化的癌症，细胞外观最为异常。这些细胞特征上生长和扩散速度快于低级别肿瘤，属于最高级别

表 1-7 头颈癌分期

癌症阶段	描述
0 期	肿瘤在头颈部位的起始位置生长，但在深层组织、附近结构、淋巴结或远处部位没有癌细胞存在
Ⅰ 期	肿瘤直径为 2 cm 或更小，位于原发部位，且未在邻近结构、淋巴结或远处部位发现癌细胞
Ⅱ 期	肿瘤直径为 2～4 cm，邻近结构、淋巴结或远处部位没有癌细胞存在
Ⅲ 期	肿瘤直径超过 4 cm，在邻近结构、淋巴结或远处部位没有癌细胞存在 **或者**肿瘤可以是任何大小，但未侵入邻近结构或远处部位 **或者**肿瘤直径小于 3 cm，且在与原发肿瘤同侧的一个淋巴结中存在癌细胞
ⅣA 期	肿瘤为任何大小，已侵入邻近结构 　淋巴结中可能没有癌细胞，或者可能已经扩散到一个与原发肿瘤同侧的淋巴结，且该淋巴结直径小于 3 cm。然而，癌症未扩散到远处部位 **或者**肿瘤可以是任何大小，可能已侵入附近结构或未侵入 　癌细胞存在于一个与原发肿瘤同侧、直径为 3～6 cm 的淋巴结中 　癌细胞存在于与原发肿瘤相对侧的一个淋巴结中，直径小于 6 cm 　癌细胞存在于两个或更多淋巴结中，均小于 6 cm，且位于头颈部的任一侧
ⅣB 期	肿瘤已侵入头颈部更深的区域和（或）组织。癌细胞可能已扩散到淋巴结，也可能没有扩散，且未扩散到远处部位 **或者**肿瘤为任何大小，可能已侵入其他结构，也可能未侵入。已扩散至一个或多个直径大于 6 cm 的淋巴结，但未扩散到远处部位
ⅣC 期	癌细胞已扩散至远处部位 肿瘤可以是任何大小，可能已扩散至淋巴结，也可能未扩散

表 1-8 头颈癌 TNM 分期

肿瘤（T）

唇和口腔（C00～C06）

TX	原发肿瘤无法评估

续 表

T0	没有原发肿瘤的证据	
Tis	原位癌	
T1	肿瘤最大径为 2 cm 或更小	
T2	肿瘤最大径超过 2 cm 但不超过 4 cm	
T3	肿瘤最大径超过 4 cm	
T4	唇肿瘤侵入骨皮质、下颌神经、口底或面部皮肤（即下巴或鼻子）	
T4a	口腔肿瘤侵入骨皮质、深层（外在）舌肌（舌骨舌肌、舌下肌、腭舌肌和茎突舌肌）、上颌窦或面部皮肤	
T4b	肿瘤侵入咬肌间隙、翼内板或颅底，和（或）包绕颈内动脉	
大唾液腺（C07～C08）		
TX	原发肿瘤无法评估	
T0	没有原发肿瘤的证据	
T1	肿瘤最大径为 2 cm 或更小，无腺体实质外侵[a]	
T2	肿瘤最大径超过 2 cm 但不超过 4 cm，且没有腺体实质外侵[a]	
T3	肿瘤最大径超过 4 cm 和（或）具有腺体实质外侵[a]	
T4a	肿瘤侵入皮肤、下颌骨、耳道和（或）面神经	
T4b	肿瘤侵入颅底和（或）翼板和（或）包绕颈动脉	
咽喉（C09～C10）		
TX	原发肿瘤无法评估	
T0	没有原发肿瘤的证据	
Tis	原位癌	
T1	肿瘤最大径为 2 cm 或更小	
T2	肿瘤最大径超过 2 cm 但不超过 4 cm	
T3	肿瘤最大径超过 4 cm	
T4a	肿瘤侵入喉、深层/外在舌肌、翼内肌、硬腭或下颌骨	
T4b	肿瘤侵入翼外肌、翼板、鼻咽侧壁或颅底，或包绕颈动脉	
鼻咽（C11）		
TX	原发肿瘤无法评估	
T0	没有原发肿瘤的证据	
Tis	原位癌	
T1	肿瘤局限于鼻咽	
T2	肿瘤扩展至软组织	
T2a	肿瘤扩展至口咽和（或）鼻腔，无咽旁间隙侵犯[b]	
T2b	任何具有咽旁间隙侵犯[b]的肿瘤	
T3	肿瘤涉及骨结构和（或）鼻窦	
T4	肿瘤有颅内扩展和（或）涉及脑神经、翼下窝、下咽、眼眶或咬肌间隙	

续　表

下咽（C12～C13）

	TX	原发肿瘤无法评估
	T0	无原发肿瘤证据
	Tis	原位癌
	T1	肿瘤限于下咽的一个亚部位，最大直径为 2 cm 或更小
	T2	肿瘤侵袭下咽的多个亚部位或邻近部位，或最大直径超过 2 cm 但不超过 4 cm 且无半喉固定
	T3	肿瘤最大直径超过 4 cm 或半喉固定
	T4a	肿瘤侵袭甲状软骨/环状软骨、舌骨、甲状腺、食管或中央区软组织
	T4b	肿瘤侵袭椎前筋膜、包绕颈动脉或累及纵隔结构

原发肿瘤（T）：鼻窦（C30）

鼻窦：上颌窦

	TX	原发肿瘤无法评估
	T0	无原发肿瘤证据
	Tis	原位癌
	T1	肿瘤限于上颌窦黏膜，没有骨质侵蚀或破坏
	T2	肿瘤导致骨质侵蚀或破坏，包括延伸到硬腭和（或）中鼻道，但不包括延伸到上颌窦后壁和翼板
	T3	肿瘤侵袭下列任意部位：上颌窦后壁骨、皮下组织、眼眶底或内侧壁、翼下窝、筛窦
	T4a	肿瘤侵袭前眼眶内容物、面颊皮肤、翼板、下颌窝、筛板、蝶窦或额窦
	T4b	肿瘤侵袭下列任意部位：眶尖、硬脑膜、脑、颅中窝、除三叉神经上颌分支（V_2）以外的脑神经、鼻咽或斜坡

鼻窦：鼻腔和筛窦

	TX	原发肿瘤无法评估
	T0	无原发肿瘤证据
	Tis	原位癌
	T1	肿瘤限于任何一个亚部位，有或无骨侵袭
	T2	肿瘤侵袭同一区域的两个亚部位或扩展到鼻-筛复合体的邻近区域，有或无骨侵袭
	T3	肿瘤扩展侵袭眼眶内侧壁或底、上颌窦、腭或筛板
	T4a	肿瘤侵袭下列任意部位：前眼眶内容物、鼻子或面颊皮肤、少量扩展到颅前窝、翼板、蝶窦或额窦
	T4b	肿瘤侵袭下列任意部位：眶尖、硬脑膜、脑、颅中窝、除三叉神经上颌分支（V_2）以外的脑神经、鼻咽或斜坡

喉（C32）

声门

	TX	原发肿瘤无法评估
	T0	无原发肿瘤证据
	Tis	原位癌
	T1	肿瘤限于声带，且活动正常
	T1a	肿瘤限于一侧声带
	T1b	肿瘤侵犯双侧声带

续 表

T2	肿瘤侵犯至声门上方和（或）声门下方，或声带活动受限	
T3	肿瘤限于喉，伴声带固定，和（或）侵袭声门旁间隙，和（或）轻度甲状软骨侵犯（例如内板）	
T4a	肿瘤侵袭甲状软骨和（或）侵袭喉外组织	
T4b	肿瘤侵袭椎前间隙、包绕颈动脉或侵袭纵隔结构	
声门上型		
TX	原发肿瘤无法评估	
T0	无原发肿瘤证据	
Tis	原位癌	
T1	肿瘤限于声门上方的一个亚部位，且声带活动正常	
T2	肿瘤侵袭多个相邻的声门上方亚部位或声门，或侵犯到声门上方以外的区域，且无喉固定	
T3	肿瘤局限于喉内，伴声带固定，和（或）侵袭以下任意部位：环后区、会厌前间隙、声门旁间隙，和（或）轻度甲状软骨侵犯（例如内板）	
T4a	肿瘤侵透甲状软骨和（或）侵及喉外组织	
T4b	肿瘤侵及椎前间隙、包绕颈动脉或侵及纵隔结构	
区域淋巴结（N）		
嘴唇和口腔、咽部、喉部、下咽部、主要唾液腺和鼻窦		
NX	区域淋巴结无法评估	
N0	无区域淋巴结转移	
N1	单侧淋巴结转移，最大直径为 3 cm 或更小	
N2	单侧淋巴结转移，最大直径超过 3 cm 但不超过 6 cm；或多个单侧淋巴结转移，均不超过 6 cm；或双侧或对侧淋巴结转移，均不超过 6 cm	
N2a	单侧淋巴结转移，最大直径超过 3 cm 但不超过 6 cm	
N2b	多个单侧淋巴结转移，均不超过 6 cm	
N2c	双侧或对侧淋巴结转移，最大直径均不超过 6 cm	
N3	至少有一个淋巴结转移，最大直径超过 6 cm	
鼻咽部		
NX	区域淋巴结无法评估	
N0	无区域淋巴结转移	
N1	单侧淋巴结转移，最大直径为 6 cm 或更小，位于锁骨上窝上方	
N2	双侧淋巴结转移，最大直径为 6 cm 或更小，位于锁骨上窝上方	
N3	至少有一个淋巴结转移，超过 6 cm，和（或）转移至锁骨上窝	
N3a	最大直径超过 6 cm	
N3b	转移至锁骨上窝	
转移（M）		
MX	无法评估远处转移	
M0	无远处转移	
M1	远处转移	

注：源自参考文献[156]。
[a] 腺体实质外侵：指肿瘤侵犯软组织的临床或大体证据，仅存在显微镜下证据不足以作为分期分类依据。
[b] 咽旁间隙侵犯：指肿瘤向后外侧方向浸润突破咽颅底筋膜。

表 1-9 头颈癌的 TNM 分期分组

阶段	T	N	M	阶段	T	N	M
唇和口腔（C00～C06）				口咽（C09～C10）和下咽（C12～C13）			
0	Tis	N0	M0	0	Tis	N0	M0
Ⅰ	T1	N0	M0	Ⅰ	T1	N0	M0
Ⅱ	T2	N0	M0	Ⅱ	T2	N0	M0
Ⅲ	T3	N0	M0	Ⅲ	T3	N0	M0
Ⅲ	T1	N1	—	Ⅲ	T1	N1	—
Ⅲ	T2	N1	—	Ⅲ	T2	N1	—
Ⅲ	T3	N1	—	Ⅲ	T3	N1	—
ⅣA	T4a	N0	M0	ⅣA	T4a	N0	M0
ⅣA	T4a	N1	—	ⅣA	T4a	N1	—
ⅣA	T1	N2	—	ⅣA	T1	N2	—
ⅣA	T2	N2	—	ⅣA	T2	N2	—
ⅣA	T3	N2	—	ⅣA	T3	N2	—
ⅣB	任意 T	N3	M0	ⅣA	T4a	N2	—
ⅣB	T4b	任意 N	—	ⅣB	T4b	任意 N	M0
大唾液腺（C07～C08）				ⅣB	任意 T	N3	—
Ⅰ	T1	N0	M0	ⅣC	任意 T	任意 N	M1
Ⅱ	T2	N0	M0	鼻咽（C11）			
Ⅲ	T3	N0	M0	0	Tis	N0	M0
Ⅲ	T1	N1	—	Ⅰ	T1	N0	M0
Ⅲ	T2	N1	—	ⅡA	T2a	N0	M0
Ⅲ	T3	N1	—	ⅡB	T1	N1	M0
ⅣA	T4a	N0	M0	ⅡB	T2	N1	—
ⅣA	T4a	N1	—	ⅡB	T2a	N1	—
ⅣA	T1	N2	—	ⅡB	T2b	N0	—
ⅣA	T2	N2	—	ⅡB	T2b	N1	—
ⅣA	T3	N2	—	Ⅲ	T1	N2	M0
ⅣA	T4a	N2	—	Ⅲ	T2a	N2	—
ⅣB	T4b	任意 N	M0	Ⅲ	T2b	N2	—
ⅣB	任意 T	N3	—	Ⅲ	T3	N0	—
ⅣC	任意 T	任意 N	M1	Ⅲ	T3	N1	—

续 表

阶段	T	N	M	阶段	T	N	M
Ⅲ	T3	N2	—	ⅣB	T4b	任意 N	M0
	T4	N0	M0		任意 T	N3	—
ⅣA	T4	N1	—	ⅣC	任意 T	任意 N	M1
	T4	N2	—	喉（超声门、声门、亚声门）（C32）			
ⅣB	任意 T	N3	M0	0	Tis	N0	M0
ⅣC	任意 T	任意 N	M1	Ⅰ	T1	N0	M0
鼻腔和鼻旁窦（C30）				Ⅱ	T2	N0	M0
0	Tis	N0	M0	Ⅲ	T3	N0	M0
Ⅰ	T1	N0	M0		T1	N1	—
Ⅱ	T2	N0	M0		T2	N1	—
	T3	N0	M0		T3	N1	—
Ⅲ	T1	N1	—	ⅣA	T4a	N0	M0
	T2	N1	—		T4a	N1	—
	T3	N1	—		T1	N2	—
	T4a	N0	M0		T2	N2	—
	T4a	N1	—		T3	N2	—
ⅣA	T1	N2	—		T4a	N2	—
	T2	N2	—	ⅣB	T4b	任意 N	M0
	T3	N2	—		任意 T	N3	—
	T4a	N2	—	ⅣC	任意 T	任意 N	M1

注：源自参考文献［156］。

预 防

目前没有确凿的方法可以完全预防头颈癌，但它是潜在可预防的。预防是长期控制疾病的主要潜在策略，而在短期内改善死亡率可能仅限于早期发现和治疗。通过政府支持的项目向公众传播有关头颈癌危险因素的信息将促进大众健康[18,132]。

多种因素可诱发不同类型的头颈癌。通过养成健康习惯可以降低患癌风险，包括停止使用任何形式的烟草和戒酒，因为这两者是导致各种类型头颈癌的主要因素。

疫苗可保护免受与头颈癌相关的 HPV 毒株感染。HPV 疫苗（Cervarix 和 Gardasil）现已上市，可帮助减少先前接触 HPV 的年轻女性中各种头颈癌的发生率[38]。然而，HPV 疫苗接种尚未纳入一些国家的国家免疫计划。在澳大利亚，针对 12～13 岁女性的 HPV 疫苗接种计划于 2007 年推出，但在澳大利亚男性中使用 HPV 疫苗存在争议。HPV 疫苗接种可能会降低这些癌症的未来发生率[18, 157]。通过限制性伴侣的数量，也可以避免 HPV 感染，因为多个性伴侣增加了 HPV 感染的风险，而避孕套无法完全防护 HPV 传播。

使用具有适当防晒系数（SPF）的润唇膏可以降低唇癌的风险。维护和妥善护理假牙可以降低头颈癌风险，因为不合适的假牙可能会捕获致癌物质，如烟草和酒精。

一些研究表明，定期食用富含复杂碳水化合物、植物油、鱼类、水果、蔬菜、植物雌激素和瘦肉的饮食可将口腔癌的风险降低 50%。还观察到，与食用黄油和豆类相比，食用水果和绿叶蔬菜将头颈癌的风险降低了 50%[18, 20, 38, 115, 158-160]。Zheng 等（1996）报告称，定期饮食中加入深黄色蔬菜和动物肝脏可降低唾液腺癌的风险[80]。

深黄色蔬菜含有丰富的类胡萝卜素（β-胡萝卜素），这是维生素 A 的主要前体，而肝脏则含有高水平的视黄醇。已有研究报告称，使用高剂量的视黄醇补充剂可减少头颈癌患者二次原发癌的发生率[161]。Rowe 等（1970）报告称，维生素 A 缺乏增加了唾液腺癌发生的风险[162]。深黄色蔬菜还富含维生素 C 和许多其他类胡萝卜素，是有效的抗氧化剂，可以防止自由基引起的脂质过氧化对染色体、酶和细胞膜的损害[163]。膳食中的维生素 C、酚类、芳香异硫氰酸酯和黄酮类成分在实验研究中被报道有抑制癌变的作用[80, 163, 164]。抗氧化剂可保护细胞和分子免受活性氧（ROS）和活性氮（RNS）造成的损害[13]。

目前，由于缺乏对头颈癌的认识以及缺少癌症预防项目，公众并不重视预防措施[165]。各国及地区相关机构应主动采取措施来消除导致头颈癌的原因，如中国台湾地区早已启动了槟榔管控计划，通过提供补贴鼓励农民种植替代物以打击槟榔咀嚼习惯[166]，此外，健康保险机构还宣布计划对槟榔征收健康税[166]。加拿大已禁止销售槟榔产品[26]。美国食品药品监督管理局（FDA）也发出了进口警报，并禁止槟榔的州际交易[26]。发展中国家在宣传普及与头颈癌相关的风险因素方面更需要采取切实措施，因为该癌症在低社会经济群体中普遍存在。

治 疗

用于头颈癌的治疗方法包括手术、放射治疗（RT）、化学治疗（ChT）、靶向治疗（TT）和免疫治疗（IT）[45, 167]。针对不同类型和分期的头颈癌，所采用的治疗方法取决于癌症的类型、可能产生的副作用以及患者的整体健康状况。根据具体情况，通常会联合采用多种治疗方法。

■ 手术
该过程会切除肿瘤及周围一些健康组织。根据患者的状况，可能需要进行多次手术[118]。

■ 放射治疗（RT）
通常推荐使用这种治疗作为手术的替代方案。有时，该疗法在手术后也会用于消灭残留的癌细胞[118]。

■ 化学治疗（ChT）
这种治疗可在手术前或手术后使用，或与放射治疗结合使用。顺铂和氟尿嘧啶（5-FU）是用于治疗头颈癌的化疗药物[118]。

■ 靶向治疗（TT）
尽管目前有多种先进的治疗方法用于头颈部鳞状细胞癌（HNSCC），但其生存率、功能结局和治疗毒性仍不甚明了[168]。目前已经获得批准或正在研究的靶向药物包括表皮生长因子受体（EGFR）单克隆抗体（西妥昔单抗、帕尼单抗、扎芦木单抗和尼妥珠单抗）、EGFR 酪氨酸激酶抑制剂（吉非替尼、厄洛替尼、拉帕替尼、阿法替尼和达克替尼）、血管内皮生长因子受体（VEGFR）抑制剂（贝伐单抗、索拉非尼、舒尼替尼和凡德他尼），以及磷脂酰肌醇 3 激酶（PI3K）/AKT/ 哺乳动物雷帕霉素靶点（mTOR）、MET 和胰岛素样生长因子受体（IGF-1R）等其他途径的各种抑制剂。临床试验正在评估这些新兴药物及其组合用于治疗 HNSCC 的效果[168]。

- **免疫治疗（IT）**

免疫治疗是针对晚期头颈癌患者的一个选择。

- **饮食**

Brookes（1985）报告称，接受放射治疗的营养不良头颈癌患者在 2 年内的生存率（7.5%）与营养良好的患者（57.5%）之间存在显著差异[18, 169]。

头颈癌的分期治疗

早期头颈癌的治疗涉及手术和根治性放射治疗（RT）。手术和放射治疗在控制局部肿瘤方面具有可比的效果，似乎都能提供等效的局部肿瘤控制。然而，治疗类型的选择基于多个因素，包括肿瘤部位、治疗结果、治疗机构的专业水平、患者健康状况以及患者偏好。所有这些因素都需要评估，以提高患者的治疗效果。

手术包括切除原发肿瘤和（或）淋巴结清扫，通常在早期治疗口腔癌时优先选择，而在患者拒绝手术或肿瘤因医学原因无法手术时，则倾向于采用根治性放疗。在这种情况下，放射治疗与手术相比，能够提供更好的功能结果。对于放疗后仍有残余病灶的患者，建议进行挽救性手术；而对于切缘邻近或阳性、淋巴血管或神经侵犯，或发现淋巴结转移导致肿瘤分期升级的患者，则建议进行术后放疗[126]。

化疗（ChT）是推荐用于 HNC 的另一种治疗方法。在化疗期间，患者会接受顺铂治疗，并需具备静脉输注的能力，同时提供足够的静脉补液和止吐药。必须在化疗前、期间及完成后维持足够的水合、营养和镇痛。整个治疗过程中，监测血细胞计数和患者的健康状况至关重要，因为化疗会产生多种副作用。与治疗相关的晚期毒性，如口干症、吞咽困难、语言功能障碍、胃管依赖、长期气管切开、神经病变、抑郁以及外观畸形，都会对患者的社会心理健康产生重大影响，因此必须提供必要的护理[126]。

- **早期头颈癌**

早期头颈癌（Ⅰ期和Ⅱ期）在局部治疗下可治愈 60%～95% 的患者[170]。治愈率取决于肿瘤的大小和位置以及提供必要治疗的能力。几乎所有的头颈肿瘤都是通过外科手术治疗的，唯一例外的是鼻咽癌，由于其解剖位置复杂，手术难度较大，因此采用放射治疗进行治疗[171]。因此，Ⅰ期和Ⅱ期头颈癌选择放疗还是手术取决于多个因素，包括肿瘤位置、由治疗引发长期疾病的可能性、医生的治疗技能、患者的偏好、合并症以及既往放疗史或对未来可能需要放疗的预期[118]。

对于口腔肿瘤，可以采用手术或放疗进行治疗。接受口腔肿瘤手术的患者恢复较慢，但相对功能较好，因此与放疗相比，手术治疗患者表现出较低的发病率，因为放疗会产生急性黏膜炎、舌部不适、牙齿腐烂及可能的长期饮食习惯改变等不良反应[118]。

在治疗咽部的早期肿瘤时，更常采用放疗，因为手术通常比放疗引发更高的复发率。因此，尽管放疗存在口干、轻度至中度吞咽功能障碍等风险，这种方法仍被考虑使用[118]。

对于鼻咽部肿瘤，手术难度较大，因此Ⅰ期或Ⅱ期（相对少见）的肿瘤通常仅用放疗进行处理[118]。

- **Ⅲ期/Ⅳ期头颈癌**

Ⅲ期或Ⅳ期头颈癌（局部区域晚期头颈癌）患者通常伴有较大或局部进展的 T3 或 T4 肿瘤，或颈部淋巴结受累。值得注意的是，大约 60% 的头颈癌患者在被诊断时已为局部区域晚期的Ⅲ期和Ⅳ期肿瘤[172, 173]。在这两个阶段中，大多数患者被诊断为Ⅳ期（ⅣA 期）肿瘤[118]。Ⅳ期头颈癌患者通常不能治愈，尤其是伴有转移性和局部区域晚期头颈癌的患者，平均生存期约为 6 个月，但非转移性Ⅳ期头颈癌是可以治愈的[118]。

局部区域晚期头颈癌的治疗存在一定争议，依赖于外科医生、机构以及患者是否愿意失去重要器官（如舌头、下颌、咽喉和喉部）[118]。对于Ⅲ期和Ⅳ期肿瘤，接受原发部位手术的患者的生存结果似乎更好，这些患者通常也会接受术后放疗，而仅接受放疗的患者则结果较差。化疗（ChT）被整合入大多数Ⅲ期和Ⅳ期鼻咽肿瘤的治疗中，而Ⅲ/Ⅳ期喉癌和下咽癌则采用序贯或同步化放疗而非手术治疗[118]。

在放疗中，改变分割剂量的放疗方法包括超分割放疗（HRT，即将每日剂量分成小剂量而不缩短治疗时间）和加速放疗（ART，即在短时间内提供高剂量的放疗）。HRT 在治疗咽部癌症时被发现可以提高局部区域控制率和生存率，优于标准分次放疗。然而，HRT 也表现出显著更高的副作用。ART 并未显现出与 HRT 一致的获益[118]。

结合化疗和放疗的联合治疗始于 20 世纪 70 年代末到 80 年代初。术前化疗几乎总是导致肿瘤的显著反应。使用顺铂和 5-FU 进行化疗与单独的局部区域治疗相比，显示出轻微的生存获益[118]。

20 世纪 80 年代，同时进行化疗和放疗（同步化疗放疗，CRT）被研究用于克服头颈癌的放射抵抗。无法手术切除的头颈癌患者被随机分为仅接受放疗与同时接受化放疗的临床试验。初期的研究通常使用单一药物化疗，但后来改用了多药物化疗（MCT）。研究发现，MCT 显示出比单一药物化疗更大的总体生存获益。CRT 可以作为挽救手段，前提是无法手术。接受初始放疗的患者在经过挽救手术后有治愈的可能性。同样，少数患者，特别是那些仅接受手术的早期头颈癌患者，可以通过放疗或 CRT 进行挽救[118]。

- **转移性疾病**

对于局部区域复发、不可治愈或转移性头颈癌患者，其预后较差，未接受化疗的平均生存期为 3～4 个月，而接受化疗的患者的平均生存期为 5～6 个月[174]。几种单药化疗药物（如顺铂、卡铂、紫杉醇、多西他赛、5-FU 和甲氨蝶呤）显示出 15%～25% 的反应率[118, 175]。联合化疗通常包括顺铂/卡铂与紫杉醇/多西他赛或 5-FU 的组合，这种治疗可以将反应率提高到 30%～35%。然而，无论是单药化疗还是多药化疗，生存率均保持不变[118]。

目前正在评估用于头颈癌的新治疗方法，包括各种生物靶向治疗。$EGFR$ 在大多数头颈癌中表现出过表达，因此 $EGFR$ 被用作头颈癌治疗的靶点，通过使用针对 $EGFR$ 的单克隆抗体或 $EGFR$ 的关键下游靶点进行治疗。头颈癌患者通常过表达 $p53$ 或表达突变型 $p53$。因此，$p53$ 也被视为基因治疗的靶点。腺病毒被用作载体，可以制作成具有复制能力的或无复制能力的，用于传递突变或野生型 $p53$ 进行基因治疗。根据初步的Ⅰ期和Ⅱ期研究中观察到的利用 $p53$ 基因转移的疗效和可行性，大规模Ⅲ期临床试验已经开展，以测试当基因转移疗法添加到标准化疗中时对局部晚期头颈部癌的效果[118]。

展　望

头颈癌的流行病学数据显示，发展中国家的头颈癌发病率相比于其他癌症更高。其主要原因可能是头颈癌的症状与常见口腔疾病的症状重叠，这些症状常常被个人或医疗工作者忽视。这种延误主要源于对症状缺乏意识，导致诊断延迟，从而造成更高的发病率和死亡率。此外，意识不足也可能导致致癌物质的使用增加。在各种头颈癌中，唇部和口腔癌占据了最多的病例，这可能与普遍的生活方式习惯有关，例如吸烟和饮酒。许多发展中国家的人们消费粗制的烟草或酒精，且不进行定期的口腔护理，这可能比他们在发达国家使用的精炼产品更加危险。工人未配备口罩以防护职业性灰尘也是头颈癌发病率上升的原因之一。

为了降低头颈癌的发生率，提高发展中国家对保持口腔卫生、使用烟草和酒精的危害、各种暴露因素及其引发头颈癌严重性的认识至关重要。由于这种癌症大多数情况下在晚期被发现,因此可以通过短信向个人发送其症状和预防方法的信息,并通过学校的展板、电视广告和电影院的宣传等方式利用当地语言进行传播。

参 考 文 献

[1] Black RJ, Bray F, Ferlay J, Parkin DM. Cancer incidence and mortality in the European Union: cancer registry data and estimates of national incidence for 1990. Eur J Cancer. 1997; 33(7): 1075–107.

[2] Hoffman HT, Karnell LH, Funk GF, Robinson RA, Menck HR. The National Cancer Data Base report on cancer of the head and neck. Arch Otolaryngol Head Neck Surg. 1998; 124(9): 951–62.

[3] Levi F, Lucchini F, La Vecchia C, Negri E. Trends in mortality from cancer in the European Union, 1955–94. Lancet. 1999; 354(9180): 742–3.

[4] Stoyanov GS, Kitanova M, Dzhenkov DL, Ghenev P, Sapundzhiev N. Demographics of head and neck cancer patients: a single institution experience. Cureus. 2017; 9(7): e1418.

[5] Royster HP. Surgical diagnosis in cancer of the head and neck. Surg Clin North Am. 1952; 32(6): 1599–616.

[6] Lynch P.J. CBhcolb. https: //upload.wikimedia.org/wikipedia/commons/5/51/Head_lateral_ mouth_anatomy.jpg.

[7] Shaikh MH, Khan AI, Sadat A, Chowdhury AH, Jinnah SA, Gopalan V, et al. Prevalence and types of high-risk human papillomaviruses in head and neck cancers from Bangladesh. BMC Cancer. 2017; 17(1): 792.

[8] Siegel RL, Miller KD, Jemal A. Cancer statistics, 2020. CA Cancer J Clin. 2020; 70(1): 7–30.

[9] NIH. National cancer institute 2020. Available from: https: //seer.cancer.gov/statfacts/html/lip.html.

[10] Sankaranarayanan R, Masuyer E, Swaminathan R, Ferlay J, Whelan S. Head and neck cancer: a global perspective on epidemiology and prognosis. Anticancer Res. 1998; 18(6B): 4779–86.

[11] Addala L, Pentapati CK, Reddy Thavanati PK, Anjaneyulu V, Sadhnani MD. Risk factor profiles of head and neck cancer patients of Andhra Pradesh, India. Indian J Cancer. 2012; 49(2): 215–9.

[12] Turner MC, Nieuwenhuijsen M, Anderson K, Balshaw D, Cui Y, Dunton G, et al. Assessing the exposome with external measures: commentary on the state of the science and research recommendations. Annu Rev Public Health. 2017; 38: 215–39.

[13] Khalili J. Oral cancer: risk factors, prevention and diagnostic. Exp Oncol. 2008; 30(4): 259–64.

[14] Khan Z, Tonnies J, Muller S. Smokeless tobacco and oral cancer in South Asia: a systematic review with meta-analysis. J Cancer Epidemiol. 2014; 2014: 394696.

[15] Gupta PC, Ray CS. Epidemiology of betel quid usage. Ann Acad Med Singap. 2004; 33(4 Suppl): 31–6.

[16] Proia NK, Paszkiewicz GM, Nasca MA, Franke GE, Pauly JL. Smoking and smokeless tobacco-associated human buccal cell mutations and their association with oral cancer – a review. Cancer Epidemiol Biomark Prev. 2006; 15(6): 1061–77.

[17] Gupta PC, Sinor PN, Bhonsle RB, Pawar VS, Mehta HC. Oral submucous fibrosis in India: a new epidemic? Natl Med J India. 1998; 11(3): 113–6.

[18] Singh SP, Eisenberg R, Hoffman G. An overview and comparative evaluation of head and neck cancer risk factors in India and Australia. Int J Otolaryngol Head Neck Surg. 2018; 7(5): 254–67.

[19] Elwood JM, Pearson JC, Skippen DH, Jackson SM. Alcohol, smoking, social and occupational factors in the aetiology of cancer of the oral cavity, pharynx and larynx. Int J Cancer. 1984; 34(5): 603–12.

[20] Warnakulasuriya S. 14 – Food, nutrition and oral cancer. In: Wilson M, editor. Food constituents and oral health. Cambridge: Woodhead Publishing; 2009. p. 273–95.

[21] Garavello W, Bertuccio P, Levi F, Lucchini F, Bosetti C, Malvezzi M, et al. The oral cancer epidemic in central and eastern Europe. Int J Cancer. 2010; 127(1): 160–71.

[22] Gupta B, Johnson NW, Kumar N. Global epidemiology of head and neck cancers: a continuing challenge. Oncology. 2016; 91(1): 13–23.

[23] Gupta N, Gupta R, Acharya AK, Patthi B, Goud V, Reddy S, et al. Changing trends in oral cancer – a global scenario. Nepal J Epidemiol. 2016; 6(4): 613–9.

[24] Warnakulasuriya S. Global epidemiology of oral and oropharyngeal cancer. Oral Oncol. 2009; 45(4–5): 309–16.

[25] Boffetta P, Hecht S, Gray N, Gupta P, Straif K. Smokeless tobacco and cancer. Lancet Oncol. 2008; 9(7): 667–75.

[26] Pankaj C. Areca nut or betel nut control is mandatory if India wants to reduce the burden of cancer especially cancer of the oral cavity. Int J Head Neck Surg. 2010; 1(1): 17–20.

[27] Mahboubi E. The epidemiology of oral cavity, pharyngeal and esophageal cancer outside of North America and Western Europe. Cancer. 1977; 40(4 Suppl): 1879–86.

[28] Sapkota A, Gajalakshmi V, Jetly DH, Roychowdhury S, Dikshit RP, Brennan P, et al. Smokeless tobacco and increased risk of hypopharyngeal and laryngeal cancers: a multicentric case-control study from India. Int J Cancer. 2007; 121(8): 1793–8.

[29] Mahdavifar N, Ghoncheh M, Mohammadian-Hafshejani A, Khosravi B, Salehiniya H. Epidemiology and inequality in the incidence and mortality of nasopharynx cancer in Asia. Osong Public Health Res Perspect. 2016; 7(6): 360–72.

[30] Yu MC, Yuan JM. Epidemiology of nasopharyngeal carcinoma. Semin Cancer Biol. 2002; 12(6): 421–9.

[31] Horn-Ross PL, Ljung BM, Morrow M. Environmental factors and the risk of salivary gland cancer. Epidemiology. 1997; 8(4): 414–9.

[32] La Vecchia C, Tavani A, Franceschi S, Levi F, Corrao G, Negri E. Epidemiology and prevention of oral cancer. Oral Oncol. 1997; 33(5): 302–12.

[33] Maier H, Sennewald E, Heller GF, Weidauer H. Chronic alcohol consumption – the key risk factor for pharyngeal cancer. Otolaryngol Head Neck Surg. 1994; 110(2): 168–73.

[34] Tuyns AJ, Esteve J, Raymond L, Berrino F, Benhamou E, Blanchet F, et al. Cancer of the larynx/hypopharynx, tobacco and alcohol: IARC international case-control study in Turin and Varese (Italy), Zaragoza and Navarra (Spain), Geneva (Switzerland) and Calvados (France). Int J Cancer. 1988; 41(4): 483–91.

[35] Guenel P, Chastang JF, Luce D, Leclerc A, Brugere J. A study of the interaction of alcohol drinking and tobacco smoking among French cases of laryngeal cancer. J Epidemiol Community Health. 1988; 42(4): 350–4.

[36] Laforest L, Luce D, Goldberg P, Begin D, Gerin M, Demers PA, et al. Laryngeal and hypopharyngeal cancers and occupational exposure to formaldehyde and various dusts: a case-control study in France. Occup Environ Med. 2000; 57(11): 767–73.

[37] Blot WJ, McLaughlin JK, Winn DM, Austin DF, Greenberg RS, Preston-Martin S, et al. Smoking and drinking in relation to oral and pharyngeal cancer. Cancer Res. 1988; 48(11): 3282–7.

[38] Warnakulasuriya S. Causes of oral cancer – an appraisal of controversies. Br Dent J. 2009; 207(10): 471–5.

[39] Smith EM, Rubenstein LM, Haugen TH, Pawlita M, Turek LP. Complex etiology underlies risk and survival in head and neck cancer human papillomavirus, tobacco, and alcohol: a case for multifactor disease. J Oncol. 2012; 2012: 571862.

[40] Perdomo S, Martin Roa G, Brennan P, Forman D, Sierra MS. Head and neck cancer burden and preventive measures in Central and South America. Cancer Epidemiol. 2016; 44(Suppl 1): S43–52.

[41] Gillison ML, Koch WM, Capone RB, Spafford M, Westra WH, Wu L, et al. Evidence for a causal association between human papillomavirus and a subset of head and neck cancers. J Natl Cancer Inst. 2000; 92(9): 709–20.

[42] Näsman A, Attner P, Hammarstedt L, Du J, Eriksson M, Giraud G, et al. Incidence of human papillomavirus (HPV) positive tonsillar carcinoma in Stockholm, Sweden: an epidemic of viral-induced carcinoma? Int J Cancer. 2009; 125(2): 362–6.

[43] Mehanna H, Beech T, Nicholson T, El-Hariry I, McConkey C, Paleri V, et al. Prevalence of human papillomavirus in oropharyngeal and nonoropharyngeal head and neck cancer – systematic review and meta-analysis of trends by time and region. Head Neck. 2013; 35(5): 747–55.

[44] Mehanna H, Evans M, Beasley M, Chatterjee S, Dilkes M, Homer J, et al. Oropharyngeal cancer: United Kingdom national multidisciplinary guidelines. J Laryngol Otol. 2016; 130(S2): S90–S6.

[45] Chi AC, Day TA, Neville BW. Oral cavity and oropharyngeal squamous cell carcinoma – an update. CA Cancer J Clin. 2015; 65(5): 401–21.

[46] Chang ET, Adami HO. The enigmatic epidemiology of nasopharyngeal carcinoma. Cancer Epidemiol Biomark Prev. 2006; 15(10): 1765–77.

[47] Lawal AO, Adisa AO, Kolude B, Adeyemi BF. Malignant salivary gland tumours of the head and neck region: a single institutions review. Pan Afr Med J. 2015; 20: 121.

[48] Levi F, Pasche C, La Vecchia C, Lucchini F, Franceschi S, Monnier P. Food groups and risk of oral and pharyngeal cancer. Int J Cancer. 1998; 77(5): 705–9.

[49] Kreimer AR, Randi G, Herrero R, Castellsague X, La Vecchia C, Franceschi S, et al. Diet and body mass, and oral and oropharyngeal squamous cell carcinomas: analysis from the IARC multinational case-control study. Int J Cancer. 2006; 118(9): 2293–7.

[50] Lucenteforte E, Garavello W, Bosetti C, La Vecchia C. Dietary factors and oral and pharyngeal cancer risk. Oral Oncol. 2009; 45(6): 461–7.

[51] Forrest J, Campbell P, Kreiger N, Sloan M. Salivary gland cancer: an exploratory analysis of dietary factors. Nutr Cancer. 2008; 60(4): 469–73.

[52] Dasanayake AP, Silverman AJ, Warnakulasuriya S. Mate drinking and oral and oro-pharyngeal cancer: a systematic review and meta-analysis. Oral Oncol. 2010; 46(2): 82–6.

[53] Otoh EC, Johnson NW, Danfillo IS, Adeleke OA, Olasoji HA. Primary head and neck cancers in North Eastern Nigeria. West Afr J Med. 2004; 23(4): 305–13.

[54] da Lilly-Tariah OB, Somefun AO, Adeyemo WL. Current evidence on the burden of head and neck cancers in Nigeria. Head Neck Oncol. 2009; 1: 14.

[55] Yu MC, Ho JH, Lai SH, Henderson BE. Cantonese-style salted fish as a cause of nasopharyngeal carcinoma: report of a case-control study in Hong Kong. Cancer Res. 1986; 46(2): 956–61.

[56] Ning JP, Yu MC, Wang QS, Henderson BE. Consumption of salted fish and other risk factors for nasopharyngeal carcinoma (NPC) in Tianjin, a low-risk region for NPC in the People's Republic of China. J Natl Cancer Inst. 1990; 82(4): 291–6.

[57] Armstrong RW, Imrey PB, Lye MS, Armstrong MJ, Yu MC, Sani S. Nasopharyngeal carcinoma in Malaysian Chinese: salted fish and other dietary exposures. Int J Cancer. 1998; 77(2): 228–35.

[58] Her C. Nasopharyngeal cancer and the Southeast Asian patient. Am Fam Physician. 2001; 63(9): 1776–82.
[59] Jia WH, Luo XY, Feng BJ, Ruan HL, Bei JX, Liu WS, et al. Traditional Cantonese diet and nasopharyngeal carcinoma risk: a large-scale case-control study in Guangdong, China. BMC Cancer. 2010; 10: 446.
[60] Zou XN, Lu SH, Liu B. Volatile N-nitrosamines and their precursors in Chinese salted fish – a possible etological factor for NPC in China. Int J Cancer. 1994; 59(2): 155–8.
[61] Huang DP, Ho JH, Webb KS, Wood BJ, Gough TA. Volatile nitrosamines in salt-preserved fish before and after cooking. Food Cosmet Toxicol. 1981; 19(2): 167–71.
[62] Hildesheim A, West S, DeVeyra E, De Guzman MF, Jurado A, Jones C, et al. Herbal medicine use, Epstein-Barr virus, and risk of nasopharyngeal carcinoma. Cancer Res. 1992; 52(11): 3048–51.
[63] Divaris K, Olshan AF, Smith J, Bell ME, Weissler MC, Funkhouser WK, et al. Oral health and risk for head and neck squamous cell carcinoma: the Carolina Head and Neck Cancer Study. Cancer Causes Control. 2010; 21(4): 567–75.
[64] Meyer MS, Joshipura K, Giovannucci E, Michaud DS. A review of the relationship between tooth loss, periodontal disease, and cancer. Cancer Causes Control. 2008; 19(9): 895–907.
[65] Holmes L Jr, DesVignes-Kendrick M, Slomka J, Mahabir S, Beeravolu S, Emani SR. Is dental care utilization associated with oral cavity cancer in a large sample of community-based United States residents? Community Dent Oral Epidemiol. 2009; 37(2): 134–42.
[66] Zheng TZ, Boyle P, Hu HF, Duan J, Jian PJ, Ma DQ, et al. Dentition, oral hygiene, and risk of oral cancer: a case-control study in Beijing, People's Republic of China. Cancer Causes Control. 1990; 1(3): 235–41.
[67] Albrecht M, Banoczy J, Dinya E, Tamas G Jr. Occurrence of oral leukoplakia and lichen planus in diabetes mellitus. J Oral Pathol Med. 1992; 21(8): 364–6.
[68] van Leeuwen MT, Grulich AE, McDonald SP, McCredie MR, Amin J, Stewart JH, et al. Immunosuppression and other risk factors for lip cancer after kidney transplantation. Cancer Epidemiol Biomark Prev. 2009; 18(2): 561–9.
[69] Li AC, Warnakulasuriya S, Thompson RP. Neoplasia of the tongue in a patient with Crohn's disease treated with azathioprine: case report. Eur J Gastroenterol Hepatol. 2003; 15(2): 185–7.
[70] Zhao H, Chu M, Huang Z, Yang X, Ran S, Hu B, et al. Variations in oral microbiota associated with oral cancer. Sci Rep. 2017; 7(1): 11773.
[71] Faggiano F, Partanen T, Kogevinas M, Boffetta P. Socioeconomic differences in cancer incidence and mortality. IARC Sci Publ. 1997; 138: 65–176.
[72] Conway DI, Petticrew M, Marlborough H, Berthiller J, Hashibe M, Macpherson LM. Socioeconomic inequalities and oral cancer risk: a systematic review and meta-analysis of case-control studies. Int J Cancer. 2008; 122(12): 2811–9.
[73] McDonald JT, Johnson-Obaseki S, Hwang E, Connell C, Corsten M. The relationship between survival and socio-economic status for head and neck cancer in Canada. J Otolaryngol Head Neck Surg. 2014; 43: 2.
[74] Tiyuri A, Mohammadian-Hafshejani A, Iziy E, Gandomani H, Salehiniya H. The incidence and mortality of lip and oral cavity cancer and its relationship to the 2012 Human Development Index of Asia. BMRAT. 2017; 4(02): 1147–65.
[75] Wake M. The urban/rural divide in head and neck cancer – the effect of atmospheric pollution. Clin Otolaryngol Allied Sci. 1993; 18(4): 298–302.
[76] Dietz A, Senneweld E, Maier H. Indoor air pollution by emissions of fossil fuel single stoves: possibly a hitherto underrated risk factor in the development of carcinomas in the head and neck. Otolaryngol Head Neck Surg. 1995; 112(2): 308–15.
[77] Pintos J, Franco EL, Kowalski LP, Oliveira BV, Curado MP. Use of wood stoves and risk of cancers of the upper aero-digestive tract: a case-control study. Int J Epidemiol. 1998; 27(6): 936–40.
[78] Williams RR, Stegens NL, Goldsmith JR. Associations of cancer site and type with occupation and industry from the Third National Cancer Survey Interview. J Natl Cancer Inst. 1977; 59(4): 1147–85.
[79] Flanders WD, Rothman KJ. Occupational risk for laryngeal cancer. Am J Public Health. 1982; 72(4): 369–72.
[80] Zheng W, Shu XO, Ji BT, Gao YT. Diet and other risk factors for cancer of the salivary glands: a population-based case-control study. Int J Cancer. 1996; 67(2): 194–8.
[81] Paget-Bailly S, Guida F, Carton M, Menvielle G, Radoi L, Cyr D, et al. Occupation and head and neck cancer risk in men: results from the ICARE study, a French population-based case-control study. J Occup Environ Med. 2013; 55(9): 1065–73.
[82] Comba P, Barbieri PG, Battista G, Belli S, Ponterio F, Zanetti D, et al. Cancer of the nose and paranasal sinuses in the metal industry: a case-control study. Br J Ind Med. 1992; 49(3): 193–6.
[83] Binazzi A, Ferrante P, Marinaccio A. Occupational exposure and sinonasal cancer: a systematic review and meta-analysis. BMC Cancer. 2015; 15: 49.
[84] Cauvin JM, Guenel P, Luce D, Brugere J, Leclerc A. Occupational exposure and head and neck carcinoma. Clin Otolaryngol Allied Sci. 1990; 15(5): 439–45.
[85] Dietz A, Ramroth H, Urban T, Ahrens W, Becher H. Exposure to cement dust, related occupational groups and laryngeal cancer risk: results of a population based case-control study. Int J Cancer. 2004; 108(6): 907–11.
[86] Pukkala E, Soderholm AL, Lindqvist C. Cancers of the lip and oropharynx in different social and occupational groups in Finland. Eur J Cancer B Oral Oncol. 1994; 30B(3): 209–15.
[87] Gustavsson P, Jakobsson R, Johansson H, Lewin F, Norell S, Rutkvist LE. Occupational exposures and squamous cell carcinoma of the

oral cavity, pharynx, larynx, and oesophagus: a case-control study in Sweden. Occup Environ Med. 1998; 55(6): 393–400.

[88] Boukheris H, Curtis RE, Land CE, Dores GM. Incidence of carcinoma of the major salivary glands according to the WHO classification, 1992 to 2006: a population-based study in the United States. Cancer Epidemiol Biomark Prev. 2009; 18(11): 2899–906.

[89] Langevin SM, McClean MD, Michaud DS, Eliot M, Nelson HH, Kelsey KT. Occupational dust exposure and head and neck squamous cell carcinoma risk in a population-based case-control study conducted in the greater Boston area. Cancer Med. 2013; 2(6): 978–86.

[90] Elwood JM. Wood exposure and smoking: association with cancer of the nasal cavity and paranasal sinuses in British Columbia. Can Med Assoc J. 1981; 124(12): 1573–7.

[91] Purdue MP, Järvholm B, Bergdahl IA, Hayes RB, Baris D. Occupational exposures and head and neck cancers among Swedish construction workers. Scand J Work Environ Health. 2006; 32(4): 270–5.

[92] Straif K, Benbrahim-Tallaa L, Baan R, Grosse Y, Secretan B, El Ghissassi F, et al. A review of human carcinogens – Part C: Metals, arsenic, dusts, and fibres. Lancet Oncol. 2009; 10(5): 453–4.

[93] Menvielle G, Fayosse A, Radoi L, Guida F, Sanchez M, Carton M, et al. The joint effect of asbestos exposure, tobacco smoking and alcohol drinking on laryngeal cancer risk: evidence from the French population-based case-control study, ICARE. Occup Environ Med. 2016; 73(1): 28–33.

[94] Carton M, Barul C, Menvielle G, Cyr D, Sanchez M, Pilorget C, et al. Occupational exposure to solvents and risk of head and neck cancer in women: a population-based case-control study in France. BMJ Open. 2017; 7(1): e012833.

[95] Schottenfeld D, Fraumeni JF Jr. Cancer epidemiology and prevention. New York: Oxford University Press; 2006.

[96] Land CE, Saku T, Hayashi Y, Takahara O, Matsuura H, Tokuoka S, et al. Incidence of salivary gland tumors among atomic bomb survivors, 1950–1987. Evaluation of radiation-related risk. Radiat Res. 1996; 146(1): 28–36.

[97] Dong C, Hemminki K. Second primary neoplasms among 53 159 haematolymphoproliferative malignancy patients in Sweden, 1958–1996: a search for common mechanisms. Br J Cancer. 2001; 85(7): 997–1005.

[98] Perea-Milla Lopez E, Minarro-Del Moral RM, Martinez-Garcia C, Zanetti R, Rosso S, Serrano S, et al. Lifestyles, environmental and phenotypic factors associated with lip cancer: a case-control study in southern Spain. Br J Cancer. 2003; 88(11): 1702–7.

[99] Vukadinovic M, Jezdic Z, Petrovic M, Medenica LM, Lens M. Surgical management of squamous cell carcinoma of the lip: analysis of a 10-year experience in 223 patients. J Oral Maxillofac Surg. 2007; 65(4): 675–9.

[100] Ariyawardana A, Johnson NW. Trends of lip, oral cavity and oropharyngeal cancers in Australia 1982–2008: overall good news but with rising rates in the oropharynx. BMC Cancer. 2013; 13: 333.

[101] Belsky JL, Takeichi N, Yamamoto T, Cihak RW, Hirose F, Ezaki H, et al. Salivary gland neoplasms following atomic radiation: additional cases and reanalysis of combined data in a fixed population, 1957–1970. Cancer. 1975; 35(2): 555–9.

[102] Spitz MR, Tilley BC, Batsakis JG, Gibeau JM, Newell GR. Risk factors for major salivary gland carcinoma. A case-comparison study. Cancer. 1984; 54(9): 1854–9.

[103] Khlifi R, Hamza-Chaffai A. Head and neck cancer due to heavy metal exposure via tobacco smoking and professional exposure: a review. Toxicol Appl Pharmacol. 2010; 248(2): 71–88.

[104] Llewellyn CD, Linklater K, Bell J, Johnson NW, Warnakulasuriya S. An analysis of risk factors for oral cancer in young people: a case-control study. Oral Oncol. 2004; 40(3): 304–13.

[105] Hussein AA, Helder MN, de Visscher JG, Leemans CR, Braakhuis BJ, de Vet HCW, et al. Global incidence of oral and oropharynx cancer in patients younger than 45 years versus older patients: a systematic review. Eur J Cancer. 2017; 82: 115–27.

[106] Russell JL, Chen NW, Ortiz SJ, Schrank TP, Kuo YF, Resto VA. Racial and ethnic disparities in salivary gland cancer survival. JAMA Otolaryngol Head Neck Surg. 2014; 140(6): 504–12.

[107] Dahlstrom KR, Little JA, Zafereo ME, Lung M, Wei Q, Sturgis EM. Squamous cell carcinoma of the head and neck in never smoker-never drinkers: a descriptive epidemiologic study. Head Neck. 2008; 30(1): 75–84.

[108] Subapriya R, Thangavelu A, Mathavan B, Ramachandran CR, Nagini S. Assessment of risk factors for oral squamous cell carcinoma in Chidambaram, Southern India: a case-control study. Eur J Cancer Prev. 2007; 16(3): 251–6.

[109] Gheit T, Anantharaman D, Holzinger D, Alemany L, Tous S, Lucas E, et al. Role of mucosal high-risk human papillomavirus types in head and neck cancers in Central India. Int J Cancer. 2017; 141(1): 143–51.

[110] Tsao SW, Tsang CM, Lo KW. Epstein-Barr virus infection and nasopharyngeal carcinoma. Philos Trans R Soc Lond B Biol Sci. 2017; 372(1732): 20160270.

[111] King GN, Healy CM, Glover MT, Kwan JT, Williams DM, Leigh IM, et al. Increased prevalence of dysplastic and malignant lip lesions in renal-transplant recipients. N Engl J Med. 1995; 332(16): 1052–7.

[112] Tavani A, Gallus S, La Vecchia C, Talamini R, Barbone F, Herrero R, et al. Diet and risk of oral and pharyngeal cancer. An Italian case-control study. Eur J Cancer Prev. 2001; 10(2): 191–5.

[113] Petridou E, Zavras AI, Lefatzis D, Dessypris N, Laskaris G, Dokianakis G, et al. The role of diet and specific micronutrients in the etiology of oral carcinoma. Cancer. 2002; 94(11): 2981–8.

[114] Llewellyn CD, Johnson NW, Warnakulasuriya S. Factors associated with delay in presentation among younger patients with oral cancer. Oral Surg Oral Med Oral Pathol Oral Radiol Endod. 2004; 97(6): 707–13.

[115] Freedman ND, Park Y, Subar AF, Hollenbeck AR, Leitzmann MF, Schatzkin A, et al. Fruit and vegetable intake and head and neck cancer risk in a large United States prospective cohort study. Int J Cancer. 2008; 122(10): 2330–6.

[116] Talamini R, Vaccarella S, Barbone F, Tavani A, La Vecchia C, Herrero R, et al. Oral hygiene, dentition, sexual habits and risk of oral cancer. Br J Cancer. 2000; 83(9): 1238–42.

[117] Preston-Martin S, Henderson BE, Bernstein L. Medical and dental x rays as risk factors for recently diagnosed tumors of the head. Natl Cancer Inst Monogr. 1985; 69: 175–9.

[118] Brockstein B, Masters G. Head and neck cancer. New York: Springer-Verlag New York Inc.; 2003.

[119] Diz P, Meleti M, Diniz-Freitas M, Vescovi P, Warnakulasuriya S, Johnson NW, et al. Oral and pharyngeal cancer in Europe: incidence, mortality and trends as presented to the Global Oral Cancer Forum. Transl Res Oral Oncol. 2017; 2: 2057178X17701517.

[120] Epstein JB, Kish RV, Hallajian L, Sciubba J. Head and neck, oral, and oropharyngeal cancer: a review of medicolegal cases. Oral Surg Oral Med Oral Pathol Oral Radiol. 2015; 119(2): 177–86.

[121] Cancer Research UK. Together we will beat cancer. 2018 [updated 10 May 2018]. Available from: https: //www.cancerresearchuk.org/about-cancer/mouth-cancer/symptoms.

[122] Koivunen P, Rantala N, Hyrynkangas K, Jokinen K, Alho OP. The impact of patient and professional diagnostic delays on survival in pharyngeal cancer. Cancer. 2001; 92(11): 2885–91.

[123] Argiris A, Karamouzis MV, Raben D, Ferris RL. Head and neck cancer. Lancet. 2008; 371(9625): 1695–709.

[124] Davies L, Welch HG. Epidemiology of head and neck cancer in the United States. Otolaryngol Head Neck Surg. 2006; 135(3): 451–7.

[125] Mehanna H, Paleri V, West CM, Nutting C. Head and neck cancer – Part 1: Epidemiology, presentation, and prevention. BMJ. 2010; 341: c4684.

[126] WHO Expert Committee on the Selection UoEMaWHO. The selection and use of essential medicines: report of the WHO Expert Committee, 2013 (including the 18th WHO model list of essential medicines and the 4th WHO model list of essential medicines for children), WHO technical report series; no. 985. Geneva: World Health Organization; 2014.

[127] Rumboldt Z, Gordon L, Gordon L, Bonsall R, Ackermann S. Imaging in head and neck cancer. Curr Treat Options in Oncol. 2006; 7(1): 23–34.

[128] Abraham J. Imaging for head and neck cancer. Surg Oncol Clin N Am. 2015; 24(3): 455–71.

[129] Knappe M, Louw M, Gregor RT. Ultrasonography-guided fine-needle aspiration for the assessment of cervical metastases. Arch Otolaryngol Head Neck Surg. 2000; 126(9): 1091–6.

[130] Righi PD, Kopecky KK, Caldemeyer KS, Ball VA, Weisberger EC, Radpour S. Comparison of ultrasound-fine needle aspiration and computed tomography in patients undergoing elective neck dissection. Head Neck. 1997; 19(7): 604–10.

[131] Brockstein B, Masters G. Head and neck cancer. New York: Springer Science & Business Media; 2006.

[132] Argiris A, Eng C. Epidemiology, staging, and screening of head and neck cancer. Cancer Treat Res. 2003; 114: 15–60.

[133] Cancer.net. 2018. Available from: https: //www.cancer.net/cancer-types/nasal-cavity-and-paranasal-sinus-cancer/diagnosis.

[134] Knowles SM, Wu AM. Advances in immuno-positron emission tomography: antibodies for molecular imaging in oncology. J Clin Oncol. 2012; 30(31): 3884–92.

[135] Nimmagadda S, Ford EC, Wong JW, Pomper MG. Targeted molecular imaging in oncology: focus on radiation therapy. Semin Radiat Oncol. 2008; 18(2): 136–48.

[136] Lewis-Jones H, Colley S, Gibson D. Imaging in head and neck cancer: United Kingdom National Multidisciplinary Guidelines. J Laryngol Otol. 2016; 130(S2): S28–31.

[137] Nordsmark M, Overgaard J. A confirmatory prognostic study on oxygenation status and loco-regional control in advanced head and neck squamous cell carcinoma treated by radiation therapy. Radiother Oncol. 2000; 57(1): 39–43.

[138] Bratasz A, Pandian RP, Deng Y, Petryakov S, Grecula JC, Gupta N, et al. In vivo imaging of changes in tumor oxygenation during growth and after treatment. Magn Reson Med. 2007; 57(5): 950–9.

[139] Tanay A, Regev A. Scaling single-cell genomics from phenomenology to mechanism. Nature. 2017; 541(7637): 331–8.

[140] (https: //creativecommons.org/licenses/by/3.0) DCB.

[141] (https: //creativecommons.org/licenses/by/2.0) kCB.

[142] (https: //creativecommons.org/licenses/by-sa/4.0) PCB-S.

[143] (https: //creativecommons.org/licenses/by-sa/4.0) NCB-S.

[144] (https: //creativecommons.org/licenses/by-sa/4.0) mCB-S.

[145] (https: //creativecommons.org/licenses/by-sa/3.0) SCB-S.

[146] (https: //creativecommons.org/licenses/by-sa/3.0) NDCB-S.

[147] https: //www.59mdw.af.mil/News/Photos/igphoto/2000074686/.

[148] CDC (Centers for Disease Control and Prevention) – Public Health Image Library (PHIL) – ID#: 10189.

[149] Goodyear M. p. Transverse plane enhancing CT scan viewed in the caudo-cephalic direction showing a right tonsillar enhancing squamous cell carcinoma (HPV positive). 2017.

[150] Institute NC. Oncogenes. p. This graphic illustrates the stages of how a normal cell is converted to a cancer cell, when an oncogene becomes activated.

[151] Albano PM, Lumang-Salvador C, Orosa J 3rd, Racelis S, Leano M, Angeles LM, et al. Overall survival of Filipino patients with squamous cell carcinoma of the head and neck: a single-institution experience. Asian Pac J Cancer Prev. 2013; 14(8): 4769–74.

[152] Agarwal N, Singh D, Verma M, Sharma S, Spartacus RK, Chaturvedi M. Possible causes for delay in diagnosis and treatment in head

and neck cancer: an institutional study. Int J Commun Med Public Health. 2018; 5(6): 2291−5.

[153] McGurk M, Chan C, Jones J, O'Regan E, Sherriff M. Delay in diagnosis and its effect on outcome in head and neck cancer. Br J Oral Maxillofac Surg. 2005; 43(4): 281−4.

[154] NHS. 2018. Available from: https: //www.nhs.uk/common-health-questions/operations-tests-and-procedures/what-do-cancer-stages-and-grades-mean/.

[155] Cancer Treatment Centers of America. 2020[09.06.2020]. Available from: https: //www.cancercenter. com/cancer-types/head-and-neck-cancer/stages.

[156] Shah NP, Workman RB Jr, Coleman RE. PET and PET/CT in head and neck cancer. In: Workman Jr RB, Coleman RE, editors. PET/CT essentials for clinical practice. New York: Springer; 2006.

[157] Shefer A, Markowitz L, Deeks S, Tam T, Irwin K, Garland SM, et al. Early experience with human papillomavirus vaccine introduction in the United States, Canada and Australia. Vaccine. 2008; 26(Suppl 10): K68−75.

[158] Sinha R, Anderson DE, McDonald SS, Greenwald P. Cancer risk and diet in India. J Postgrad Med. 2003; 49(3): 222−8.

[159] Negri E, Franceschi S, Bosetti C, Levi F, Conti E, Parpinel M, et al. Selected micronutrients and oral and pharyngeal cancer. Int J Cancer. 2000; 86(1): 122−7.

[160] Potter JD, Steinmetz K. Vegetables, fruit and phytoestrogens as preventive agents. IARC Sci Publ. 1996; 139: 61−90.

[161] Hong WK, Lippman SM, Itri LM, Karp DD, Lee JS, Byers RM, et al. Prevention of second primary tumors with isotretinoin in squamous-cell carcinoma of the head and neck. N Engl J Med. 1990; 323(12): 795−801.

[162] Rowe NH, Grammer FC, Watson FR, Nickerson NH. A study of environmental influence upon salivary gland neoplasia in rats. Cancer. 1970; 26(2): 436−44.

[163] Steinmetz KA, Potter JD. Vegetables, fruit, and cancer. II. Mechanisms. Cancer Causes Control. 1991; 2(6): 427−42.

[164] Block G. Vitamin C and cancer prevention: the epidemiologic evidence. Am J Clin Nutr. 1991; 53(1 Suppl): 270S−82S.

[165] Bhattacharjee A, Chakraborty A, Purkaystha P. Prevalence of head and neck cancers in the north east-an institutional study. Indian J Otolaryngol Head Neck Surg. 2006; 58(1): 15−9.

[166] IARC Working Group on the Evaluation of Carcinogenic Risks to Humans. Betel-quid and areca-nut chewing and some areca-nut derived nitrosamines. IARC Monogr Eval Carcinog Risks Hum. 2004; 85: 1−334.

[167] Steuer CE, El-Deiry M, Parks JR, Higgins KA, Saba NF. An update on larynx cancer. CA Cancer J Clin. 2017; 67(1): 31−50.

[168] Dorsey K, Agulnik M. Promising new molecular targeted therapies in head and neck cancer. Drugs. 2013; 73(4): 315−25.

[169] Brookes GB. Nutritional status − a prognostic indicator in head and neck cancer. Otolaryngol Head Neck Surg. 1985; 93(1): 69−74.

[170] Worsham MJ. Identifying the risk factors for late-stage head and neck cancer. Expert Rev Anticancer Ther. 2011; 11(9): 1321−5.

[171] Yeh SA. Radiotherapy for head and neck cancer. Semin Plast Surg. 2010; 24(2): 127−36.

[172] Kim DH, Kim WT, Lee JH, Ki YK, Nam JH, Lee BJ, et al. Analysis of the prognostic factors for distant metastasis after induction chemotherapy followed by concurrent chemoradiotherapy for head and neck cancer. Cancer Res Treat. 2015; 47(1): 46−54.

[173] Lee JH, Song JH, Lee SN, Kang JH, Kim MS, Sun DI, et al. Adjuvant postoperative radiotherapy with or without chemotherapy for locally advanced squamous cell carcinoma of the head and neck: the importance of patient selection for the postoperative chemoradiotherapy. Cancer Res Treat. 2013; 45(1): 31−9.

[174] Brockstein B, Vokes E. Treatment of metastatic and recurrent head and neck cancer UpToDate: UpToDate; 2013. Available from: uptodate.com/contents/treatment-of-metastatic-and-recurrent-head-and-neck-cancer/print.

[175] Molin Y, Fayette J. Current chemotherapies for recurrent/metastatic head and neck cancer. Anti-Cancer Drugs. 2011; 22(7): 621−5.

第 2 章

Hamzah Alkofahi and Mehdi Ebrahimi

口腔潜在恶性病变
Potentially Malignant Disorders of the Oral Cavity

引 言

头颈癌，包括口腔癌，会对患者的生活质量造成严重影响，早期发现和治疗头颈癌或潜在恶性病变可以大大降低癌症的发病率和死亡率[1]，因此，在癌变前对头颈部潜在恶性病变进行早期干预至关重要。

口腔癌发生前，口腔黏膜可以出现明显的临床变化，表现为患癌风险增加的临床中间状态。1972年，"癌前病变"（precancer）一词首次被世界卫生组织（WHO）认可，此后，这一概念又进一步分为两类：癌前病变和癌前状态。随着对口腔癌前病变过程的不断了解，2007年，WHO专家小组引入了"口腔潜在恶性病变"（oral potentially malignant disorders, OPMDs）一词[2]。随后，该术语又在2017年被WHO纳入头颈部肿瘤分类[3]。

文献报道中也曾有其他相关术语，如癌前病变（precancer）、恶变前的（premalignant）、瘤变前的（preneoplastic）、有癌变倾向（carcinoma prone）、上皮先驱病变（epithelial precursor）、上皮内瘤变（intraepithelial neoplasia）和上皮内癌（intraepithelial carcinoma），用以描述"口腔黏膜"向"口腔鳞状细胞癌"（oral squamous cell carcinoma，OSCC）的转化，后者是一种严重危害头颈部和全身健康的恶性病变。全球OPMDs的患病率约为4.47%（95% CI：2.43%～7.08%），亚洲人和男性的患病率更高[4]。将口腔黏膜的某些疾病或病变称为"癌前的"概念是基于OPMDs与癌性病损在临床表现、形态学和细胞学观察、基因组或分子改变存在相似性[1]。

根据WHO的定义，"癌前病变"定义为"与正常的对应组织相比，更易发生口腔癌的一种形态学改变的组织"。例如：① 口腔白斑（OL）；② 口腔红斑（OE）；③ 舌下角化症；④ 慢性增生性念珠菌病。但是，并不是所有的潜在癌前病变都会转变为恶性肿瘤，一般来说，白色病变比红色病变更为常见，恶变风险也更低。

WHO将"癌前状态"定义为"与癌症风险

H. Alkofahi
Division of Plastic & Reconstructive Surgery, Department of Surgery, Stanford University School of Medicine, Stanford, CA, USA

Department of Oral and Maxillofacial Surgery, Jordanian Royal Medical Services, Irbid, Jordan

M. Ebrahimi (✉)
Prince Philip Dental Hospital, The University of Hong Kong, Pok Fu Lam, Hong Kong, China
e-mail: ebrahimi@connect.hku.hk

显著增加相关的一种全身状态"，常见的如口腔黏膜下纤维性变（OSMF），其他不太常见且癌变风险较小的有扁平苔藓、缺铁性吞咽困难、胼胝症、先天性角化不良和吸烟相关角化病。表2-1总结了临床相关的OPMDs、种类、临床特征、好发部位和癌变率。本章简要概述了最常见的OPMDs，详细讨论了OPMDs早期发现和恶变检测的现有筛查方法，包括传统的（即染色、光基检测系统、光学诊断技术）和最近有应用前景的分子生物标志物分析技术。

表2-1 OPMDs的特征

病 变	临 床 特 征	部 位	累积恶变率（99% CI）
口腔白斑病	通常是无症状的白色斑块，不能擦掉	脸颊，嘴唇，牙龈	8.6%（5.1%～13.0%）
口腔红斑病	有明显症状的红色斑片，边缘清晰	口底，舌，磨牙后垫，软腭	33.1%（13.6%～56.2%）
增殖性疣状白斑（PVL）	多发性皱纹状白色斑片或斑块，复发率高	牙龈，牙槽突，腭	49.5%（26.7%～72.4%）
Viadent相关白斑病	白色斑片或斑块	牙龈，颊侧和唇部前庭	无数据
念珠菌性白斑	坚硬的白色皮革状斑块	脸颊，唇，腭	无数据
无烟烟草角化病	白色斑块	颊侧或唇侧前庭	无数据
与反吸烟相关的腭角化病	白色斑片和斑块	腭，舌	83%异常增生
疣状增生	广泛的厚白色斑块	颊黏膜	无数据
口腔疣状癌	广泛的厚白色斑块	颊黏膜	无数据
先天性角化不良	口腔白斑	颊黏膜，舌，口咽	无数据
光化性唇干裂	弥漫性，界限不清萎缩性，糜烂性，溃疡性或角化性斑块	下唇	无数据
角化棘皮瘤	坚硬，无蒂，无压痛的结节+中央角蛋白栓	嘴唇，舌头，舌下区	无数据
口腔黏膜下纤维性变	黏膜僵硬，张嘴受限	颊黏膜，磨牙后垫，舌，软腭	5.2%（2.9%～8.0%）
口腔苔藓样病变	白色和红色病变，呈网状条纹状	位于致敏物旁边	3.8%（1.6%～7.0%）
口腔扁平苔藓	有症状的，网状，环状，线状，糜烂性，萎缩性，大疱性，溃疡性，流行性，斑块样	后牙颊黏膜，舌，牙龈，腭，朱红色缘	1.4%（0.9%～1.9%）
盘状红斑狼疮	白色斑块，边界隆起，放射白色条纹和毛细血管扩张	脸颊，唇，腭	无数据
表皮松解大疱	轻度创伤后形成大疱和水疱	脸颊，舌，腭	无数据
疣状黄瘤	黄白色或红色，乳突状或疣状表面，界限清晰的肿块	牙龈，舌，颊，前庭，口底	无数据
移植物抗宿主病	萎缩，红斑，糜烂，溃疡，苔藓样病变	脸颊，舌，嘴唇，颊侧和唇部前庭	无数据

注：源自参考文献［5，6］。

口腔潜在恶性病变（OPMDs）

口腔白斑

口腔白斑（oral leukoplakia, OL；leuko 即白色，plakia 即斑）是最常见的口腔癌前病变。OL 被定义为与特定诊断无关的白色斑片或斑块[7]。在大多数情况下，口腔白色病变的病因较为明确，可能是真菌感染、创伤、白色水肿、白色海绵状斑痣或慢性刺激等，因此，只有排除其他白色病变后才能确诊。口腔白斑的全球患病率为 1.49%~2.60%[8]，癌变率为 0.1%~17.5%[9]。尽管白斑可发生于任何年龄，但相较而言，40 岁以下的男性更为多见[10]。OL 的全球发病率存在显著差异，可能与年龄、不良习惯和种族多样性有关。OL 的主要病因尚不明确，但许多诱发因素（如吸烟/无烟烟草、酒精、人乳头瘤病毒、慢性刺激和流电反应）可以增加 OL 的发生及癌变风险。吸烟或无烟烟草可导致 OL 发生风险增加 6 倍[11]。有趣的是，与不使用烟草的患者相比，烟草相关的白斑癌变概率似乎更低[12]。

临床上，OL 可分为两大类：① 均质型：无症状、均匀扁平的白色斑片，表面可有皲裂（图 2-1）；② 非均质型。非均匀型通常有症状，临床又可以分为三种亚型：① 斑点型，以白色病损为主，间杂红色斑点，如红白斑；② 结节型，小而圆，红色/白色，边缘不规则的赘生物；③ 疣状型或外生型，病损表面不平整呈波纹状或皱纹状，并伴有乳头状突起，与疣状癌难以区分[11]。虽然颊黏膜是白斑最好发部位，但白斑可发生在口腔的任何部位，包括牙龈、舌和口底。软腭和舌下区 OL 癌变风险最高。OL 的显微镜下特征是：① 过度角化或过度正角化（由角蛋白分泌引起的上皮增厚）；② 上皮棘层增生。上皮固有层有不同程度的慢性炎症浸润。

增殖性疣状白斑（PVL）是一种特殊类型的 OL，表现为多发，界限分明，疣状、斑点状分布的白色斑块，更易发展成为侵袭性的恶性肿瘤，如鳞癌或疣状癌。诊断 PVL 的主要临床标准包括：① OL 累及两个以上口腔部位，好发于牙龈、牙槽嵴和腭；② 部分区域呈疣状外观；③ 疾病持续进展；④ 治疗过的部位复发[13]。Carrard 等人（2013）[14] 介绍了 PVL 的组织学诊断标准，包括：① 存在疣状或类疣样外观，涉及两个以上的口腔位点；② 病损区域至少 3 cm；③ 病程 5 年以上，并不断扩大，且在原治疗区复发；④ 至少 1 次活检，排除疣状癌（VC）或 OSCC。

目前研究证实高龄、女性、病损面积大于 200 mm^2、非均质型（如红白斑）、合并白色念珠菌感染、较高级别的上皮异常增生程度是 OL 癌变的重要决定因素[15]。OL 的疾病进展和癌变并无规律可循，因此，应对患者密切随访，观察病变外观的均质性、面积大小的变化情况和有无新发病损。OL 的治疗策略主要是消除相关危险

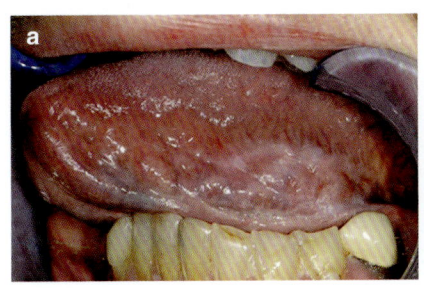 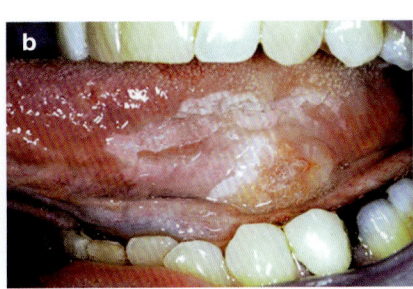 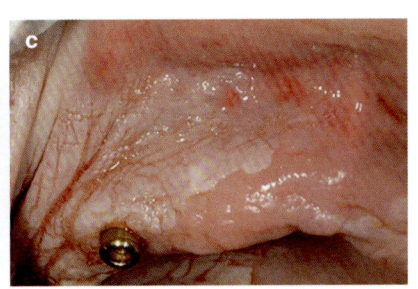

图 2-1 白斑类型。a. 均质型白斑，呈扁平、薄而均匀的白色外观。b. 非均质型白斑发生癌变。c. 累及牙龈、牙槽和颊黏膜的增殖性疣状白斑（经允许引自参考文献 [11]）

因素，以及手术干预（如传统外科手术、激光治疗、冷冻和光动力治疗）。

细胞外基质（extracellular matrix, ECM）通路[16]的下调可以促进 OL 的恶性转变，这一转变过程可以是隐匿的，无明显临床变化的。最新研究表明，上皮和间充质表型之间的动态转化在疾病进展和癌变形成中发挥了重要作用。细胞从上皮状态向间充质状态的转变过程被称为上皮-间充质转化（epithelial-mesenchymal transition, EMT），可通过改变细胞表达的黏附分子，赋予细胞转移和侵袭能力。目前，对 EMT 通路及其相关蛋白（Snail、Twist、E-cadherin、N-cadherin 和 Vimentin）以及聚义转化过程仍不明确，需要进一步深入了解，以获得更好的生存预后和管理策略[17,18]。

口腔红斑

口腔红斑是一种鲜红色天鹅绒样病变，平坦或略凹陷，边缘清晰但不规则，且不能诊断为任何其他特定疾病（图 2-2）。红斑病通常无症状，但一些患者在进食时可能会有烧灼疼痛感[19]。红斑最常见于软腭和口底，舌和颊黏膜次之，与念珠菌病或系统性狼疮多发性病损不同，红斑多呈现为单个独立的病变[20]。

虽然红斑不如白斑常见，但其恶变概率更高[7]。口腔红斑常被认为是早期浸润性口腔癌的一部分，活检时多表现为"原位癌"或"浸润性癌"[2,21]。全球不同地区的红斑发病率为 0.02%~0.8%，中老年人群中男女发病率相近[20]。口腔红斑的病因尚不清楚，但与吸烟和饮酒密切相关[22]。

组织病理学上，红斑通常表现为上皮从异常增生到浸润性癌的一系列改变[23]。显微镜下，萎缩的口腔黏膜上皮细胞不能产生角蛋白，因而在临床上表现为红色病损。上皮下结缔组织可见炎细胞浸润。对单纯红斑病变来说，异常增生程度越严重，恶变的风险越大[24]。因此，对红斑病损的体征和症状进行充分的临床检查是必不可少的，同时，还需要管理不良生活行为，包括戒烟戒酒，必要时可以进行活检和长期随访以追踪可能的复发。一旦活检确定病变的性质和范围后，手术切除是治疗红斑的首选方法[25]。早期发现可预防恶变，提高生存率和生活质量[26]。

口腔黏膜下纤维性变

口腔黏膜下纤维性变（OSMF）是一种慢性不可逆病变，其特征是固有层和深层结缔组织的炎症以及伴随的纤维性变（图 2-3）。早期临床症状多表现为黏膜发白、进食辛辣食物后有烧灼感、正常色素沉着丧失[27]。进展期可表现为纤维弹性丧失、上皮萎缩以及显著张口受限[28]。

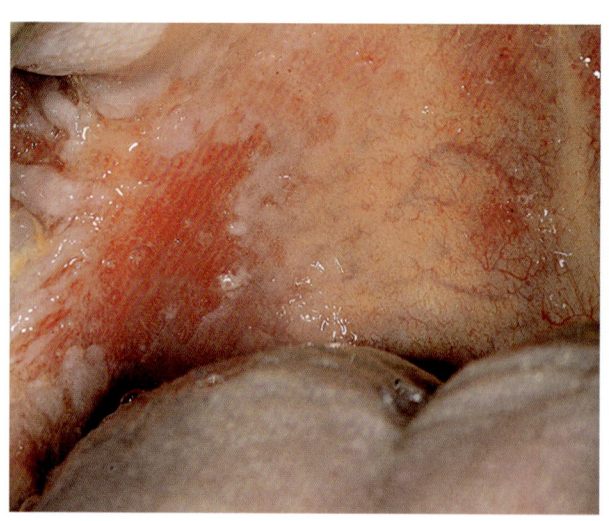

图 2-2　软腭口腔红斑。该红色斑块处活检观察到上皮重度异常增生（经允许引自参考文献[11]）

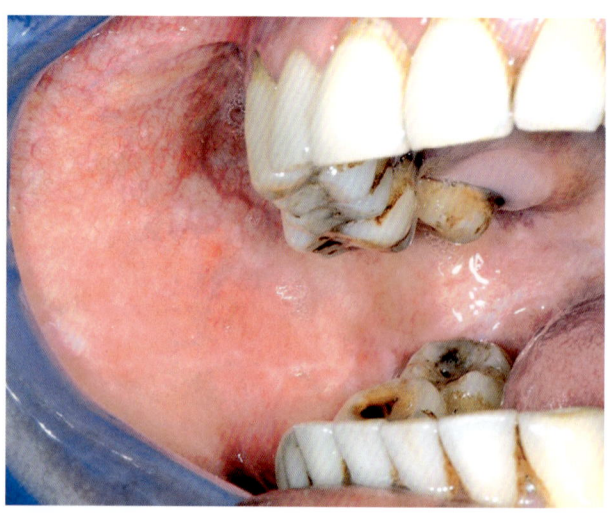

图 2-3　OSMF 早期，颊黏膜苍白（经允许引自参考文献[11]）

尽管 OSMF 可以累及上消化道黏膜的任何部位，但颊黏膜最常被报道[29]。OSMF 的发生主要与咀嚼槟榔有关[30]，咀嚼槟榔是东南亚和印度的一种习惯，类似于西方国家的咀嚼烟草。

OSMF 的发病机制尚不清楚，但普遍认为是多因素的，包括咀嚼槟榔、辣椒刺激、遗传和免疫因素以及营养缺乏等[31,32]。OSMF 的发病率很高，且常会出现进行性张口受限，导致进食困难和营养缺乏。

OSMF 以恶变为鳞状细胞癌而闻名，恶变率可高达10%[33]。多种分子和基因途径可诱发 OSMF 癌变，如细胞周期、DNA、血管生成、EMT 和组织缺氧的改变[30,31]。有研究提出包括转化生长因子-β（TGF-β）[31,34]、白细胞介素-6（IL-6）[35]、骨形态发生蛋白7（BMP7）[36]和胶原蛋白亚型[36]在内的基因途径的激活在 OSMF 的癌变过程中发挥了重要作用。

OSMF 的不同病程发展阶段，其组织学表现也不同（图2-3）[37]。组织病理学上，OSMF 通常表现为致密的胶原纤维束、上皮下延伸至黏膜下的玻璃样变性带（取代脂肪或纤维血管组织）、血管减少、上皮和下层肌肉萎缩[38,39]。

OSMF 患者治疗方案的选择取决于疾病的病程发展阶段。疾病早期属于可逆阶段，需要对患者进行卫生宣教和习惯管理；疾病后期属于不可逆阶段，治疗的主要目的是恢复正常的口腔功能。已有研究报道使用类固醇、胎盘提取物[40]、透明质酸酶[41]、IFN-γ[42]、番茄红素[43]和己酮可可碱[44]等药物用于 OSMF 的治疗。对于严重张口受限患者和有异常增生或癌变的患者，手术干预是必要的。手术方式包括单纯切除纤维病变组织、双侧颞肌切开术或喙突切除术后移植中厚皮片，以及使用激光治疗（如 KTP-532 激光和 ErCr: YSGG 激光）[38,45,46]。

口腔潜在恶性病变（OPMDs）的诊断和筛查

口腔黏膜癌变前通常存在 OPMDs[47]；然而，由于 OPMDs 类型和特点不同，很难评估单个病例的恶变风险[15,48]。恰恰因为 OPMDs 恶变风险难以预测，早期诊断极其重要。早期发现癌变可以降低治疗相关的并发症和死亡率，显著提高生活质量。有数据表明，如果早期发现局部癌变，患者生存率可提高到82%（图2-4）[49]。

据报道，因致癌刺激导致的癌变大多发生在 OPMDs 被发现的前2年，而且在之后的10～15年癌变风险仍会持续上升[50,51]，这些致癌风险可诱发细胞学改变并最终导致癌变，这种现象称为"区域癌变"（field cancerization），由 Slaughter 于1953年首次提出，在最近的分子研究中也得到了证实[52]。因此，在随访期间，应仔细筛查和监测高危人群（如大量吸烟、咀嚼槟榔、饮酒者）和高危 OPMDs（红斑、红白斑、增殖性疣状白斑、OSMF）[53]。

对头颈部进行系统性的口内口外视诊和触诊是口腔癌前病变临床诊断的关键，也是筛查和随访 OPMDs 潜在恶变倾向的最常用方法。该方法简便易行，敏感性可以达到84%，特异性可以达到96%[54]。但是，这种方式只在可视诊和触诊区域可行，并存在假阴性结果的风险，因此，一些辅助检查技术手段已被开发并应用于相关临床和研究领域[54,55]。这些检查技术大致分为两种：有创性（即细胞刷、活检）和无创性（即染色、基于光的检测系统、光学诊断方法和分子标志物）。

无创性技术

■ 活体染色

活体染色是指使用染料对口腔黏膜组织进行染色，以便更好地观察 OPMDs 和恶性肿瘤。已有多种染色方法，如甲苯胺蓝或亚甲基蓝染色[57,58]、孟加拉玫瑰红染色[59,60]和卢戈氏碘染色[61]，应用于临床诊疗和基础研究。染色

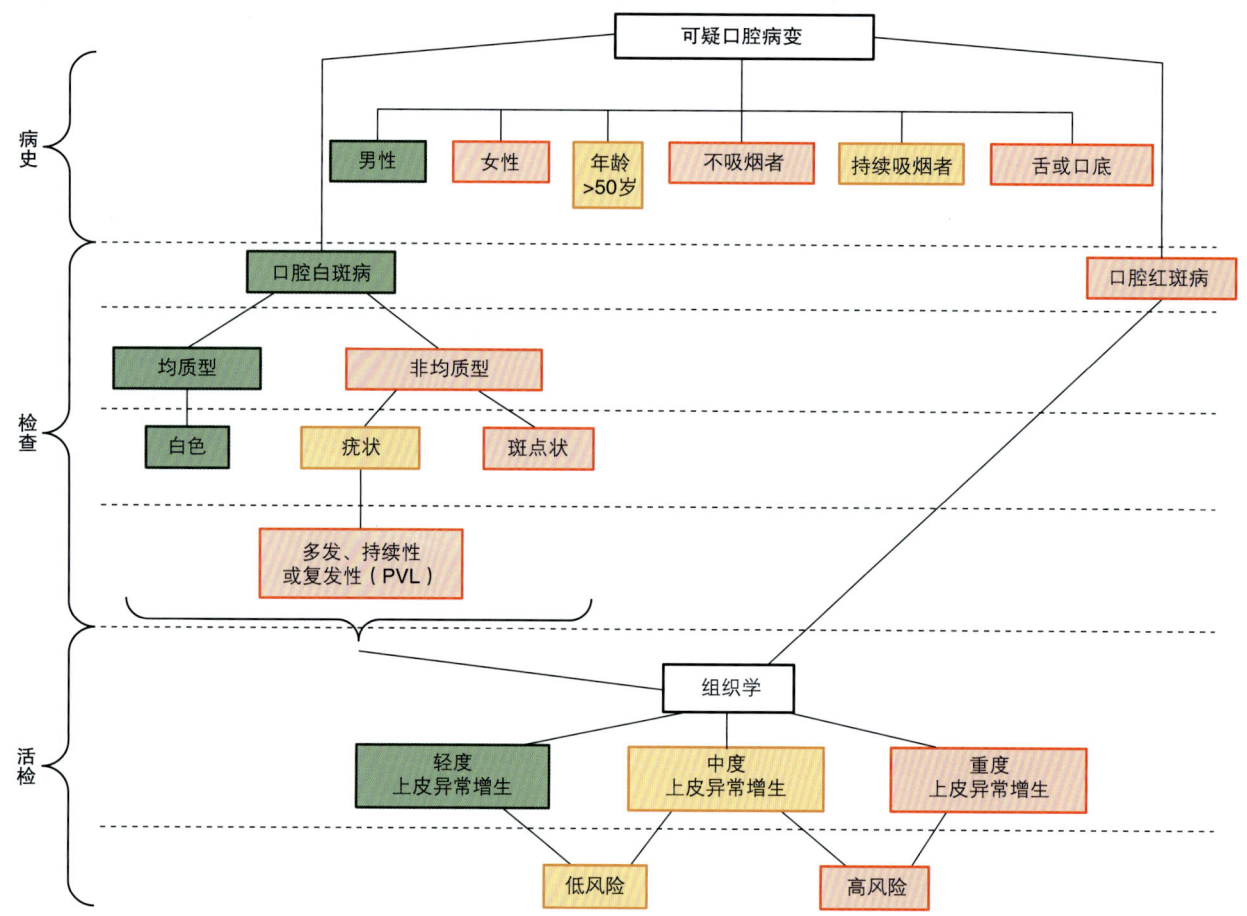

图 2-4　口腔潜在恶性病变（OPMDs）临床癌变风险的简易评估法。临床医生评估可疑的口腔病变时，每一评估阶段单个要素的风险用绿色（低风险）、黄色（中风险）或红色（高风险）表示（经允许引自参考文献[56]）

前，先用乙酸预处理，然后用水冲洗口腔黏膜，如果观察到组织染色，则测试结果为阳性，否则为阴性。例如，甲苯胺蓝或亚甲基蓝对酸性成分（即核酸）具有很高的亲和力，染色后呈深色（阳性）或淡宝蓝色（可疑）[62-64]。

活体染色是一种简单、廉价、便利的方法，能够明确临床表现不明显的病变，也可用于评估OPMDs活检的切除范围；其缺点是可能因为良性炎性病变而导致假阳性结果，在一些癌变和异常增生的病损中灵敏度较差。因此，由于活体染色的假阳性结果比例相对较高[65]，在应用时可以联合其他检测方法（如细胞学和基于光的检测方法）[66]。

- **基于光的检测系统**
  - *化学发光法*

化学发光法是指发射特定波长（430 nm、540 nm 和 580 nm）的光（luminescence），用于区分正常和异常组织，应用化学发光技术的商品化仪器有 ViziLite、ViziLite Plus、Microlux/DL 和 Orascoptic DK。ViziLite™ 是最常用的检测系统，包括：① ViziLite（OralLite），一次性化学发光荧光棒；② ViziLite 蓝色口腔病变识别和标记系统，这是一种辅助 ViziLite 测试的三组分拭子系统[67]。使用 ViziLite 时，首先需要患者用 1% 的柠檬酸漱口以清洁附着的糖蛋白并使黏膜脱水，然后施加光源，如果上皮表面呈浅蓝白色，则检测结果为阴性，如果呈明显的白色（醋酸白色）则为阳性[68]。然而，目前的研究报道仍没有足够的证据证实应用化学发光技术可以有效区分炎症、创伤、OPMDs 和恶性病变[69-71]。

  - *组织自体荧光*

组织自体荧光是指细胞内的内源性荧光分子

暴露于特定波长（365 nm）的光下会产生荧光发射的现象[72]。由于组织结构和荧光分子浓度的变化，异常的黏膜组织可以改变光的吸收和散射特性[73]。由于自体荧光缺失，异常组织呈现暗区，而正常组织呈现淡绿色荧光[74]。虽然该系统有助于OPMDs和口腔癌的筛查，但不能有效地区分两者[75]。此外，由于假阳性率过高，对于检测结果应仔细甄别，例如，黏膜色素沉着、溃疡、牙龈炎、局部刺激和血肿等情况可能会降低荧光，导致外观变暗。因此，对于可疑的阳性病变需要谨慎随访[76]。

- 光动力技术

光动力技术是一种冷光化学过程，不产生热量，而且它对底层和周围组织以及重要结构的损伤风险最小。因此，与热激光方法和其他有创性方法相比，它更为安全[77]，是用于诊断和治疗OPMDs以及其他口腔癌的一种替代性微创方法。

该技术有三个基本要素：组织氧、光敏剂和特定波长的可见光[78]。光敏剂在光照射下被激活，导致一系列基于光源类型的光化学和光生物学反应。使用短波长的光源激活光敏剂时，可达到诊断目的，被激发的电子进行"内部转换"并以荧光的形式释放能量，可用于病变的可视化[79]；使用长波长的光源激活光敏剂时，被激活的光敏剂发生"系间窜越"（intersystem crossing）导致Ⅰ型或Ⅱ型反应，同时释放出活性氧，从而用于治疗[79]。

关键的系统性文献回顾的结果表明，光动力疗法是治疗OPMDs的一种有效的无创治疗方案[80-82]。常用的光敏剂有氨基酮戊酸（ALA）、替莫波芬、Foscan、血卟啉衍生物、Photofrin、Photosan、亚甲基蓝和Ce6（二氢卟吩e6）。激光照射（例如波长420～660 nm，功率密度50～500 mW/cm^2）适当时间（1～15分钟，间隔7天）的完全响应率为23.58%～100%[77,80,82]。根据目前文献报道，最具应用前景的光动力疗法是局部应用20% ALA，并以二极管激光作为光源的最佳选择[81]。但是，仍需要更深入的随机临床研究，包括中期和长期随访，以验证该方法在OPMDs治疗中的有效性。

- 光学诊断技术

不断创新的光学诊断系统和试剂有望作为组织病理学和显微镜检查的替代辅助手段，用于诊断和筛查癌前（即OPMDs）和癌性病变。这些系统能够通过实时成像结果追踪组织内的微小变化，例如拉曼光谱、漫反射光谱、光学相干断层成像、激光共聚焦显微镜、高分辨率显微内镜和窄带成像技术[83]。然而，由于技术限制，穿透深度有限，成本较高，关于这些技术在OPMDs中的应用仍缺乏强有力的研究结果支持。此外，作为其他筛查方法的潜在替代方案，其可靠性还需要进一步研究[84-87]。

近年来，纳米技术和纳米颗粒（如纳米珠、金纳米阵列、纳米生物芯片）的发展有助于获得更高的图像对比度和分辨率，检测灵敏度也得到明显提高，这使得早期发现并准确地监测潜在的上皮内恶变得以实现[88]。而且，基于纳米技术的诊断方法可以通过分子靶向成像在纳米尺度上分析生物标志物，使得术中确定手术边缘成为可能[88]。然而，这项技术在检测潜在癌前和癌性病变的应用尚处于早期发展阶段，要将该技术成功地应用于临床实践还需要进一步的研究。

预后判断的分子标志物

OPMDs的治疗计划取决于对单位目标人群恶变风险的评估和相关卫生保健制度。低风险病变可通过改变不良习惯、口腔卫生指导和密切监测来治疗，高风险病变则需要有创治疗（手术或激光），并密切随访观察[89,90]。遗憾的是，尽管口腔肿瘤治疗取得了一些进展，但口腔鳞状细胞癌的生存率却并没有显著提高，这主要还是与诊断过晚有关[91]。

这种情况下，理想的方法是根据精确识别恶变风险的预后分子生物标志物制订个体化治疗计划，为OPMDs和其他恶性病变提供包括诊断、癌变风险评估、无创性和有创性干预以及随访在内的个性化治疗方案，也有助于降低全球癌症发病率[92,93]。

p53（肿瘤抑制基因TP53的产物，在细胞周期调节、细胞凋亡和DNA修复中起重要作用[94])是最常被报道的免疫组织化学生物标志物，然而，关于p53与OPMDs恶变之间的关系，目前的研究报道仍存在矛盾[95]。

另一个常见的生物标志物是Ki-67蛋白，它在有丝分裂期的细胞核中表达[96]，因此，Ki-67被认为是不同肿瘤侵袭性水平的重要表达指标[97,98]。据文献报道，约50%的研究中Ki-67过表达与癌变相关，但Ki-67并不是OPMDs癌变的独立预测因素[99]。

Podoplanin是另一种潜在的OPMDs恶变的独立预测因子，也是一种有临床应用前景的生物标志物[99]。Podoplanin是一种跨膜糖蛋白，可通过ErBb3结合蛋白-1（Ebp1）的转录激活诱导口腔肿瘤发生[100]。此外，Podoplanin也可通过下调E-cadherin，促进上皮-间充质转化（epithelial-mesenchymal transition, EMT）[17,101]；并且，Podoplanin还可能与血小板聚集有关，从而促进细胞迁移和恶性进展[102]。然而，关于其在癌变中的作用仍需要进一步的全面深入研究。

其他仍在研究且有应用前景的预后生物标志物包括DNA倍体[103-105]、DNA含量异常（DNA异倍体）[106,107]、表皮生长因子受体（EGFR）基因拷贝数增加[108,109]，以及3p/9p杂合性（LOH）缺失[110,111]。

随着细胞学和基因组学领域的不断进步，一些新的生物标志物已经被发现，但这些新标志物的具体机制及其临床应用尚存疑问[112]。目前关于分子生物标志物监测OPMDs恶变的预后判断的证据尚不明确[113]，因此，迄今为止，还没有单个的生物标志物被证实具有真正的临床应用价值[56,99]。未来在不同人群中设计的纵向研究将有助于填补关于生物标志物在OPMDs恶变中的预后价值的知识空白。此外，因为不同的人群面临着不同的影响癌变概率和程度的危险因素，因此在研究OPMDs的预后生物标志物时，应考虑到种族多样性和人口因素的重要性。为避免可能的发表偏倚，在研究方案设计和报告研究结果时应遵守国际准则，如观察性研究的《加强流行病学中观察性研究报告指南》（STROBE）[114]和临床试验的《临床试验报告统一标准》（CONSORT）[115]。

有创性检测技术

■ 切取活检

目前，手术切取活检和镜下的组织病理学评估仍然是OPMDs临床诊断的金标准[53,116]，可以减少误诊风险，排除隐匿恶变，确定上皮存在的异常增生，并有助于合理恰当的治疗。然而在实际临床工作中，由于活检取样的偏差，有可能会造成结果的偏差或误诊，因此，标准活检应包括病变的所有可疑区域（即白色和红色斑块），以确定是否存在上皮异常增生或鳞状细胞癌[53]。此外，组织病理学评估应根据WHO病理报告指南分为标准的上皮异常增生三级系统（即轻度、中度或重度），或根据Kujan等人[117]分为两级系统（即低风险和高风险）。也有人提出双层系统在临床诊疗中可能更具可重复性和操作性[118]。

■ 口腔细胞刷检（OBC）

OBC是一种微创、简单、安全、相对无痛的方法，可以从口腔黏膜可疑病变中获取样本细胞[119]。自1963年口腔细胞学临床应用以来，OBC技术得到了显著发展。近年来，由于现代OBC技术在OPMDs和口腔癌的筛查和早期检测以及口腔生物标志物筛检方面的潜在作用，其成为众多研究的焦点[47,66]。

刷检技术主要有两种类型：传统的脱落细胞学（如Cytobrush, OralCDx, Toothbrush）和液基细胞学（如Cytobrush, Orcellex）。例如，OralCDx®是一种计算机辅助的脱落细胞学上皮样本分析技术，可检测口腔黏膜所有上皮层的异常细胞[120]。但是，任何可疑病变最终都需要手术活检进一步确认。

液基细胞学的引入为传统的OBC技术增加了更多的应用价值，这种方法可维持良好细胞的形态和染色质量，使得观察背景更为干净[66]。鉴于OBC具有较高的特异度和敏感度，该方法似乎是最准确辅助检测技术[66,121]。然而，仍需要进一步完善研究设计来评估该方法和其他联合辅助技术的准确性[47]。

有学者对41项关于OPMDs不同筛查方法的横断面研究进行系统回顾和meta分析，结果发现尚无任何筛查方法的可靠性能够替代常规切取活检[66]，因此，手术切取活检仍然是诊断和筛查OPMDs的金标准。但OBC作为一种替代辅助检测方法已经显示出较好的应用前景（表2-2）。

表2-2 OPMDs和口腔癌筛查及诊断技术

分类	技 术	灵敏度（%）	特异度（%）	优 势	劣 势	适 应 证
活体染色	甲苯胺蓝，氯化甲苯	38～100	9～100	• 灵敏 • 椅旁 • 快速 • 低成本	• 假阳性率高 • 失败可能性大 • 碘过敏禁忌证	有助于确定异常的不可见区域和评估活检的切除部位
	亚甲基蓝染色	90～91.4	66.6～69		无数据	在OPMDs检测方面文献缺乏，疗效不明
	孟加拉玫瑰红染色	90～100	73.7～89.09		无数据	
	卢戈氏碘染色	87.5～94.7	83.8～84.2	无数据	无数据	无数据
基于光的检测系统	化学发光 ViziLite	71～100	0～84.6	• 有效的 • 快速 • 椅旁，简单	• 特异度低 • 需黑暗环境 • 初始设置成本高 • 无法客观测量可视化结果	能通过组织反射率提高白色显像
	化学发光 ViziLite Plus	77.3	27.8			
	化学发光 Microlux/DL	77.8～94.3	70.7～99.6			
	化学发光 Orascoptic DK	无数据	无数据			
	VELscope	30～100	15～100	• 快速 • 椅旁 • 操作方便	• 中等假阳性率	有助于更好地识别OPMDs
	光动力诊断	79～100	50～99	• 实时 • 性价比高	• 严格的患者管理 • 假阳性率高	临床应用较少
光学诊断技术	拉曼光谱	97.44～100	77～100	• 实时	• 信号微弱 • 耗时，频谱获取速度相对较慢	捕获弱组织拉曼信号困难
	弹性散射光谱	72～98	68～75	• 实时	无数据	很少应用
	漫反射光谱	76～100	76～97	• 简单 • 低成本 • 实时	无数据	有助于发现口腔黏膜的异常组织形态
	窄带成像技术	84.62～96	88.2～100	• 实时 • 易于管理	• 中等假阳性率	可以增强黏膜表面和微血管的显像

续表

分类	技术	灵敏度（%）	特异度（%）	优势	劣势	适应证
光学诊断技术	光学相干断层成像	73～100	78～98	• 实时 • 灵敏度高 • 特异度高	• 需要组织病理学家解释和评估 • 每次只检查很小的区域	用于体外或体内 OPMDs 评估和成像
	激光共聚焦内镜	80	100	• 实时 • "光学活检"		
	反射式共聚焦显微镜	73	88			用于黏膜的三维成像
口腔细胞刷检	常规剥脱（即 OralCDx），液体细胞学（即 Orcellex）	91	91	• 能够发现大的或多个病变 • 能够从口腔黏膜的所有三个上皮层进入基底膜收集细胞 • 液体细胞学提供了更好的细胞形态学	• 可能无法发现较小或不太明显的病变 • 难以发现坏死或血栓病变	样本细胞的显微评估和解释
分子生物标志物分析	Podoplanin, p53, Ki-67, EGFR, DNA 非整倍性, LOH, miRNA	无数据	无数据	• 快速 • 操作方便，微创（血液），无创（唾液）	• 早期发展阶段 • 缺乏扎实的有效性知识	利用血液或唾液中的生物标志物进行 OPMDs 的早期检测和动态监测

注：源自参考文献［99，122］。

小 结

准确预测 OPMDs 的癌变风险是当前研究的主要目标，最终目的是降低 OPMDs 的发病率和死亡率，提高患者的生存率和生活质量。尽管近年来 OPMDs 的检测技术有所进步，但现有辅助诊断技术的准确性仍然不高，假阳性率出现频繁，因此，切取活检和组织学评估仍是目前 OPMDs 的诊断金标准。虽然使用液基的口腔细胞刷检技术显示了良好的应用前景，但在 OPMDs 的癌变风险预测方面仍是一个临床挑战。令人欣喜的是，近年来，基于基因组学和分子生物学领域确定癌变的预后生物标志物的研究为 OPMDs 的癌变风险预测及预后评估带来了新的希望。

参 考 文 献

[1] Dhanuthai K, Rojanawatsirivej S, Thosaporn W, Kintarak S, Subarnbhesaj A, Darling M, Kryshtalskyj E, Chiang C-P, Shin H-I, Choi S-Y, Lee S-S, Aminishakib P. Oral cancer: a multicenter study. Med Oral Patol Oral Cir Bucal. 2018; 23: e23–9. https://doi.org/10.4317/medoral.21999.

[2] Warnakulasuriya S, Johnson NW, van der Waal I. Nomenclature and classification of potentially malignant disorders of the oral mucosa. J Oral Pathol Med. 2007; 36: 575–80. https://doi.org/10.1111/j.1600-0714.2007.00582.x.

[3] Müller S. Update from the 4th edition of the World Health Organization of head and neck tumours: tumours of the oral cavity and mobile tongue. Head Neck Pathol. 2017; 11: 33–40. https://doi.org/10.1007/s12105-017-0792-3.

[4] Mello FW, Miguel AFP, Dutra KL, Porporatti AL, Warnakulasuriya S, Guerra ENS, Rivero ERC. Prevalence of oral potentially malignant disorders: a systematic review and meta-analysis. J Oral Pathol Med. 2018; 47: 633–40. https://doi.org/10.1111/jop.12726.

[5] Iocca O, Sollecito TP, Alawi F, Weinstein GS, Newman JG, De Virgilio A, Di Maio P, Spriano G, Pardiñas López S, Shanti RM.

Potentially malignant disorders of the oral cavity and oral dysplasia: a systematic review and meta-analysis of malignant transformation rate by subtype. Head Neck. 2020; 42: 539–55. https: //doi.org/10.1002/hed.26006.

[6] Mortazavi H, Baharvand M, Mehdipour M. Oral potentially malignant disorders: an overview of more than 20 entities. J Dent Res Dent Clin Dent Prospects. 2014; 8: 6–14. https: //doi. org/10.5681/joddd.2014.002.

[7] van der Waal I. Potentially malignant disorders of the oral and oropharyngeal mucosa; terminology, classification and present concepts of management. Oral Oncol. 2009; 45: 317–23. https: //doi.org/10.1016/j.oraloncology.2008.05.016.

[8] Petti S. Pooled estimate of world leukoplakia prevalence: a systematic review. Oral Oncol. 2003; 39: 770–80. https: //doi.org/10.1016/S1368-8375(03)00102-7.

[9] Kumar Srivastava V. To study the prevalence of premalignancies in teenagers having betel, gutkha, khaini, tobacco chewing, beedi and ganja smoking habit and their association with social class and education status. Int J Clin Pediatr Dent. 2014; 7: 86–92. https: //doi.org/10.5005/jp-journals-10005-1243.

[10] Vazquez-Alvarez R, Fernandez-Gonzalez F, Gandara-Vila P, Reboiras-Lopez D, Garcia-Garcia A, Gandara-Rey J. Correlation between clinical and pathologic diagnosis in oral leukoplakia in 54 patients. Med Oral Patol Oral Cir Bucal. 2010; 15: e832–8. https: //doi.org/10.4317/medoral.15.e832.

[11] Warnakulasuriya S. Clinical features and presentation of oral potentially malignant disorders. Oral Surg Oral Med Oral Pathol Oral Radiol. 2018; 125: 582–90. https: //doi.org/10.1016/j. oooo.2018.03.011.

[12] Haya-Fernández MC, Bagán JV, Murillo-Cortés J, Poveda-Roda R, Calabuig C. The prevalence of oral leukoplakia in 138 patients with oral squamous cell carcinoma. Oral Dis. 2004; 10: 346–8. https: //doi.org/10.1111/j.1601-0825.2004.01031. x.

[13] Cerero-Lapiedra R, Baladé-Martínez D, Moreno-López L-A, Esparza-Gómez G, Bagán JV. Proliferative verrucous leukoplakia: a proposal for diagnostic criteria. Med Oral Patol Oral Cir Bucal. 2010; 15: e839–45. http: //www.ncbi.nlm.nih.gov/pubmed/20173704.

[14] Carrard VC, Brouns EREA, van der Waal I. Proliferative verrucous leukoplakia; a critical appraisal of the diagnostic criteria. Med Oral Patol Oral Cir Bucal. 2013; 18: e411–3. https: //doi.org/10.4317/medoral.18912.

[15] Warnakulasuriya S, Ariyawardana A. Malignant transformation of oral leukoplakia: a systematic review of observational studies. J Oral Pathol Med. 2016; 45: 155–66. https: //doi. org/10.1111/jop.12339.

[16] Farah CS, Fox SA. Dysplastic oral leukoplakia is molecularly distinct from leukoplakia without dysplasia. Oral Dis. 2019; 25: 1715–23. https: //doi.org/10.1111/odi.13156.

[17] Nieto MA, Huang RY-J, Jackson RA, Thiery JP. EMT: 2016. Cell. 2016; 166: 21–45. https: //doi.org/10.1016/j.cell.2016.06.028.

[18] Liu P-F, Kang B-H, Wu Y-M, Sun J-H, Yen L-M, Fu T-Y, Lin Y-C, Liou H-H, Lin Y-S, Sie H-C, Hsieh I-C, Tseng Y-K, Shu C-W, Hsieh Y-D, Ger L-P. Vimentin is a potential prognostic factor for tongue squamous cell carcinoma among five epithelial–mesenchymal transition-related proteins. PLoS One. 2017; 12: e0178581. https: //doi.org/10.1371/journal. pone.0178581.

[19] Holmstrup P. Oral erythroplakia-what is it? Oral Dis. 2018; 24: 138–43. https: //doi. org/10.1111/odi.12709.

[20] Reichart PA, Philipsen HP. Oral erythroplakia – a review. Oral Oncol. 2005; 41: 551–61. https: //doi.org/10.1016/j.oraloncology.2004.12.003.

[21] Lapthanasupkul P, Poomsawat S, Punyasingh J. A clinicopathologic study of oral leukoplakia and erythroplakia in a Thai population. Quintessence Int. 2007; 38: e448–55. http: //www.ncbi. nlm.nih.gov/pubmed/17823667.

[22] Villa A, Villa C, Abati S. Oral cancer and oral erythroplakia: an update and implication for clinicians. Aust Dent J. 2011; 56: 253–6. https: //doi.org/10.1111/j.1834-7819.2011.01337. x.

[23] van der Waal I. Potentially malignant disorders of the oral and oropharyngeal mucosa; present concepts of management. Oral Oncol. 2010; 46: 423–5. https: //doi.org/10.1016/j. oraloncology.2010.02.016.

[24] Warnakulasuriya S, Reibel J, Bouquot J, Dabelsteen E. Oral epithelial dysplasia classification systems: predictive value, utility, weaknesses and scope for improvement. J Oral Pathol Med. 2008; 37: 127–33. https: //doi.org/10.1111/j.1600-0714.2007.00584. x.

[25] Yang SW, Lee YS, Chang LC, Hsieh TY, Chen TA. Outcome of excision of oral erythroplakia. Br J Oral Maxillofac Surg. 2015; 53: 142–7. https: //doi.org/10.1016/j.bjoms.2014.10.016.

[26] Mignogna MD, Fedele S. Oral cancer screening: 5 minutes to save a life. Lancet. 2005; 365: 1905–6. https: //doi.org/10.1016/S0140-6736(05)66635-4.

[27] Zain RB, Ikeda N, Gupta PC, Warnakulasuriya S, van Wyk CW, Shrestha P, Axéll T. Oral mucosal lesions associated with betel quid, areca nut and tobacco chewing habits: consensus from a workshop held in Kuala Lumpur, Malaysia, November 25–27, 1996. J Oral Pathol Med. 1999; 28: 1–4. https: //doi.org/10.1111/j.1600-0714.1999. tb01985.x.

[28] Cox SC, Walker DM. Oral submucous fibrosis. A review. Aust Dent J. 1996; 41: 294–9. https: //doi.org/10.1111/j.1834-7819.1996. tb03136.x.

[29] Paissat DK. Oral submucous fibrosis. Int J Oral Surg. 1981; 10: 307–12. https: //doi. org/10.1016/s0300-9785(81)80026-9.

[30] Chattopadhyay A, Ray JG. Molecular pathology of malignant transformation of oral submucous fibrosis. J Environ Pathol Toxicol Oncol. 2016; 35: 193–205. https: //doi.org/10.1615/JEnvironPatholToxicolOncol.2016014024.

[31] Pant I, Rao SG, Kondaiah P. Role of areca nut induced JNK/ATF2/Jun axis in the activation of TGF-β pathway in precancerous Oral Submucous Fibrosis. Sci Rep. 2016; 6: 34314. https: //doi.org/10.1038/srep34314.

[32] Hernandez BY, Zhu X, Goodman MT, Gatewood R, Mendiola P, Quinata K, Paulino YC. Betel nut chewing, oral premalignant lesions, and the oral microbiome. PLoS One. 2017; 12: e0172196. https: //doi.org/10.1371/journal.pone.0172196.

[33] Lian I-B, Tseng Y-T, Su C-C, Tsai K-Y. Progression of precancerous lesions to oral cancer: results based on the Taiwan Health Insurance Database. Oral Oncol. 2013; 49: 427–30. https: //doi.org/10.1016/j.oraloncology.2012.12.004.

[34] Haque MF, Harris M, Meghji S, Barrett AW. Immunolocalization of cytokines and growth factors in oral submucous fibrosis. Cytokine. 1998; 10: 713–9. https: //doi.org/10.1006/cyto.1997.0342.

[35] Chang M-C, Wu H-L, Lee J-J, Lee P-H, Chang H-H, Hahn L-J, Lin B-R, Chen Y-J, Jeng J-H. The induction of prostaglandin E2 production, interleukin-6 production, cell cycle arrest, and cytotoxicity in primary oral keratinocytes and KB cancer cells by areca nut ingredients is differentially regulated by MEK/ERK activation. J Biol Chem. 2004; 279: 50676–83. https: //doi.org/10.1074/jbc.M404465200.

[36] Khan I, Agarwal P, Thangjam GS, Radhesh R, Rao SG, Kondaiah P. Role of TGF-β and BMP7 in the pathogenesis of oral submucous fibrosis. Growth Factors. 2011; 29: 119–27. https: //doi.org/10.3109/08977194.2011.582839.

[37] Agarwal RK, Hebbale M, Mhapuskar A, Tepan M. Correlation of ultrasonographic measurements, histopathological grading, and clinical staging in oral submucous fibrosis. Indian J Dent Res. 2017; 28: 476–81. https: //doi.org/10.4103/ijdr.IJDR_517_16.

[38] Canniff JP, Harvey W, Harris M. Oral submucous fibrosis: its pathogenesis and management. Br Dent J. 1986; 160: 429–34. https: //doi.org/10.1038/sj.bdj.4805876.

[39] Kadani M, Satish BNVS, Maharudrappa B, Prashant KM, Hugar D, Allad U, Prabhu PS. Evaluation of plasma fibrinogen degradation products and total serum protein concentration in oral submucous fibrosis. J Clin Diagn Res. 2014; 8: ZC54–7. https: //doi.org/10.7860/JCDR/2014/9061.4385.

[40] Sur TK, Biswas TK, Ali L, Mukherjee B. Anti-inflammatory and anti-platelet aggregation activity of human placental extract. Acta Pharmacol Sin. 2003; 24: 187–92. http: //www.ncbi.nlm.nih.gov/pubmed/12546729.

[41] Kakar PK, Puri RK, Venkatachalam VP. Oral submucous fibrosis – treatment with hyalase. J Laryngol Otol. 1985; 99: 57–9. https: //doi.org/10.1017/s0022215100096286.

[42] Haque MF, Meghji S, Nazir R, Harris M. Interferon gamma (IFN-gamma) may reverse oral submucous fibrosis. J Oral Pathol Med. 2001; 30: 12–21. https: //doi.org/10.1034/j.1600-0714.2001.300103.x.

[43] Kumar A, Bagewadi A, Keluskar V, Singh M. Efficacy of lycopene in the management of oral submucous fibrosis. Oral Surg Oral Med Oral Pathol Oral Radiol Endod. 2007; 103: 207–13. https: //doi.org/10.1016/j.tripleo.2006.07.011.

[44] Liu J, Chen F, Wei Z, Qiu M, Li Z, Dan H, Chen Q, Jiang L. Evaluating the efficacy of pentoxifylline in the treatment of oral submucous fibrosis: a meta-analysis. Oral Dis. 2018; 24: 706–16. https: //doi.org/10.1111/odi.12715.

[45] Nayak DR, Mahesh SG, Aggarwal D, Pavithran P, Pujary K, Pillai S. Role of KTP-532 laser in management of oral submucous fibrosis. J Laryngol Otol. 2009; 123: 418–21. https: //doi. org/10.1017/S0022215108003642.

[46] Chaudhry Z, Gupta SR, Oberoi SS. The efficacy of ErCr: YSGG laser fibrotomy in management of moderate oral submucous fibrosis: a preliminary study. J Maxillofac Oral Surg. 2014; 13: 286–94. https: //doi.org/10.1007/s12663-013-0511-x.

[47] Alsarraf AH, Kujan O, Farah CS. The utility of oral brush cytology in the early detection of oral cancer and oral potentially malignant disorders: a systematic review. J Oral Pathol Med. 2018; 47: 104–16. https: //doi.org/10.1111/jop.12660.

[48] Fitzpatrick SG, Hirsch SA, Gordon SC. The malignant transformation of oral lichen planus and oral lichenoid lesions. J Am Dent Assoc. 2014; 145: 45–56. https: //doi.org/10.14219/jada.2013.10.

[49] Gómez I, Seoane J, Varela-Centelles P, Diz P, Takkouche B. Is diagnostic delay related to advanced-stage oral cancer? A meta-analysis. Eur J Oral Sci. 2009; 117: 541–6. https: //doi. org/10.1111/j.1600-0722.2009.00672. x.

[50] Silverman S, Gorsky M, Lozada F. Oral leukoplakia and malignant transformation. A follow-up study of 257 patients. Cancer. 1984; 53: 563–8. https: //doi.org/10.1002/1097-0142(19840201)53: 3<563: : aid-cncr2820530332> 3.0.co; 2-f.

[51] Warnakulasuriya S, Kovacevic T, Madden P, Coupland VH, Sperandio M, Odell E, Møller H. Factors predicting malignant transformation in oral potentially malignant disorders among patients accrued over a 10-year period in South East England. J Oral Pathol Med. 2011; 40: 677–83. https: //doi.org/10.1111/j.1600-0714.2011.01054. x.

[52] Torezan LAR, Festa-Neto C. Cutaneous field cancerization: clinical, histopathological and therapeutic aspects. An Bras Dermatol. 2013; 88: 775–86. https: //doi.org/10.1590/abd1806-4841.20132300.

[53] Warnakulasuriya S. Oral potentially malignant disorders: a comprehensive review on clinical aspects and management. Oral Oncol. 2020; 102: 104550. https: //doi.org/10.1016/j. oraloncology.2019.104550.

[54] Downer MC, Moles DR, Palmer S, Speight PM. A systematic review of test performance in screening for oral cancer and precancer. Oral Oncol. 2004; 40: 264–73. https: //doi. org/10.1016/j.oraloncology.2003.08.013.

[55] Awan KH, Morgan PR, Warnakulasuriya S. Assessing the accuracy of autofluorescence, chemiluminescence and toluidine blue as diagnostic tools for oral potentially malignant disorders – a clinicopathological evaluation. Clin Oral Investig. 2015; 19: 2267–72. https: //doi. org/10.1007/s00784-015-1457-9.

[56] Speight PM, Khurram SA, Kujan O. Oral potentially malignant disorders: risk of progression to malignancy. Oral Surg Oral Med Oral Pathol Oral Radiol. 2018; 125: 612–27. https: //doi. org/10.1016/j.oooo.2017.12.011.

[57] Seoane Lestón J, Diz Dios P. Diagnostic clinical aids in oral cancer. Oral Oncol. 2010; 46: 418–22. https: //doi.org/10.1016/j.oraloncology.2010.03.006.

[58] Lingen MW, Kalmar JR, Karrison T, Speight PM. Critical evaluation of diagnostic aids for the detection of oral cancer. Oral Oncol. 2008; 44: 10–22. https: //doi.org/10.1016/j. oraloncology.2007.06.011.

[59] Du G-F, Li C-Z, Chen H-Z, Chen X-M, Xiao Q, Cao Z-G, Shang S-H, Cai X. Rose Bengal staining in detection of oral precancerous and malignant lesions with colorimetric evaluation: a pilot study. Int J Cancer. 2007; 120: 1958–63. https: //doi.org/10.1002/ijc.22467.

[60] Mittal N, Palaskar S, Shankari M. Rose Bengal staining – diagnostic aid for potentially malignant and malignant disorders: a pilot study. Indian J Dent Res. 2012; 23: 561–4. https: //doi.org/10.4103/0970-9290.107326.

[61] Chaudhari A, Hegde-Shetiya S, Shirahatti R, Agrawal D. Comparison of different screening methods in estimating the prevalence of precancer and cancer amongst male inmates of a jail in Maharashtra, India. Asian Pac J Cancer Prev. 2013; 14: 859–64. https: //doi.org/10.7314/apjcp.2013.14.2.859.

[62] Pallagatti S, Sheikh S, Aggarwal A, Gupta D, Singh R, Handa R, Kaur S, Mago J. Toluidine blue staining as an adjunctive tool for early diagnosis of dysplastic changes in the oral mucosa. J Clin Exp Dent. 2013; 5: e187–91. https: //doi.org/10.4317/jced.51121.

[63] Riaz A, Shreedhar B, Kamboj M, Natarajan S. Methylene blue as an early diagnostic marker for oral precancer and cancer. Springerplus. 2013; 2: 95. https: //doi. org/10.1186/2193-1801-2-95.

[64] Gandolfo S, Pentenero M, Broccoletti R, Pagano M, Carrozzo M, Scully C. Toluidine blue uptake in potentially malignant oral lesions in vivo: clinical and histological assessment. Oral Oncol. 2006; 42: 89–95. https: //doi.org/10.1016/j.oraloncology.2005.06.016.

[65] Driemel O, Kunkel M, Hullmann M, von Eggeling F, Müller-Richter U, Kosmehl H, Reichert TE. Diagnosis of oral squamous cell carcinoma and its precursor lesions. J Dtsch Dermatol Ges. 2007; 5: 1095–100. https: //doi.org/10.1111/j.1610-0387.2007.06397. x.

[66] Macey R, Walsh T, Brocklehurst P, Kerr AR, Liu JLY, Lingen MW, Ogden GR, Warnakulasuriya S, Scully C. Diagnostic tests for oral cancer and potentially malignant disorders in patients presenting with clinically evident lesions. Cochrane Database Syst Rev. 2015; 2015(5): CD010276. https: //doi.org/10.1002/14651858.CD010276.pub2.

[67] Sambandham T, Masthan KMK, Kumar MS, Jha A. The application of vizilite in oral cancer. J Clin Diagn Res. 2013; 7: 185–6. https: //doi.org/10.7860/JCDR/2012/5163.2704.

[68] Rajmohan M, Rao UK, Joshua E, Rajasekaran ST, Kannan R. Assessment of oral mucosa in normal, precancer and cancer using chemiluminescent illumination, toluidine blue supravital staining and oral exfoliative cytology. J Oral Maxillofac Pathol. 2012; 16: 325–9. https: //doi. org/10.4103/0973-029X. 102476.

[69] McIntosh L, McCullough MJ, Farah CS. The assessment of diffused light illumination and acetic acid rinse (Microlux/DL) in the visualisation of oral mucosal lesions. Oral Oncol. 2009; 45: e227–31. https: //doi.org/10.1016/j.oraloncology.2009.08.001.

[70] Awan KH, Morgan PR, Warnakulasuriya S. Utility of chemiluminescence (ViziLite™) in the detection of oral potentially malignant disorders and benign keratoses. J Oral Pathol Med. 2011; 40: 541–4. https: //doi.org/10.1111/j.1600-0714.2011.01048. x.

[71] Rashid A, Warnakulasuriya S. The use of light-based (optical) detection systems as adjuncts in the detection of oral cancer and oral potentially malignant disorders: a systematic review. J Oral Pathol Med. 2015; 44: 307–28. https: //doi.org/10.1111/jop.12218.

[72] Farah CS, McIntosh L, Georgiou A, McCullough MJ. Efficacy of tissue autofluorescence imaging (VELscope) in the visualization of oral mucosal lesions. Head Neck. 2012; 34: 856–62. https: //doi.org/10.1002/hed.21834.

[73] Bhatia N, Lalla Y, Vu AN, Farah CS. Advances in optical adjunctive AIDS for visualisation and detection of oral malignant and potentially malignant lesions. Int J Dent. 2013; 2013: 194029. https: //doi.org/10.1155/2013/194029.

[74] Balevi B. Evidence-based decision making: should the general dentist adopt the use of the VELscope for routine screening for oral cancer? J Can Dent Assoc. 2007; 73: 603–6. http: //www.ncbi.nlm.nih.gov/pubmed/17868507.

[75] Moro A, Di Nardo F, Boniello R, Marianetti TM, Cervelli D, Gasparini G, Pelo S. Autofluorescence and early detection of mucosal lesions in patients at risk for oral cancer. J Craniofac Surg. 2010; 21: 1899–903. https: //doi.org/10.1097/SCS.0b013e3181f4afb4.

[76] Mercadante V, Paderni C, Campisi G. Novel non-invasive adjunctive techniques for early oral cancer diagnosis and oral lesions examination. Curr Pharm Des. 2012; 18: 5442–51. https: //doi.org/10.2174/138161212803307626.

[77] Figueira JA, Veltrini VC. Photodynamic therapy in oral potentially malignant disorders-critical literature review of existing protocols. Photodiagn Photodyn Ther. 2017; 20: 125–9. https: //doi.org/10.1016/j.pdpdt.2017.09.007.

[78] Hopper C. Photodynamic therapy: a clinical reality in the treatment of cancer. Lancet Oncol. 2000; 1: 212–9. https: //doi.org/10.1016/s1470-2045(00)00166-2.

[79] Zhu TC, Finlay JC. The role of photodynamic therapy (PDT) physics. Med Phys. 2008; 35: 3127–36. https: //doi.org/10.1118/1.2937440.

[80] Li Y, Wang B, Zheng S, He Y. Photodynamic therapy in the treatment of oral leukoplakia: a systematic review. Photodiagn Photodyn Ther. 2019; 25: 17–22. https: //doi.org/10.1016/j. pdpdt.2018.10.023.

[81] Jin X, Xu H, Deng J, Dan H, Ji P, Chen Q, Zeng X. Photodynamic therapy for oral potentially malignant disorders. Photodiagn Photodyn Ther. 2019; 28: 146–52. https: //doi.org/10.1016/j. pdpdt.2019.08.005.

[82] Gondivkar SM, Gadbail AR, Choudhary MG, Vedpathak PR, Likhitkar MS. Photodynamic treatment outcomes of potentially-malignant lesions and malignancies of the head and neck region: a systematic review. J Investig Clin Dent. 2018; 9: e12270. https: //doi.org/10.1111/jicd.12270.

[83] Wu C, Gleysteen J, Teraphongphom NT, Li Y, Rosenthal E. In-vivo optical imaging in head and neck oncology: basic principles, clinical applications and future directions. Int J Oral Sci. 2018; 10: 10. https: //doi.org/10.1038/s41368-018-0011-4.

[84] Stephen MM, Jayanthi JL, Unni NG, Kolady PE, Beena VT, Jeemon P, Subhash N. Diagnostic accuracy of diffuse reflectance imaging for early detection of pre-malignant and malignant changes in the oral cavity: a feasibility study. BMC Cancer. 2013; 13: 278. https: //doi.org/1 0.1186/1471-2407-13-278.

[85] Green B, Tsiroyannis C, Brennan PA. Optical diagnostic systems for assessing head and neck lesions. Oral Dis. 2016; 22: 180–4. https: //doi.org/10.1111/odi.12398.

[86] Krishna H, Majumder SK, Chaturvedi P, Sidramesh M, Gupta PK. In vivo Raman spectroscopy for detection of oral neoplasia: a pilot

clinical study. J Biophotonics. 2014; 7: 690–702. https: //doi.org/10.1002/jbio.201300030.

[87] Green B, Cobb ARM, Brennan PA, Hopper C. Optical diagnostic techniques for use in lesions of the head and neck: review of the latest developments. Br J Oral Maxillofac Surg. 2014; 52: 675–80. https: //doi.org/10.1016/j.bjoms.2014.06.010.

[88] Chen X-J, Zhang X-Q, Liu Q, Zhang J, Zhou G. Nanotechnology: a promising method for oral cancer detection and diagnosis. J Nanobiotechnology. 2018; 16: 52. https: //doi.org/10.1186/s12951-018-0378-6.

[89] Wetzel SL, Wollenberg J. Oral potentially malignant disorders. Dent Clin N Am. 2020; 64: 25–37. https: //doi.org/10.1016/j.cden.2019.08.004.

[90] Dancyger A, Heard V, Huang B, Suley C, Tang D, Ariyawardana A. Malignant transformation of actinic cheilitis: a systematic review of observational studies. J Investig Clin Dent. 2018; 9: e12343. https: //doi.org/10.1111/jicd.12343.

[91] Miller KD, Siegel RL, Lin CC, Mariotto AB, Kramer JL, Rowland JH, Stein KD, Alteri R, Jemal A. Cancer treatment and survivorship statistics, 2016. CA Cancer J Clin. 2016; 66: 271–89. https: //doi.org/10.3322/caac.21349.

[92] Foy J-P, Bertolus C, Saintigny P. Oral cancer prevention worldwide: challenges and perspectives. Oral Oncol. 2019; 88: 91–4. https: //doi.org/10.1016/j.oraloncology.2018.11.008.

[93] Warnakulasuriya S. Potentially malignant disorders of the oral cavity. In: Textbook of oral cancer. Cham: Springer; 2020. p. 141–58. https: //doi.org/10.1007/978-3-030-32316-5_12.

[94] Vogelstein B, Lane D, Levine AJ. Surfing the p53 network. Nature. 2000; 408: 307–10. https: //doi.org/10.1038/35042675.

[95] Goldstein I, Marcel V, Olivier M, Oren M, Rotter V, Hainaut P. Understanding wild-type and mutant p53 activities in human cancer: new landmarks on the way to targeted therapies. Cancer Gene Ther. 2011; 18: 2–11. https: //doi.org/10.1038/cgt.2010.63.

[96] Scholzen T, Gerdes J. The Ki-67 protein: from the known and the unknown. J Cell Physiol. 2000; 182: 311–22. https: //doi.org/10.1002/(SICI)1097-4652(200003)182: 3<311: : AID-JCP1> 3.0.CO; 2-9.

[97] Pelosi G, Massa F, Gatti G, Righi L, Volante M, Birocco N, Maisonneuve P, Sonzogni A, Harari S, Albini A, Papotti M. Ki-67 evaluation for clinical decision in metastatic lung carcinoids: a proof of concept. Clin Pathol. 2019; 12: 2632010X19829259. https: //doi.org/10.1177/2632010X19829259.

[98] Niotis A, Tsiambas E, Fotiades PP, Ragos V, Polymeneas G. Ki-67 and topoisomerase IIa proliferation markers in colon adenocarcinoma. J BUON. 2018; 23: 24–7. http: //www.ncbi.nlm.nih.gov/pubmed/30722108.

[99] Mello FW, Melo G, Guerra ENS, Warnakulasuriya S, Garnis C, Rivero ERC. Oral potentially malignant disorders: a scoping review of prognostic biomarkers. Crit Rev Oncol Hematol. 2020; 153: 102986. https: //doi.org/10.1016/j.critrevonc.2020.102986.

[100] Mei Y, Zhang P, Zuo H, Clark D, Xia R, Li J, Liu Z, Mao L. Ebp1 activates podoplanin expression and contributes to oral tumorigenesis. Oncogene. 2014; 33: 3839–50. https: //doi. org/10.1038/onc.2013.354.

[101] Martin-Villar E, Megias D, Castel S, Yurrita MM, Vilaro S, Quintanilla M. Podoplanin binds ERM proteins to activate RhoA and promote epithelial-mesenchymal transition. J Cell Sci. 2006; 119: 4541–53. https: //doi.org/10.1242/jcs.03218.

[102] Suzuki-Inoue K, Osada M, Ozaki Y. Physiologic and pathophysiologic roles of interaction between C-type lectin-like receptor 2 and podoplanin: partners from in utero to adulthood. J Thromb Haemost. 2017; 15: 219–29. https: //doi.org/10.1111/jth.13590.

[103] Danielsen HE, Pradhan M, Novelli M. Revisiting tumour aneuploidy – the place of ploidy assessment in the molecular era. Nat Rev Clin Oncol. 2016; 13: 291–304. https: //doi. org/10.1038/nrclinonc.2015.208.

[104] Zaini ZM, McParland H, Møller H, Husband K, Odell EW. Predicting malignant progression in clinically high-risk lesions by DNA ploidy analysis and dysplasia grading. Sci Rep. 2018; 8: 15874. https: //doi.org/10.1038/s41598-018-34165-5.

[105] Siebers TJH, Bergshoeff VE, Otte-Höller I, Kremer B, Speel EJM, van der Laak JAWM, Merkx MAW, Slootweg PJ. Chromosome instability predicts the progression of premalignant oral lesions. Oral Oncol. 2013; 49: 1121–8. https: //doi.org/10.1016/j.oraloncology.2013.09.006.

[106] Bradley G, Odell EW, Raphael S, Ho J, Le LW, Benchimol S, Kamel-Reid S. Abnormal DNA content in oral epithelial dysplasia is associated with increased risk of progression to carcinoma. Br J Cancer. 2010; 103: 1432–42. https: //doi.org/10.1038/sj.bjc.6605905.

[107] Nayak S, Goel MM, Makker A, Bhatia V, Chandra S, Kumar S, Agarwal SP. Fibroblast growth factor (FGF-2) and its receptors FGFR-2 and FGFR-3 may be putative biomarkers of malignant transformation of potentially malignant oral lesions into oral squamous cell carcinoma. PLoS One. 2015; 10: e0138801. https: //doi.org/10.1371/journal.pone.0138801.

[108] Poh CF, Zhu Y, Chen E, Berean KW, Wu L, Zhang L, Rosin MP. Unique FISH patterns associated with cancer progression of oral dysplasia. J Dent Res. 2012; 91: 52–7. https: //doi. org/10.1177/0022034511425676.

[109] Taoudi Benchekroun M, Saintigny P, Thomas SM, El-Naggar AK, Papadimitrakopoulou V, Ren H, Lang W, Fan Y-H, Huang J, Feng L, Lee JJ, Kim ES, Hong WK, Johnson FM, Grandis JR, Mao L. Epidermal growth factor receptor expression and gene copy number in the risk of oral cancer. Cancer Prev Res (Phila). 2010; 3: 800–9. https: //doi.org/10.1158/1940-6207. CAPR-09-0163.

[110] Foy J-P, Bertolus C, Ortiz-Cuaran S, Albaret M-A, Williams WN, Lang W, Destandau S, De Souza G, Sohier E, Kielbassa J, Thomas E, Deneuve S, Goudot P, Puisieux A, Viari A, Mao L, Caux C, Lippman S, Saintigny P. Immunological and classical subtypes of oral premalignant lesions. Onco Targets Ther. 2018; 7: e1496880. https: //doi.org/10.1080/2162402X.2018.1496880.

[111] William WN, Papadimitrakopoulou V, Lee JJ, Mao L, Cohen EEW, Lin HY, Gillenwater AM, Martin JW, Lingen MW, Boyle JO, Shin DM, Vigneswaran N, Shinn N, Heymach JV, Wistuba II, Tang X, Kim ES, Saintigny P, Blair EA, Meiller T, Gutkind JS, Myers J, El-Naggar A, Lippman SM. Erlotinib and the risk of oral cancer. JAMA Oncol. 2016; 2: 209. https: //doi.org/10.1001/jamaoncol.2015.4364.

[112] Sarode GS, Sarode SC, Maniyar N, Sharma N, Yerwadekar S, Patil S. Recent trends in predictive biomarkers for determining malignant

potential of oral potentially malignant disorders. Oncol Rev. 2019; 13: 424. https: //doi.org/10.4081/oncol.2019.424.
[113] El-Sakka H, Kujan O, Farah CS. Assessing miRNAs profile expression as a risk stratification biomarker in oral potentially malignant disorders: a systematic review. Oral Oncol. 2018; 77: 57–82. https: //doi.org/10.1016/j.oraloncology.2017.11.021.
[114] von Elm E, Altman DG, Egger M, Pocock SJ, Gøtzsche PC, Vandenbroucke JP. The strengthening the reporting of observational studies in epidemiology (STROBE) statement: guidelines for reporting observational studies. Int J Surg. 2014; 12: 1495–9. https: //doi.org/10.1016/j. ijsu.2014.07.013.
[115] Moher D, Hopewell S, Schulz KF, Montori V, Gøtzsche PC, Devereaux PJ, Elbourne D, Egger M, Altman DG. CONSORT 2010 explanation and elaboration: updated guidelines for reporting parallel group randomised trials. Int J Surg. 2012; 10: 28–55. https: //doi.org/10.1016/j. ijsu.2011.10.001.
[116] McCullough MJ, Prasad G, Farah CS. Oral mucosal malignancy and potentially malignant lesions: an update on the epidemiology, risk factors, diagnosis and management. Aust Dent J. 2010; 55(Suppl 1): 61–5. https: //doi.org/10.1111/j.1834-7819.2010.01200. x.
[117] Kujan O, Oliver RJ, Khattab A, Roberts SA, Thakker N, Sloan P. Evaluation of a new binary system of grading oral epithelial dysplasia for prediction of malignant transformation. Oral Oncol. 2006; 42: 987–93. https: //doi.org/10.1016/j.oraloncology.2005.12.014.
[118] Ranganathan K, Kavitha L. Oral epithelial dysplasia: classifications and clinical relevance in risk assessment of oral potentially malignant disorders. J Oral Maxillofac Pathol. 2019; 23: 19–27. https: //doi.org/10.4103/jomfp.JOMFP_13_19.
[119] Mehrotra R, Gupta A, Singh M, Ibrahim R. Retraction: application of cytology and molecular biology in diagnosing premalignant or malignant oral lesions. Mol Cancer. 2012; 11: 57. https: //doi.org/10.1186/1476-4598-11-57.
[120] Casparis S, Borm JM, Tomic MA, Burkhardt A, Locher MC. Transepithelial brush biopsy – oral CDx® – a noninvasive method for the early detection of precancerous and cancerous lesions. J Clin Diagn Res. 2014; 8: 222–6. https: //doi.org/10.7860/JCDR/2014/7659.4065.
[121] Lingen MW, Tampi MP, Urquhart O, Abt E, Agrawal N, Chaturvedi AK, Cohen E, D'Souza G, Gurenlian J, Kalmar JR, Kerr AR, Lambert PM, Patton LL, Sollecito TP, Truelove E, Banfield L, Carrasco-Labra A. Adjuncts for the evaluation of potentially malignant disorders in the oral cavity: diagnostic test accuracy systematic review and meta-analysis-a report of the American Dental Association. J Am Dent Assoc. 2017; 148: 797–813.e52. https: //doi. org/10.1016/j.adaj.2017.08.045.
[122] Liu D, Zhao X, Zeng X, Dan H, Chen Q. Non-invasive techniques for detection and diagnosis of oral potentially malignant disorders. Tohoku J Exp Med. 2016; 238: 165–77. https: //doi. org/10.1620/tjem.238.165.

第 3 章

M. Anthony Pogrel

口内上皮异常增生的诊断和治疗

Diagnosis and Management of Intraoral Epithelial Dysplasia

引 言

根据美国癌症协会（ACS）的数据，仅在2020年，美国就诊断出了超过53 000例口腔癌和口咽癌的新病例。口腔癌的发病率与黑色素瘤一样正在由于未知原因而逐渐增加[1]。口腔癌很少由正常上皮发展而来，而是从初期的异常增生阶段演变而来。因此，如果能够在异常增生阶段根除病变，后续的癌症就不会发生。

"异常增生"是一个组织学术语，指上皮和基底层细胞的异常和不规则生长。其通常在组织学上被分为以下等级：① 轻度异常增生；② 中度异常增生；③ 重度异常增生（图3-1）；④ 原位癌。

这些病变转变为鳞状细胞癌的可能性尚不清楚。异常增生是否必须逐级进展，或者是否可以从轻度或中度异常增生直接转变为癌症也同样是未知的。轻度异常增生在五年内转变为鳞状细胞癌的概率为10%～20%[2]，而中度或重度异常增生的恶性转化率则在35%～50%。位于口底的病变（图3-2）更容易发生恶性转化，这可能与口底聚集了更多的致癌副产物有关[3]。许多研究尝试发现可以预测异常增生发生癌变的特征标志。例如，在进展为癌症的病变中，可能存在

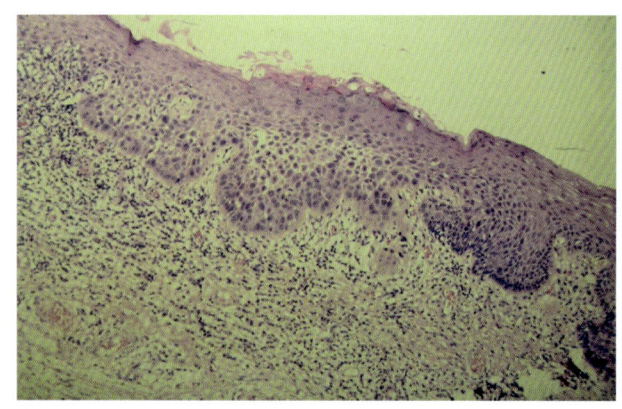

图3-1 重度上皮异常增生的组织病理学特征，显示核的深染、形态多样性，以及不规则但完整的基底膜（苏木精-伊红染色；40倍放大）

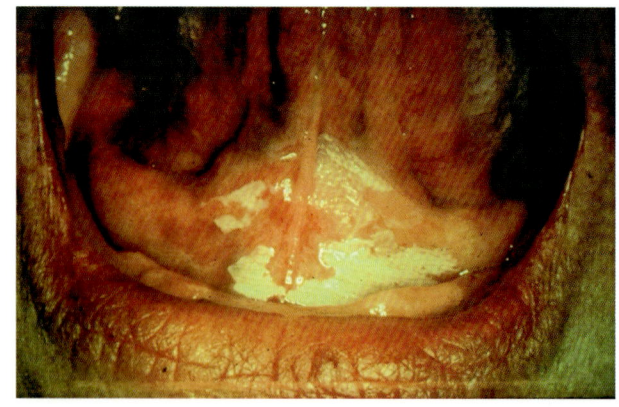

图3-2 具有较高的恶性转化倾向的口底轻度异常增生

M. A. Pogrel (✉)
Department of Oral and Maxillofacial Surgery, University of California, San Francisco, San Francisco, CA, USA
e-mail: tony.pogrel@ucsf.edu

金属蛋白酶 1 和 9 的过表达、mRNA（通过逆转录测定）过表达，以及在免疫组化中观察到的 Ki-67 的表达。在微阵列分析中观察到的基因组标志物的异常也被考虑作为预测恶性转化的一种方法[4]。然而，目前这些标志物都没有表现出稳定的可靠性或可预测性。

另一个问题是口腔黏膜异常增生的诊断缺乏标准化。研究表明，不同口腔颌面病理学家之间对组织学标本的分级并没有可靠的一致性；甚至当同一位口腔颌面病理学家在间隔 30 天后对同一标本分级时，结果也没有一致性[5]。

临床上，异常增生的表现缺乏统一性。它可以呈现为白色斑块，也就是白斑（图 3-3a），这是最轻微的异常增生形式，恶性转化率较低，为 2%～5%。它也可以表现为红白相间的斑块，通常称为红白斑（图 3-3b），其预后更加不良，恶性转化率较高，为 20%～30%[6]。然而，在临床上可能看起来完全正常的黏膜，在组织病理学检查中仍然可能存在异常增生，这使得临床检测变得具有挑战性。

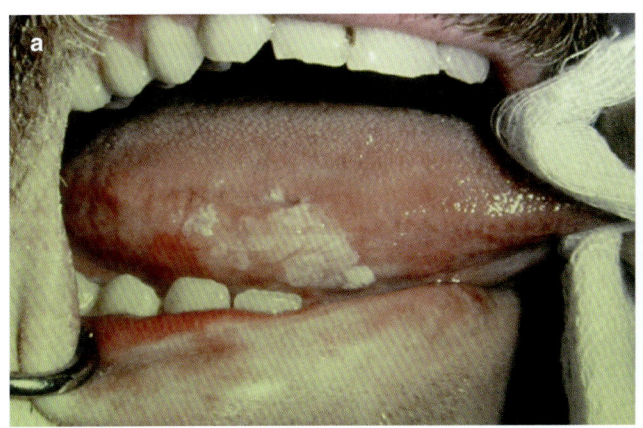 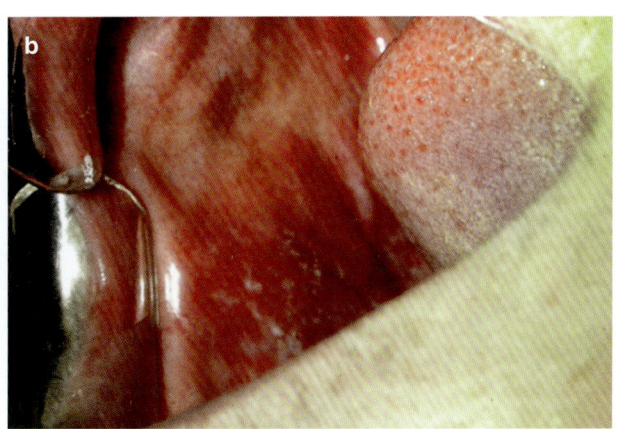

图 3-3 异常增生的临床表现缺乏统一性。a. 右侧舌缘为典型的均质型白斑，组织学上通常表现为轻度异常增生。b. 斑点状红白相间的红白斑，其恶性转化率已知高于白斑

口腔异常增生的辅助诊断方法

多年来，许多技术被用以更准确地诊断口腔异常增生，从而实现更可预测的治疗。

■ 甲苯胺蓝染色

甲苯胺蓝是一种活体染料，主要染色靠近细胞表面的细胞核。由于异常增生的组织细胞通常有这种表现，因此用甲苯胺蓝染色黏膜可以显示可能存在异常增生的区域。该技术首先使用碳酸氢钠或 1% 醋酸去除表面黏液，然后用 1% 甲苯胺蓝染色该区域，再用 1% 醋酸轻轻去色。染料仍然保留的区域很可能是异常增生，应进一步进行活检（图 3-4）。染色的区域也可以通过自然的方法脱色：染色后让患者离开 1～2 小时去喝水，黏膜会自然脱色，仍然保留染料的区域可被认为是可疑的[7]。这一技术经过了广泛的研究，结果有效[8]。该技术被推荐用来确定在哪些区域进行活检可以获得最准确的结果。然而，炎症和肉芽肿反应也会在甲苯胺蓝染色中呈现阳性结果。在欧洲，类似的染色技术利用了卢戈氏碘液，显示糖原的缺失，并取得了同样有意义的结果[9]。

■ 刷检（OralCDx）

该技术利用细胞学来寻找异常增生细胞。细胞学在早期诊断宫颈癌方面取得了很大的成功。然而，在口腔黏膜上使用时一直存在问题。这是因为口腔黏膜受到唾液、食物和其他碎屑的污

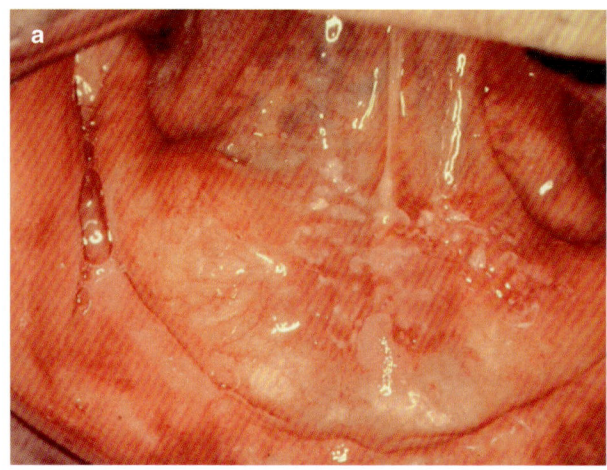 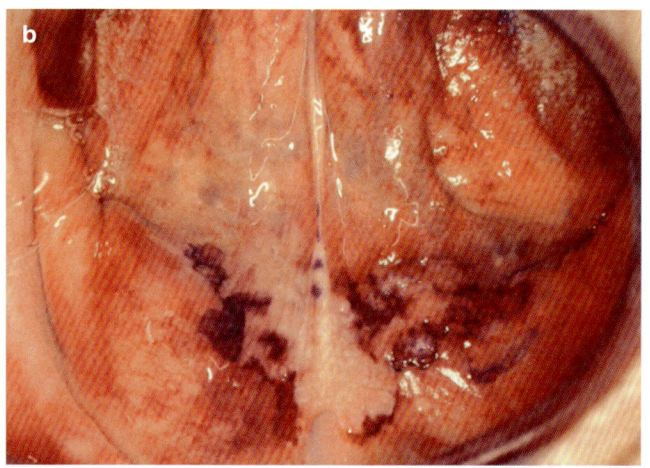

图 3-4 用甲苯胺蓝染色白斑。a. 口底白斑。b. 用甲苯胺蓝染色后的白斑病变,注意保留蓝色染料的区域,这些区域最有可能出现异常增生,并应进行活检

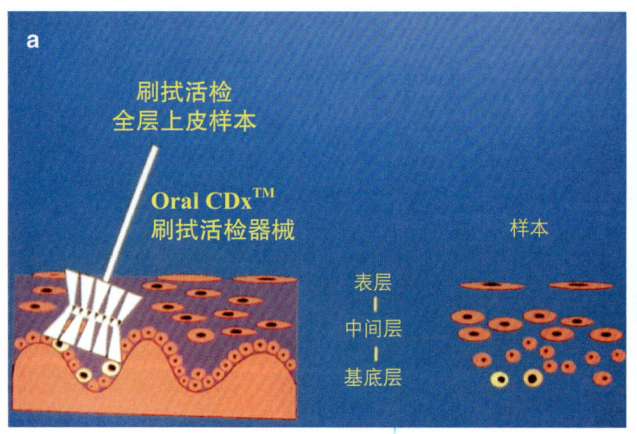 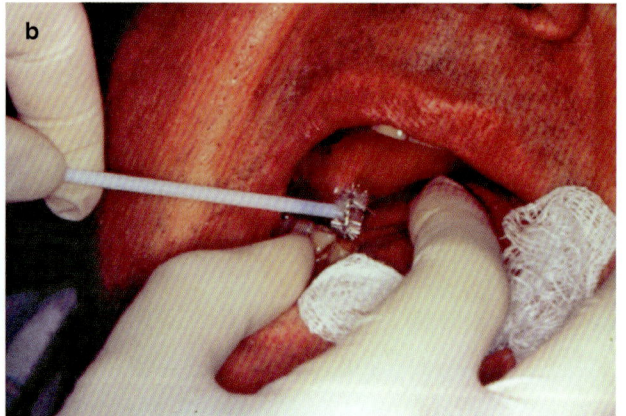

图 3-5 刷检。a. 刷检技术示意图。b. 临床图片展示了刷检应用于组织上

染,同时基底层位于深处,获取有意义的材料也更困难。最近开发的一种刷检技术能够深入到基底膜,并结合计算机检查系统,使其能够进行更准确的细胞学检查[10,11](图3-5)。但是该技术还不能替代正式的活检,常用作活检前的初步筛查,因此它并不会节省时间或减少程序。还有研究表明,仅使用刷检而不使用计算机检查系统也可以取得类似的效果[12]。

■ **ViziLite**

这项技术利用化学发光和组织反射,其基本原理是在暗室中通过化学反应发出的光可以比在自然光下的直接检查更好地显示异常增生区域。

该技术也曾与甲苯胺蓝染色联合使用[13]。尽管有相关说法,但此技术似乎并不优于在自然光下的直接检查[14]。

■ **荧光灯检查**

这种方法使用荧光灯来检查口腔黏膜。其原理是,正常组织会反射荧光,而异常增生和恶性组织会吸收荧光。因此,在正常组织中不会出现反射,区域会显得较暗[15,16]。然而,目前尚不清楚这种技术是否比使用高质量头灯进行的直接检查更有优势。该技术确实能检测到区域内血液供应的增加,因此可以检测到异常增生组织和炎症组织,所以在炎症状态下会导致假阳性结果。

特殊说明的鉴别诊断

增殖性疣状白斑

增殖性疣状白斑（proliferative verrucous leukoplakia, PVL）是一种特殊的疾病，由 Hansen 等[17]于 1985 年首次诊断。它是一种特殊形式的白斑，可以通过临床（图 3-6）和组织学手段进行诊断。如果不加以治疗，该病变几乎不可避免地会经历疣状增生阶段，进展为疣状癌，最终发展成鳞状细胞癌。去除这种病变需要相当激进的手术，且重建可能涉及硬组织和软组织的移植。即使如此，该病变也可能难以完全清除，多年后可能复发。当病变位于牙龈周围（图 3-6b）时，尤其难以去除，因为它有通过牙周膜扩散的倾向[18]，进行牙龈切除术或其他局部手术效果有限，只有进行根尖下截骨术将牙齿包含在切除骨块内才能成功（图 3-6c、d）。

扁平苔藓

关于口腔扁平苔藓（lichen planus, LP）是否应被视为一种癌前病变存在争议。口腔扁平苔藓影响 0.2%～0.3% 的人群，并且在女性中更为常见。目前的研究表明，网状型扁平苔藓（图 3-7a）可能不是癌前病变；但萎缩型（图 3-7b）或溃疡型（图 3-7c）可能是癌前病变，恶变率为 1%～2%[19, 20]。因此，应努力治疗表现为溃疡型或萎缩型的扁平苔藓。治疗通常使用类固

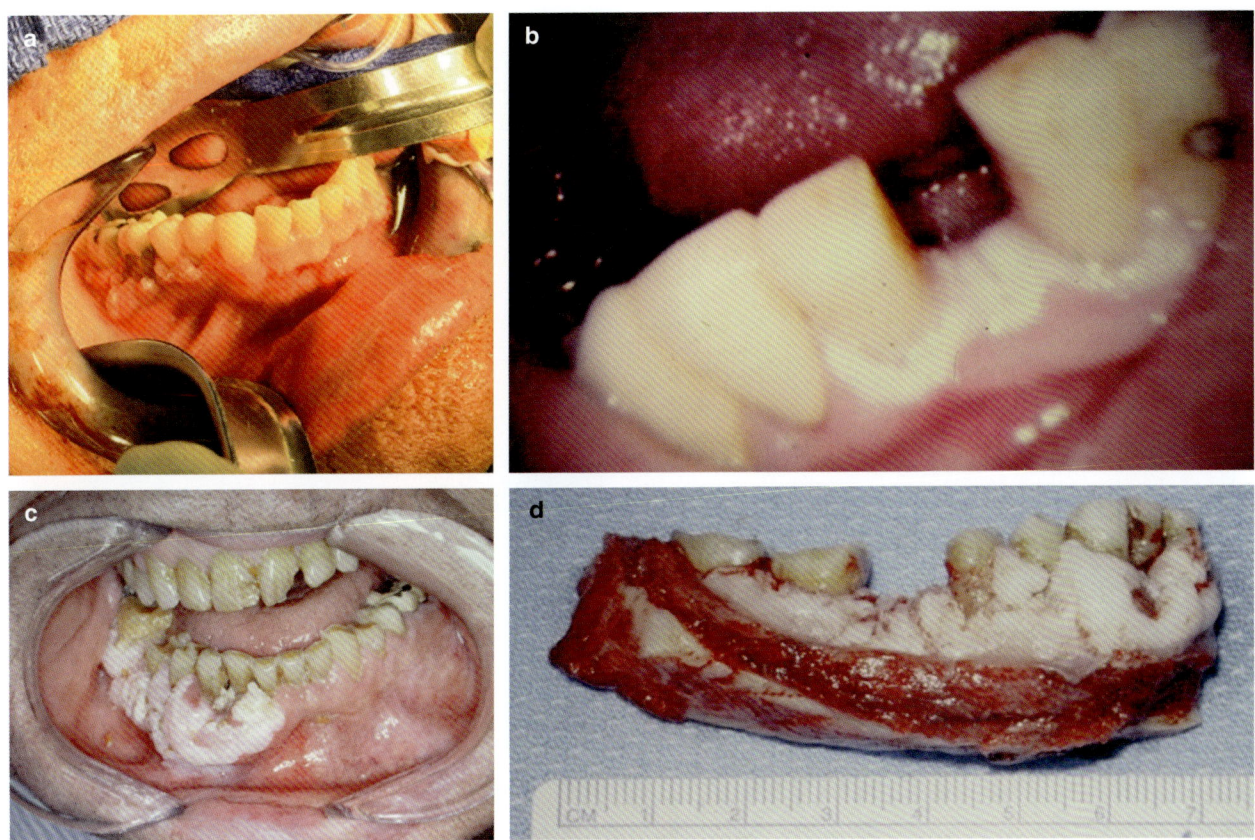

图 3-6 增殖性疣状白斑（PVL）。a. PVL 在口腔中的典型疣状外观。b. PVL 特定分布在牙龈缘区域。c、d. 更具增殖性的疣状白斑类型，只能通过下颌骨的"整体"边缘切除术去除

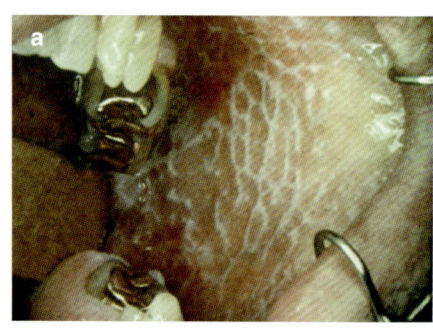 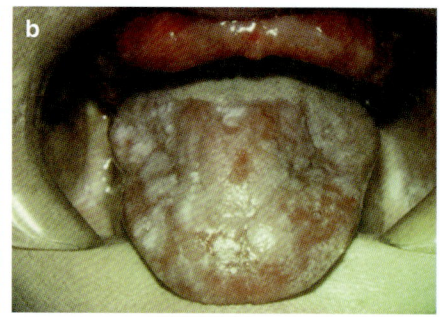 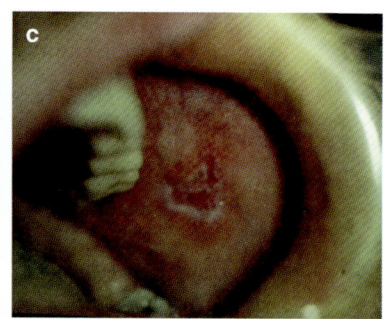

图 3-7　口腔扁平苔藓的不同类型。a. 网状型扁平苔藓，通常是良性的。b、c. 萎缩型和溃疡型扁平苔藓，可能具有恶性潜能

醇或其他免疫调节剂，对于局部病变在适当情况下则进行外科切除或激光切除。目前，WHO将扁平苔藓分类为潜在恶性疾病（potentially malignant disease, PMD），而不是癌前病变。

口腔异常增生的治疗

口腔异常增生的传统治疗为活检明确诊断后手术治疗。在可能的情况下，建议进行扩大切除，必要时进行皮肤或黏膜移植以重建术后缺损。尽管一些来自欧洲的多中心研究提供了早期手术干预在长期内可能获益的合理证据，但很难证明这种技术能改善结局并降低后续口腔癌的发生率[21, 22]。手术治疗应去除至少在基底膜下2～3 mm 深度的组织（图 3-8）。

当口腔异常增生表现为白斑或红白斑时，建议使用手术激光，如波长为 10.6 μm 的二氧化碳激光来进行切除。使用激光作为外科工具去除手术标本是可行的，但这会给口腔颌面病理学家带来更多困难，因为病理学家需要考虑激光对手术切缘的干扰，而受干扰的切缘通常延伸到三层细胞的厚度。此外，当激光用于"擦除"或汽化治疗病变区域时，其穿透深度有限。因此，异常增生往往会复发（图 3-9）。还有报道称，在使用二氧化碳激光手术"擦除"或汽化治疗的病变区域，口腔癌可能会进展，这更加令人担忧[23, 24]。虽然有说法认为激光可能刺激口腔癌的形成，但更可能癌症已经存在于异常增生的组织中，只是去除更表浅的上皮层将其显现出来了，这也进一步支持了进行更深层

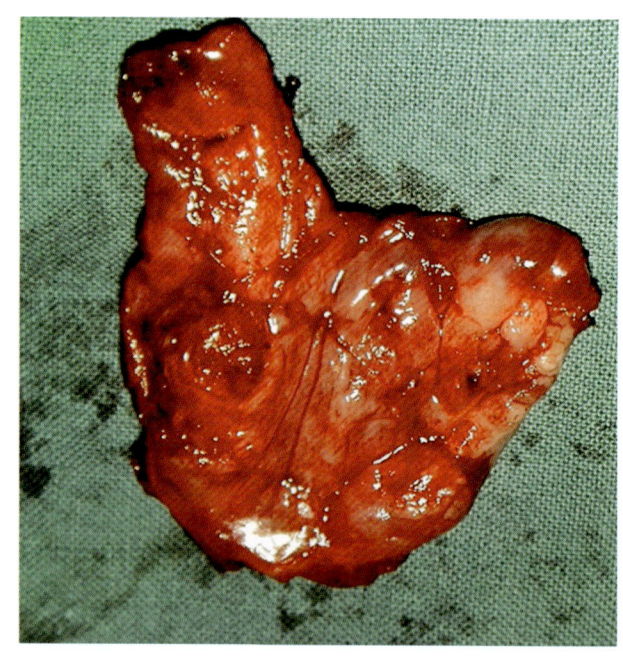

图 3-8　手术切除的红白斑病标本，切除深度为 2～3 mm，以提供最佳治愈条件

次切除的观点[23, 24]。

对于广泛的白斑区域，或对于轻度或中度的异常增生，可能需要采用"观察等待"的方案，并在适当时进行活检。该方法的理论依据是，通过定期检查，任何恶性变化都可以早期诊断，从而有助于获得更好的预后。

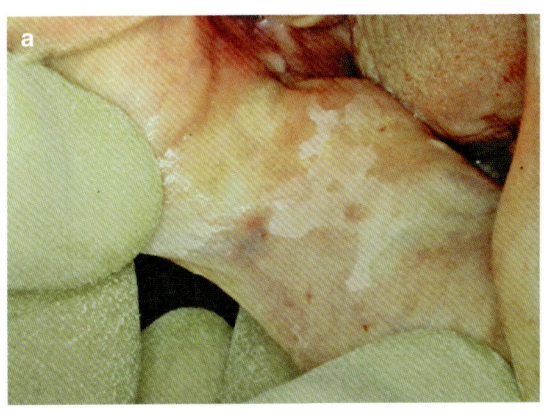
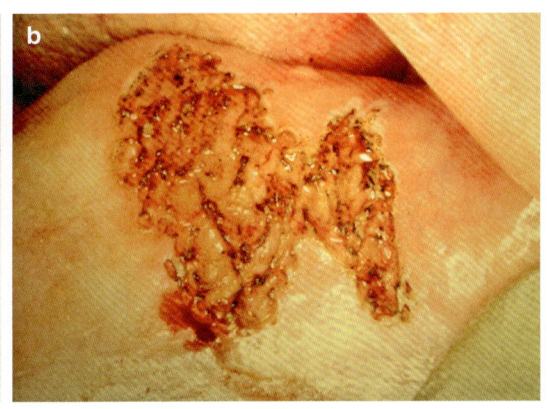

图 3-9　a.薄膜状白斑区域经过。b.二氧化碳激光表面汽化治疗。这种技术复发率高，且可能显现潜在的恶性病变

口腔异常增生和口腔癌的影响因素

吸烟

吸烟是已知的增加口腔癌发病率的习惯之一。雪茄和烟斗尽管对肺部危害更小，但它们在口腔内的烟雾温度更高，与香烟相比对口腔黏膜更具危害。无烟烟草（如嚼烟或鼻烟）的使用仍然存在争议。毫无疑问，这些习惯会导致黏膜发生变化，引起增生和疣状型病变，近期研究表明，这些病变中有些会进展为口腔癌[25]。

饮酒

烈性酒被认为会促进口腔癌的发生，可能是通过引起口腔黏膜脱水，导致黏膜萎缩，从而使其对饮食中的致癌物质更为敏感。此外，尽管饮酒和吸烟是两个独立的风险因素，但它们可能会协同作用，进一步增加口腔癌的患病风险。

嚼槟榔

在印度次大陆，嚼食槟榔被认为是口腔黏膜下纤维化的已知原因，这是一种癌前病变，可能导致口腔癌。研究表明，槟榔中的槟榔油是主要的刺激物[26]。

维生素失衡

早期关于维生素 A 及其衍生物的研究显示，高剂量维生素 A 能够使白斑和其他口腔异常增生病变逆转[27-33]。然而，一旦停止治疗，这些病变便会复发。此外，维生素 A 会导致黏膜极度变薄、开裂以及其他对大多数患者来说不可接受的系统性副作用。目前尚不清楚这种治疗是否会减少后续口腔癌的发生，但目前并未将维生素 A 用于此目的。维生素 A 的在植物中的等价成分是 β-胡萝卜素，这种物质耐受性更好，并被推荐作为预防口腔病变和预防已治疗病变复发的方法[29-32]。类胡萝卜素及其相关的类黄酮主要来自胡萝卜、红薯、生菜和羽衣甘蓝等食物[28]。每天四根胡萝卜条就足够，过量摄入会导致皮肤变成橙色。β-胡萝卜素还可以通过富含胡萝卜素的饮品或片剂形式摄入。叶酸（维生素 B_9）也可能降低口腔癌的风险，叶酸存在于菠菜、芦笋、豆类、豌豆和扁豆中[34]。酒精会产生乙醛，而乙醛会抑制叶酸，这可能是酒精促进口腔癌的另一个原因。

致癌病毒

尽管超过 50% 的口咽癌患者人乳头瘤病毒（HPV）DNA 检测阳性，但口腔癌患者中的这一比例要低得多。如果检测 P16（作为 HPV 的替代标志物），大约 25% 的口腔癌患者是阳性的，但如果检测病毒 DNA，只有大约 5% 是阳性的。这两个数字之间的差异尚未得到充分解释。几乎所有HPV阳性的口腔恶性肿瘤都发生在口底,可能与微创伤、异位唾液腺或扁桃体组织有关。因此,HPV似乎并不是导致口腔上皮异常增生或口腔恶性肿瘤的主要原因[35]。然而,像增殖性疣状白斑这样的潜在恶性病变则可能由病毒导致[18]。

药物的意外好处

某些常用药物显示出降低口腔癌发病率的有益效果,因此可能也会降低异常增生的发生率。这些药物包括烟酰胺[36]、阿司匹林[37,38]和二甲双胍[39,40]。此外,一项大型退伍军人事务管理局的研究显示,用于治疗失神发作和癫痫疾病的丙戊酸钠可能导致头颈癌的发生率降低[41,42]。这些药物在预防原发性口腔癌及其复发方面的作用机制尚不清楚,但可能与它们的抗炎作用有关。

小 结

尽管经过多年的癌症研究,我们对口腔异常增生的临床行为及背后的分子生物学机制研究仍然进展甚微。这一不幸的情况很可能是导致口腔癌五年生存率总体改善不明显的原因。未来,这个问题可以从多个方面加以解决,包括:利用经典分子标签和非经典方法(如借助人工智能/机器学习进行的数字组织形态计量分析)开发预测预后和治疗反应特异性的生物标志物;创建生物传感器,为那些与潜在疾病相关的早期生物标志物提供实时监测;进行详细的前瞻性研究,将临床进展与生物标志物相关的分子研究进展相结合;最后,加深对临床表型与分子基因型相关性的理解,从而最终实现靶向药物的开发。癌症总是能找到方法击败任何意图控制它的治疗。但针对异常增生的治疗则可以更加有效,因为与癌症相比,其基因复制调控的分子机制并没有受到太大干扰,因此抵抗治疗的可能性相对较小。

参 考 文 献

[1] Campbell BR, Netterville JL, Sinard RJ, Mannion K, Rohde SL, Langerman A, Kim YJ, Lewis JS, Lang Kuhs KA. Early onset oral tongue cancer in the United States: a literature review. Oral Oncol. 2018; 87: 1–7.

[2] Reibel J. Prognosis of oral pre-malignant lesions: significance of clinical, histopathological, and molecular biological characteristics. Crit Rev Oral Biol Med. 2003; 14: 47–62.

[3] Rock LD, Rosin MP, Zhang L, Chan B, Shariati B, Laronde DM. Characterization of epithelial oral dysplasia in non smokers: first steps towards precision medicine. Oral Oncol. 2018; 78: 119–25.

[4] Smith J, Rattay T, McConkey C, Helliwell T, Mehanna H. Biomarkers in dysplasia of the oral cavity: a systematic review. Oral Oncol. 2009; 45: 647–53.

[5] Warnakulasuriya S, Reibel J, Bouquot J, Dabelsteen E. Oral epithelial dysplasia classification systems: predictive value, utility, weaknesses and scope for improvement. J Oral Pathol Med. 2008; 37: 127–33.

[6] Awadallah M, Idle M, Patel K, Kademani D. Management update of potentially premalignant oral epithelial lesions. Oral Surg Oral Med Oral Pathol Oral Radiol. 2018; 125: 628–36.

[7] Silverman S Jr, Migliorati C, Barbosa J. Toluidine blue staining in the detection of oral precancerous and malignant lesions. Oral Surg Oral Med Oral Pathol. 1984; 57: 379–82.

[8] Chainani-Wu N, Madden E, Cox D, Sroussi H, Epstein J, Silverman S Jr. Toluidine blue aids in detection of dysplasia and carcinoma in suspicious oral lesions. Oral Dis. 2015; 21: 879–85.

[9] Elimairi I, Altay MA, Abdoun O, Elmairi A, Tozoglu S, Baur DA, Quereshy F. Clinical relevance of the utilization of vital Lugol's Iodine staining in detection and diagnosis of oral cancer and dysplasia. Clin Oral Investig. 2017; 21: 589–95.

[10] Casparis S, Borm JM, Tomic MA, Burkhardt A, Locher MC. Transepithelial brush biopsy-Oral CDx-A non invasive method for the early detection of precancerous and cancerous lesions. J Clin Diagn Res. 2014; 8: 222–6.

[11] Sciubba JJ, Larian B. Oral squamous cell carcinoma; early detection and improved 5 year survival in 102 patients. Gen Dent. 2018; 66: e11-6.

[12] Mehrotra R, Singh MK, Pandya S, Singh M. The use of an oral brush biopsy without computer-assisted analysis in the evaluation of oral lesions: a study of 94 patients. Oral Surg Oral Med Oral Pathol Oral Radiol Endod. 2008; 106: 246-53.

[13] Sambandham T, Masthan KM, Kumar MS, Jha A. The application of vizilite in oral cancer. J Clin Diagn Res. 2013; 7: 185-6.

[14] Oh ES, Laskin DM. Efficacy of the Vizilite system in the identification of oral lesions. J Oral Maxillofac Surg. 2007; 65: 424-6.

[15] Yamamoto N, Kawaguchi K, Fujihara H, Hasebe M, Kishi Y, Yasukama M, Kumagai K, Hamada Y. Detection accuracy for epithelial dysplasia using an objective autofluoroescence visualization method based on the luminance ratio. Int J Oral Sci. 2017; 9(11): e2. https://doi.org/10.1038/ijosNov2017.37.

[16] Kikuta S, Iwanaga J, Todoroki K, Shinozaki K, Tanoue R, Nakamura M, Kusukawa J. Clinical application of the illumiscan fluorescence visualization device in detecting oral mucosal lesions. Cureus. 2018; 10(8): e3111. https://doi.org/10.7759/cureus.311.

[17] Hansen LS, Olson JA, Silverman S Jr. Proliferative verrucous leukoplakia. A long term study of thirty patients. Oral Surg Oral Med Oral Pathol. 1985; 60: 285-98.

[18] Upadhyaya JD, Fitzpatrick SG, Islam MN, Bhattacharyya I, Cohen DM. A retrospective 20 year analysis of proliferative verrucous hyperplasia and its progression to malignancy and association with high risk human papillomavirus. Head Neck Pathol. 2018; 12(4): 500-10. https://doi.org/10.1007/s12105-018-0893-7.

[19] Ingafou M, Leao JC, Porter SR, Scully C. Oral lichen planus: a retrospective study of 690 British patients. Oral Dis. 2006; 12: 463-8.

[20] Speight PM, Khurram SA, Kujan O. Oral potentially malignant disorders: risk of progression to malignancy. Oral Surg Oral Med Oral Pathol Oral Radiol. 2018; 125: 612-27.

[21] Mehanna HM, Rattay T, Smith J, McConkey CC. Treatment and follow up of oral dysplasia-a systematic review and meta-analysis. Head Neck. 2009; 31: 1600-9.

[22] Balasundaram I, Payne KF, Al-Hadad I, Alibhai M, Thomas S, Bhandari R. Is there any benefit in surgery for potentially malignant disorders of the oral cavity? J Oral Pathol Med. 2014; 43: 239-44.

[23] Brouns ER, Baart JA, Karagozoglu KH, Aartman IH, Bloemena E, Van der Waal I. Treatment results of CO_2 laser vaporisation in a cohort of 35 patients with oral leukoplakia. Oral Dis. 2013; 19: 212-6.

[24] Dong Y, Chen Y, Tao Y, Hao Y, Jiang Y, Dan H, Zang X, Chen Q, Zhou Y. Malignant transformation of oral leukoplakia treated with carbon dioxide laser: a meta-analysis. Lasers Med Sci. 2018; 34(1): 209-21. https://doi.org/10.1007/s10103-018-2674-7.

[25] Gupta S, Gupta R, Sinha DN, Mehrotra R. Relationship between type of smokeless tobacco and risk of cancer: a systematic review. Indian J Med Res. 2018; 148: 56-76.

[26] Avakeri G, Patil SG, Aljabab AS, Lin KC, Merkx MAW, Gao S, Brennan PA. Oral submucous fibrosis: an update on pathophysiology of malignamnt transformation. J Orasl Pathol Med. 2017; 46: 413-7.

[27] Hong WK, Endicott J, Itri LM, Doos W, Batsakis JG, Bell R, Fofonoff S, Byers R, Atkinson EN, Vaughan C, et al. 13-cic-retinoic acid in the treatment of oral leukoplakia. N Engl J Med. 1986; 315: 1501-5.

[28] Piatelli A, Fiorini M, Santinelli A, Rubini C. blc-2 expression and apoptotic bodies in 13-cis-retinoic acid(isotretinoin)-treated oral leukoplakia: a pilot study. Oral Onc. 1999; 35: 314-20.

[29] Sankaranarayanan R, Mathew B, Varghese C, Sudhakaran PR, Menon V, Jayadeep A, Nair MK, Mathews C, Mahalingam TR, Balaram P, Nair PP. Chemoprevention of oral leukoplakia with Vitamin A and beta carotene: an assessment. Oral Onc. 1999; 33: 231-6.

[30] Stich HF, Mathew B, Sankaranarayanan R, Nair MK. Remission of oral precancerous lesions of tobacco/areca nut chewers following administration of beta-carotene or Vitamin A, and maintenance of the protective effect. Cancer Detect Prev. 1991; 15: 93-8.

[31] Stich HF, Brunnemann KD, Mathew B, Sankaranarayanan R, Nair MK. Chemoprevention trials with Vitamin A and beta carotene: some unresolved issues. Prev Med. 1989; 18: 732-9.

[32] Stich HF, Rosin MP, Hornby AP, Mathew B, Sankaranarayanan R, Nair MK. Remission of oral leukoplakias and micronuclei in tobacco/betel quid chewers treated with beta carotene and with beta carotene plus vitamin A. Int J Cancer. 1988; 15: 195-9.

[33] Stich HF, Hornby AP, Mathew B, Sankaranarayanan R, Nair MK. Response of oral leukoplakia to the administration of Vitamin A. Cancer Lett. 1988; 40: 93-101.

[34] Galeone C, Edefonti V, Parpinel M, Leoncini E, Matsuo K, Talamini O, Olshan AF, Zevallos JP, Winn DM, Jayaprakash V, Moysich K, Zhang ZF, Morgenstern H, Levi F, Bosetti C, Kelsey K, Mc Clean M, Schantz S, Yu GP, Boffetta P, Lee YC, Hashibe M, La Vecchia C, Boccia S. Folate intake and the risk of oral cavity and pharyngeal cancer: a pooled analysis within the International Head and neck Cancer Epidemiology Consortium. Int J Cancer. 2015; 136: 904-14.

[35] Hubbers CU, Akgul B. HPV and cancer of the oral cavity. Virulence. 2015; 6: 244-8.

[36] Chen AC, Martin AJ, Choy B, Fernandez-Panas P, Dalziell RA, McKenzie CA, Scolyer RA, Dhillon HM, Vardy JKL, Kricker A, St George G, Chinniah N, Halliday GM, Damian DL. A phase 3 randomized trial of nicotinamide for skin cancer chemoprotection. N Engl J Med. 2015; 373: 1618-26.

[37] Lumley CJ, Kaffenberger TM, Desale S, Tefera E, Han CJ, Rafei H, Maxwell JH. Post diagnosis aspirin use and survival in patients with head and neck cancer. Head Neck. 2018; 41(5): 1220-6. https://doi.org/10.1002/hed.25518.

[38] Zhang X, Feng H, Li Z, Guo J, Li M. Aspirin is involved in the cell cycle arrest, apoptosis, cell migration, and invasion of oral squamous cell carcinoma. Int J Med Sci. 2018; 19m12(7): E2029. https://doi.org/10.3390/ijms19072029.

[39] Saka Herran C, Jane-Salas C, Estrugo Devesa A, Lopez-Lopez J. Protective effects of metformin, statins and anti-inflammatory drugs on head and neck cancer: a systematic review. Oral Oncol. 2018; 85: 68–81.

[40] Verma A, Rich LJ, Vincent-Chong VK, Seshadri M. Visualizing the effects of metformin on tumor growth, vascularity and metabolism in head and neck cancer. J Oral Pathol Med. 2018; 47: 484–91.

[41] Kang H, Gillespie TW, Goodman M, Brodie SA, Brandes M, Ribeiro M, Ramalingam SS, Shin DM, Khuri FR, Brandes JC. Long term use of valproic acid in US veterans is associated with a reduced risk of smoking-related cases of head and neck cancer. Cancer. 2014; 120: 1394–400.

[42] Lee SH, Nam HJ, Kang HJ, Samuels TL, Johnston N, Lim YC. Valproic acid suppresses the self-renewal and proliferation of head and neck cancer stem cells. Oncol Rep. 2015; 34: 2065–71.

第 4 章

Lisa M. Evangelista

头颈肿瘤中的吞咽困难
Dysphagia in Head and Neck Cancers

引 言

在美国，头颈肿瘤治疗范式的转变反映了该病种发展趋势的变化。从 1988 年到 2004 年，由于烟草使用率的下降，喉癌和下咽癌的发病率下降了 50%，但是口咽癌的发病率却在过去的几十年里出现了惊人的上升。在美国，口咽部是头颈癌最常见的发病部位。口咽鳞状细胞癌发病率的升高与人乳头瘤病毒（HPV）直接相关。从 1988 年到 2004 年，HPV 相关口咽癌的发病率上升了 225%[1]。尽管 HPV 阳性的癌症患者的生存预期较 HPV 阴性者更为乐观，但治疗带来的副作用对患者生理功能的影响仍然较大。

头颈癌治疗进展在于既要提高肿瘤的治愈率，同时还要注重功能的保全。尽管人们已经努力减轻导致吞咽困难的治疗毒性，但在接受头颈癌治疗的患者中，吞咽困难的发生率仍在增加。吞咽困难可能在癌症治疗过程中或结束后即刻出现，也可能因为治疗剂量的累积作用远期出现并进行性加重。头颈癌患者治疗后 2 年内出现吞咽困难和肺炎的概率为 45.3%。治疗后 10 年内吞咽困难发生率上升 11.7%。进一步研究评估了头颈癌患者在接受放化疗后吞咽困难及其相关并发症的增加趋势。对于在诊断后 2～5 年和 5 年以上完成放化疗的患者，吞咽困难的发生率从 14.9% 增加到 26%。在同一时间段内，胃造瘘管置管率从 2.82% 上升到 3.32%，吸入性肺炎的发病率从 3.13% 上升到 6.75%[2]。虽然在治疗模式和方案制订方面已经做出了重大努力，以尽量减少吞咽不良的结果，但旨在降低吞咽困难发生率和严重程度的干预措施仍然是一个需要优先考虑的问题。

外 科 治 疗

头颈癌外科手术后吞咽困难的出现及其严重程度在很大程度上取决于手术切除的类型、位置和范围。传统的手术方式采用大范围的切除模式，导致严重的功能损伤。手术切除和重建影响吞咽相关的解剖结构和生理功能，从而导致吞咽困难和误吸。

L. M. Evangelista (✉)
Department of Otolaryngology/Head & Neck Surgery, University of California at Davis Medical Center, Sacramento, CA, USA
e-mail: evangelista@ucdavis.edu

在头颈癌的外科治疗中，一个重要的进展是经口机器人手术（transoral robotic surgery，TORS）的应用。TORS是一种应用内镜技术进行头颈部肿瘤切除的微创术式[3]。通过减少开放手术方法的需求，如下颌骨切开或咽切开，TORS能够保留关键吞咽结构的解剖结构。此外，与在根治性治疗需要的放射剂量相比，先使用TORS再进行辅助性放化疗可能会减少所需的放射剂量。通过限制必要的放射治疗剂量，可以减轻导致吞咽困难的放射毒性。与强度调制放射治疗（intensity-modulated radiation therapy，IMRT）治疗口咽癌相比，接受TORS治疗的患者中，需要放置饲管和依赖的比例较低[4]。随着微创手术的出现、机器人技术的使用以及外科重建技术的进步，头颈癌外科干预后的功能保留越来越重要[5]。

口腔癌

口腔癌的手术切除和重建术可在口腔预备期、口腔期和咽部期造成明显的吞咽困难[6]。手术切除嘴唇、舌头、口腔底、牙槽突和硬腭可导致以下情况。

- 唇闭合不全、口腔内容物外溢。
- 口腔容纳功能下降导致食物提前进入咽腔。
- 舌活动性下降导致食物从口腔到咽腔的前后传递效率下降。
- 硬腭缺损导致食物和液体反流进入鼻腔。
- 口底肌肉的切除导致舌骨喉复合体运动能力下降。

口咽和鼻咽癌

口咽和鼻咽的切除，包括舌根、腭扁桃体、咽扁桃体及软腭，可能导致的吞咽功能异常如下。

- 腭咽关闭不全导致鼻腔反流。
- 咽运动反射损伤导致吞咽起始延迟。
- 舌根收缩和咽收缩功能损伤导致咽腔食物清除能力下降。

喉和下咽癌

喉和下咽癌患者术后的吞咽功能主要受手术切除范围的影响。早期喉癌的治疗不一定会引起明显的或长期的吞咽困难。晚期喉癌的手术治疗往往会影响喉的闭合和咽的收缩。虽然早期下咽癌多采用保留器官的治疗模式，但晚期下咽癌的治疗需同时切除全喉和下咽。

部分喉切除术，包括垂直部分喉切除术、声门上喉切除术和肩胛上喉切除术，可能导致以下生理性损伤和吞咽困难症状[7]。

- 舌根收缩功能减退导致咽腔清除能力下降。
- 声门重建后功能不全导致喉的穿透和误吸。
- 舌骨喉复合体运动能力下降导致喉的闭合功能和咽的清除能力下降。

全喉切除手术可能应用于晚期癌症、肿瘤长期未根治及无功能喉的患者[8]。虽然全喉切除术后因为气管食管的分隔而不存在误吸的风险，但吞咽困难仍很常见，发生率高达72%[9]。吞咽功能损伤的生理机制如下。

- 舌根收缩功能的下降导致重建后的咽腔食物清除能力下降。
- 咽收缩功能的下降导致重建后的咽腔食物残留。
- 咽感觉能力下降导致咽蠕动能力下降。
- 重建后的咽食管区段狭窄或挛缩产生食物黏于喉腔的异物感。

放射治疗

放射治疗是头颈癌治疗中的常用方式。无论是根治性剂量还是辅助治疗剂量，放疗后的患者都有可能经历治疗早期或远期的吞咽相关并发症[10]。文献证明，吞咽困难的程度与吞咽相关器官接受的放疗剂量相关[11]。随着调强放疗的出现，放射肿瘤学可以通过降低受累器官的放疗剂量来保护吞咽功能，改善传统放疗模式带来的并发症。虽然随着技术的进步放疗的毒性得到控制，但吞咽困难仍然是头颈癌治疗近期和远期常见的并发症[12]。

放疗近期或急性不良反应包括口干、黏膜炎和味觉障碍。

- 口干是放疗最常见的不良反应。口干可能持续整个放疗过程以及放疗结束后。放疗期间，唾液腺分泌细胞的萎缩或慢性炎症会导致口干。长期的口干与放疗诱导的涎腺坏死相关。口干可能增加龋齿、口腔念珠菌病感染和咀嚼吞咽困难的风险[13]。

- 黏膜炎是放疗导致的常见的组织损伤（图4-1）。口腔和咽腔黏膜的炎症可能引起严重的吞咽疼痛。此外，黏膜炎也可以导致经口摄入减少及体重下降[14]。

- 味觉障碍有可能会影响生活质量。味觉改变可能导致经口摄入减少，从而引起营养不良[15]。

- 手术或放疗后可能引起头颈部组织的水肿（图4-2）。组织水肿可能导致吞咽相关肌肉的蠕动和收缩能力减退（图4-3）。

放疗的远期不良反应可导致吞咽器官不可逆的继发性功能损伤。吞咽相关肌肉的纤维化、萎

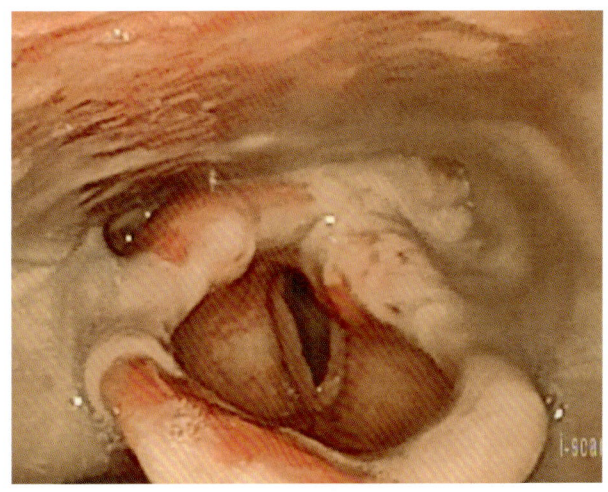

图 4-1　咽和喉的黏膜炎

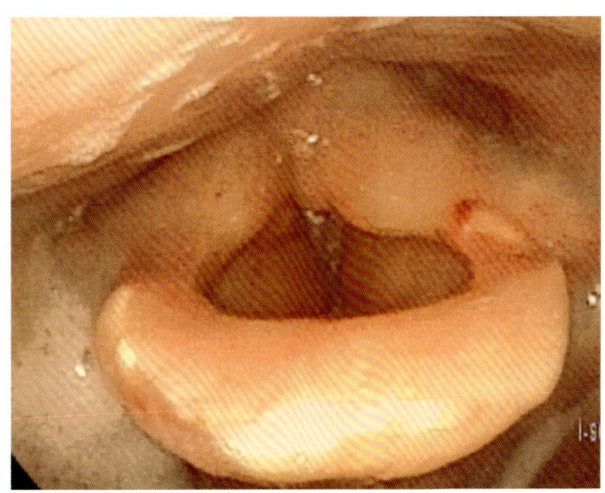

图 4-2　放疗结束后的喉水肿

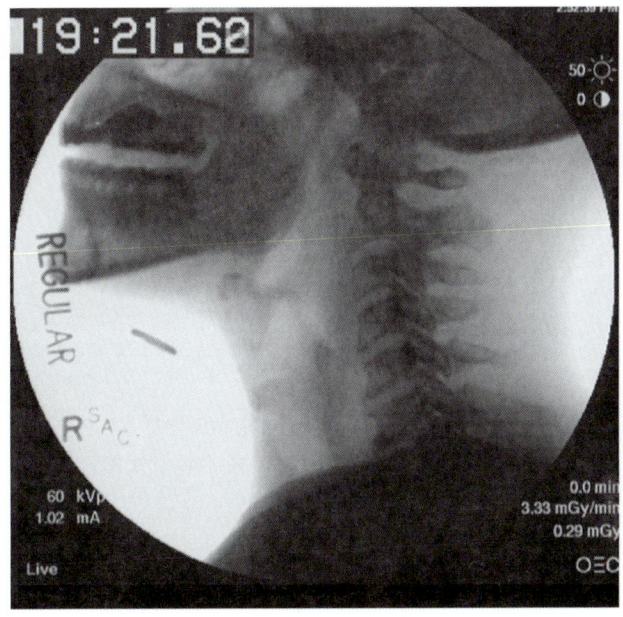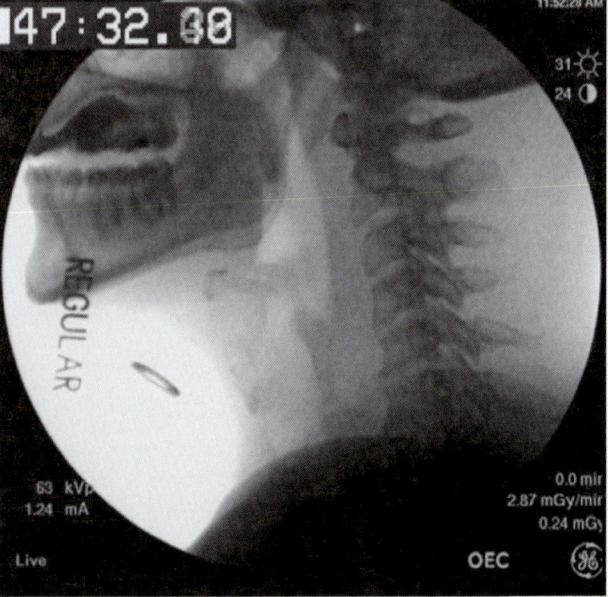

图 4-3　透视镜下放疗前和放疗后 3 个月咽后壁水肿情况的比较

缩和血管损伤均可影响吞咽的安全性和有效性。放疗诱发的吞咽困难的患者可能会有吞咽困难和喉紧绷感，或出现吸入性肺炎，甚至需要改变进食和饮水的方式[16]。

纤维化和失神经支配导致肌肉萎缩，从而影响整个吞咽肌群的活动性和收缩性，导致以下情况（图4-4和图4-5）。

- 舌和舌根的活动性减弱导致口腔和咽腔的食物清除能力下降。
- 呼吸道保护功能减弱导致喉部穿透和误吸。
- 咽肌收缩功能减弱导致咽和下咽的食物清除能力下降。
- 咽食管区段弹性减弱导致食管狭窄。

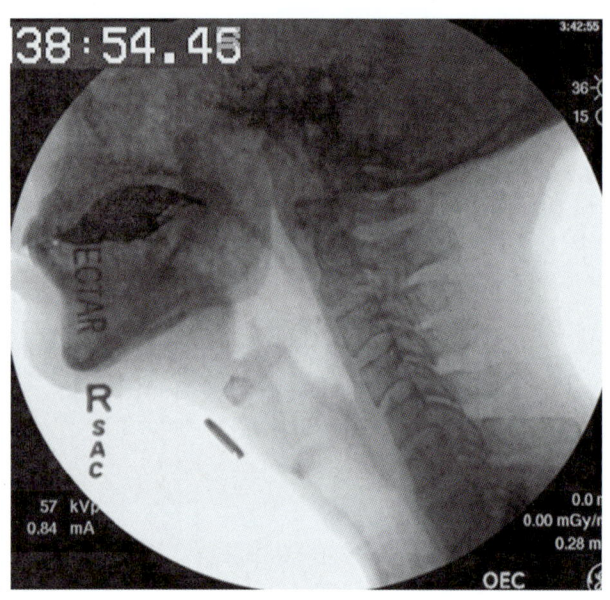

图4-4　电视透视镜下舌根萎缩影像

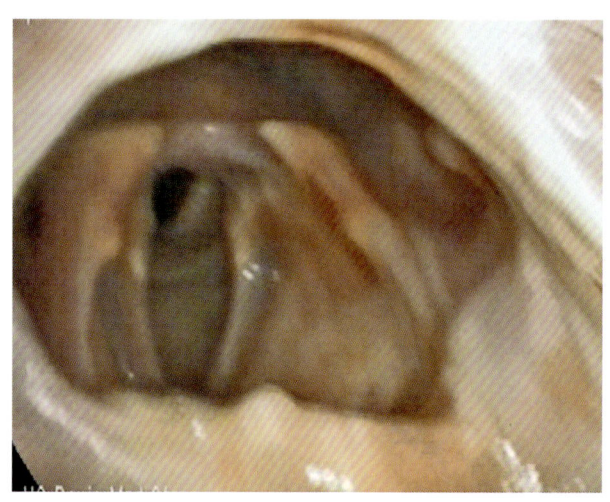

图4-5　放疗毒性引起的喉失神经支配

头颈癌中吞咽功能异常的评估

吞咽功能的综合评估包括全面的病史调查、口腔临床检查和仪器检查。吞咽功能的评估最好能在癌症治疗之前进行，以便知晓患者的基线功能[16]。

病史

一份全面的患者病历资料应包括患者的现病史和既往病史。相关病史包括如下内容。

- 肿瘤情况，包括病灶位置和肿瘤分期。
- 既往或计划的头颈癌相关的手术和药物治疗方案。
- 既往或现有的吞咽困难。
- 目前的饮食方案、是否需要更改饮食方案或进食饮水方式。
- 计划外的体重下降。
- 肺的情况，包括目前或既往是否有吸入性肺炎病史。
- 可能影响吞咽功能的合并症。
- 目前的用药情况。

临床口腔检查

临床检查可以为口腔结构的完整性和功能情况提供信息。对口面结构的感觉和运动功能的评估是发现可能影响吞咽功能的脑神经和肌肉异常的必要手段。

首先是评估静息状态下口面结构的解剖对称性和完整性。其次是评估嗅神经、三叉神经、面神经、舌咽神经、迷走神经和舌下神经的感觉与运动功能（图 4-6～图 4-8）。脑神经功能异常导致的异常运动，如松弛、痉挛、运动障碍、不自主收缩或震颤，均可能导致吞咽困难[17]。

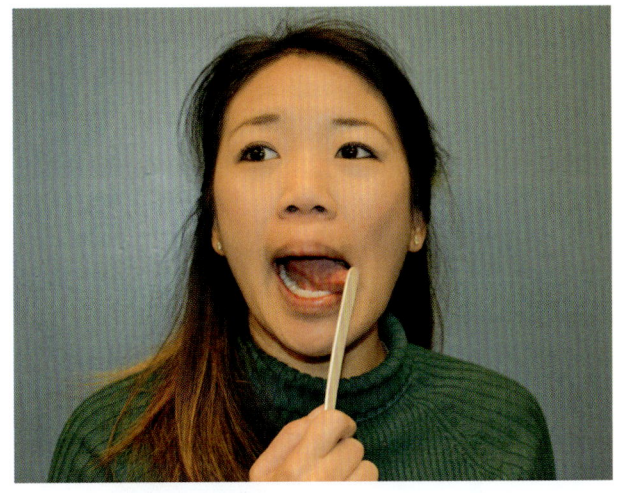

图 4-6　舌活动度

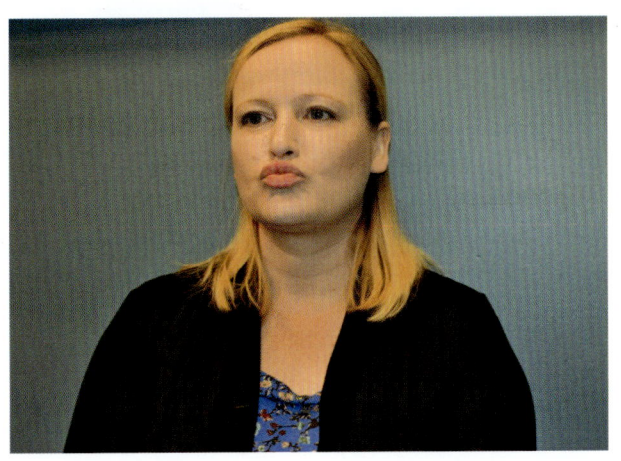

图 4-7　唇外凸时的唇活动度

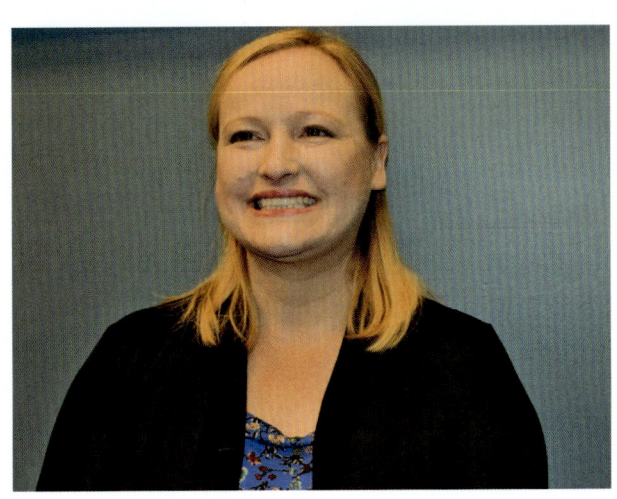

图 4-8　唇后缩时的唇活动度

仪器检查

仪器检查可以从结构和生理层面评估吞咽机制。电视透视吞咽功能检查（videofluoroscopic swallow study, VFSS）和纤维内镜吞咽功能检查（fiberoptic endoscopic evaluation of swallowing, FEES）是头颈癌中最常见的评估吞咽功能的仪器。

VFSS 将吞咽的口腔准备期、口腔期、咽腔期和食管上段期可视化。使用荧光透视技术可视化吞咽过程中的解剖结构和生理运动（图 4-9）。在做 VFSS 过程中，患者保持直立坐姿，服用一种不同浓度和剂量的不透射线的造影剂——钡剂，评估吞咽的安全性和有效性。通过侧位和前后位透视图评估口腔、咽、喉和食管上段的生物力学情况（图 4-10 和图 4-11）[18]。

VFSS 的分析包括口腔、喉、咽和食管上段的结构表现和生理功能的评估。虽然 VFSS 是一种常用的诊断方法，但在吞咽参数的分析中仍

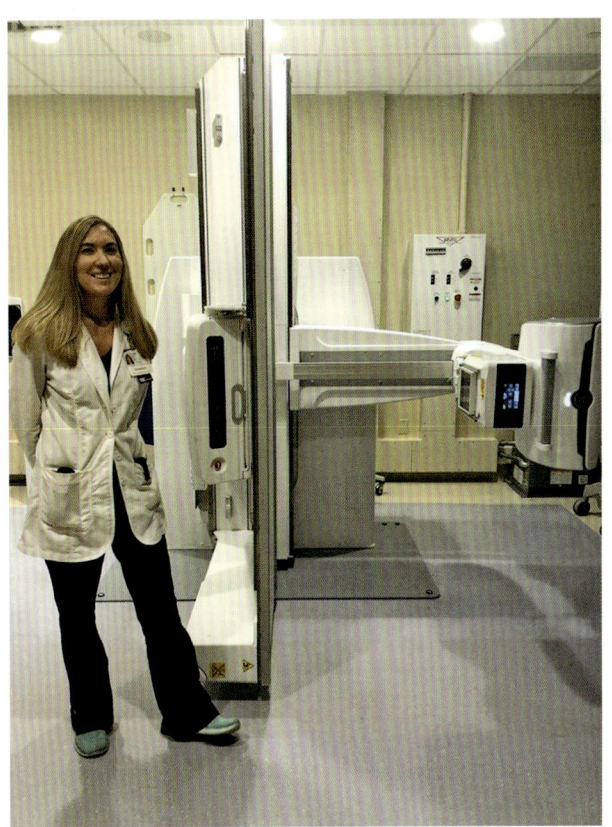

图 4-9　辐射防护室内的视频荧光透视检查仪

纤维内镜吞咽功能检查为我们提供喉和咽的直观图像。FEES 使用的内镜从鼻腔插入，经过腭帆进入咽腔（图 4-12）。软腭、舌根、口咽、喉和下咽的结构和运动被可视化展现。除了评估吞咽功能，纤维内镜还可以检查咽腔的分泌功能及病理状态[20]。对于头颈癌治疗后的患者，纤维内镜可以对术后和放疗后吞咽相关解剖结构的改变提供一个全方位的评估。在 FEES 检测过程中，为了提高内镜下的分辨率，不同浓度的食物和液体分别被染色成白色或蓝色。检查过程中可观察到喉的穿透、误吸，以及咽腔残留情况（图 4-13）。此外，FEES 还能可视化评估为提升吞咽安全性和效率的代偿性策略与动作的有效性[22]。

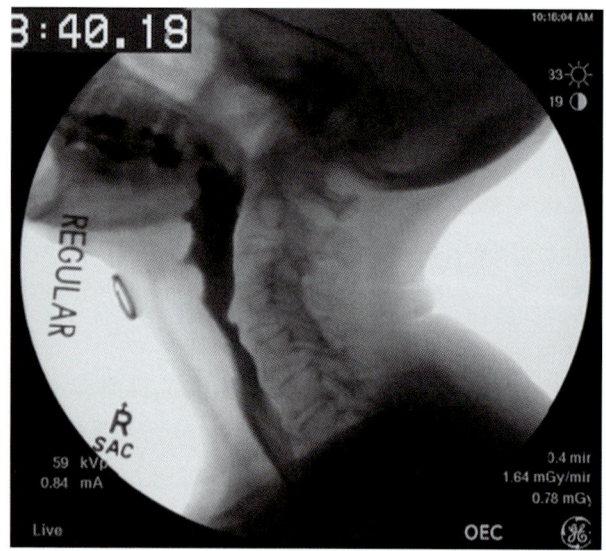

图 4-10　透视吞咽检查（侧方位）

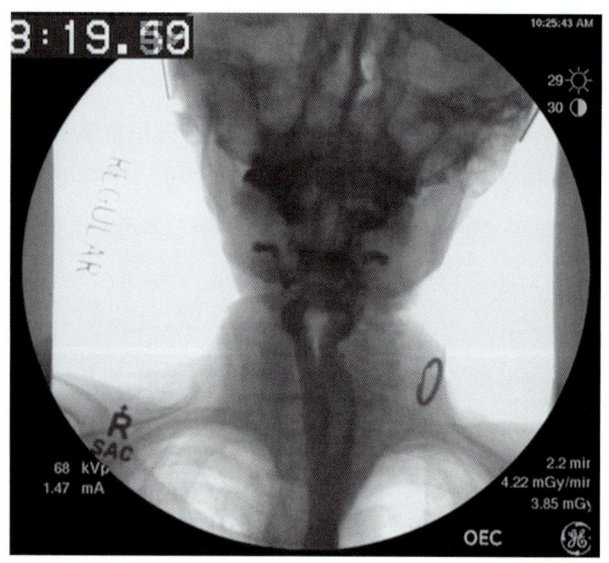

图 4-11　透视吞咽检查（前后位）

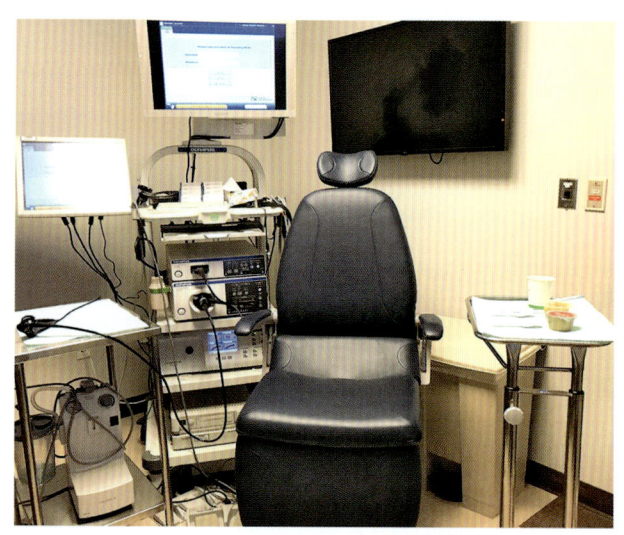

图 4-12　纤维内镜吞咽功能评估设备

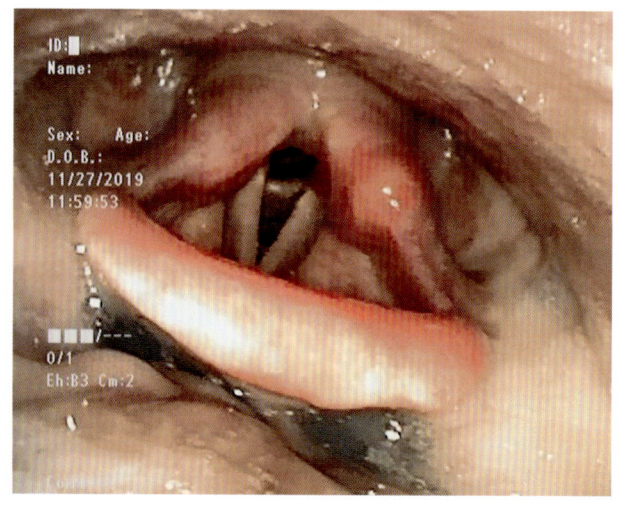

图 4-13　纤维内镜吞咽功能检查时咽腔残留物图像

然存在差异性。在过去的 20 年里，人们不断开发标准化和客观性的工具以提升 VFSS 分析结果。一个 8 分制的穿透-误吸量表可用于评估喉穿透或误吸的严重度以及患者对此类事件的反应[19]。为了量化咽部残留物，咽部滞留量表可记录吞咽后小窦和梨状窝中残留物的聚集容积[20]。随着科技进步，应用电脑分析技术可以更精细、更客观地评估吞咽的生物力学。客观的吞咽动力学评估指标能够量化评估吞咽动作的时机和结构位移。客观的评估指标降低了对生理性和病理性吞咽活动的主观解读成分[21]。

头颈癌患者吞咽困难的治疗

头颈癌治疗后吞咽困难的康复是多因素的。治疗可侧重于饮食调整,在吞咽过程中使用代偿性策略或动作,以及锻炼以改善吞咽功能。

调整饮食

为了改善吞咽的安全性和效率,患者在接受癌症治疗后有可能需要调整他们的食谱。根据吞咽困难的严重程度,患者的吞咽能力受到不同程度的损害,因此需要更改进食习惯和动作,或者更改摄取营养和水分的方式,以便预防营养不良和肺功能受损[23]。合理的食谱可以改善用餐时长、营养状况和生活质量[24]。食谱调整方案举例如下。

- 口腔咀嚼功能受损患者避免进食固体食物。
- 呼吸道保护功能受损的患者应食用黏稠的液态食物。
- 咽收缩功能受损的患者食用稀薄的液态食物。
- 更改摄取营养和水分的方式(例如,鼻胃营养管、经皮内镜下胃造口营养管)。

代偿性策略和动作

吞咽过程中使用代偿性策略或体位性动作可能会改善食团流动或气道保护。在头颈癌术后患者人群中,有81%的患者可以通过恰当的体位改变解决误吸的问题[25]。使用代偿性策略或体位性动作改善受损的生物动力性能必须首先经过透视镜(VFSS)或内镜(FEES)可视化评估其有效性。改善吞咽效率和安全性的代偿性策略、吞咽动作或体位改变如下。

■ 体位改变

- 收下巴体位(下巴压低体位或颈部弯曲,图4-14):当下巴向后移位时,舌根和会厌更靠近咽后壁,而咽腔的空间变得更宽敞。这个体位可以增加咽腔的容量,为吞咽这个动作争取更多

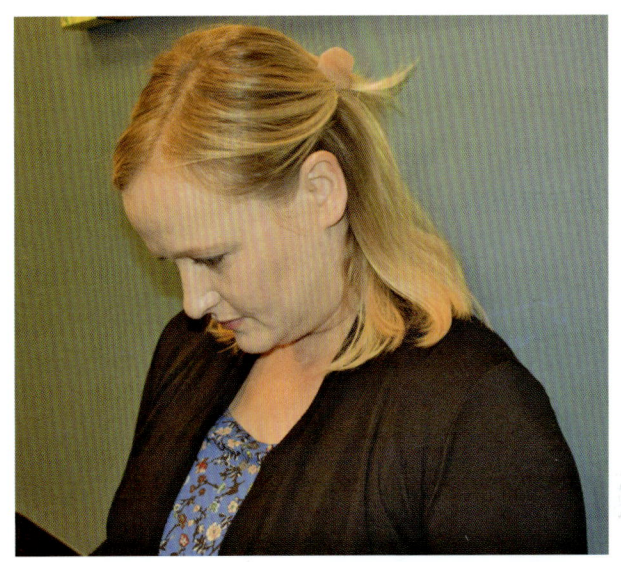

图4-14 收下巴体位

时间,也使得喉腔闭合更彻底和持久。

- 头侧方倾斜位(图4-15):头向功能好的一侧倾斜,将功能弱的一侧食物导向功能好的一侧,改善咽腔的清除能力。在单侧口腔或咽腔功能受损的情况下,利用重力的作用,改善吞咽能力。

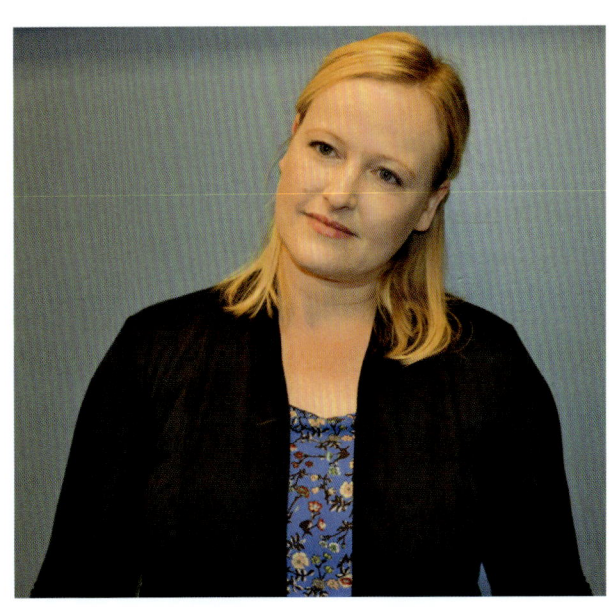

图4-15 头侧方倾斜位

• 头部旋转位（图4-16）：头部向咽和喉功能弱的一侧旋转，将食物导向对侧。食物一旦从功能弱的一侧导出，咽腔的清除能力就能得到改善。这个动作也适用于改善一侧声带麻痹导致的声门闭合不全。

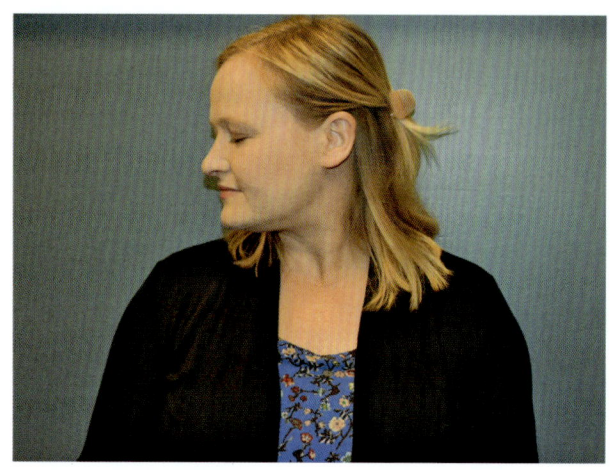

图4-16 头部旋转位

■ **代偿性策略**

• 用力吞咽：用力吞咽的动作旨在通过增强舌根收缩力和咽腔压力来改善咽和上段食管括约肌的食物清除能力。有吞咽后咽腔食物残留的患者被要求"用力"吞咽来改善食物清除能力。

• 声门上吞咽动作：声门上吞咽动作是为吞咽前或吞咽过程中出现误吸的患者设计的，旨在提升保护气道的自主能力。患者被要求首先屏气，然后继续屏气吞咽，最后吞咽后咳嗽，以便咳出可能进入喉腔的异物。

• 超声门上吞咽动作：与声门上吞咽动作相似，超声门上吞咽动作也是为了保护气道而设计的，它通过杓状软骨和会厌根部的活动关闭假声带，从而更进一步地保护气道。患者被要求屏气，向下用力，然后吞咽，最后吞咽后咳嗽以排出气道内异物。

• 门德尔松（Mendelsohn）动作：门德尔松动作旨在延长吞咽过程中喉部活动范围和上食管括约肌的开启时间。要求患者使用颈部肌肉将喉部保持在升高的位置。

吞咽练习

头颈癌治疗后因为吞咽相关肌肉的变化，如水肿、纤维化及萎缩，而出现吞咽困难。吞咽练习的目的是改善肌肉的运动和力量。负荷练习可以恢复吞咽相关肌肉的力量。预防性吞咽练习，即吞咽异常出现之前就开始进行吞咽练习，可以在放疗期间帮助维持口咽肌肉功能[26]。

■ **动作幅度和力量的练习**

• 下颌的被动和主动开合，改善门齿之间的开口度（图4-17和图4-18）。

• 舌头的伸缩和对抗阻力练习，增强舌头的

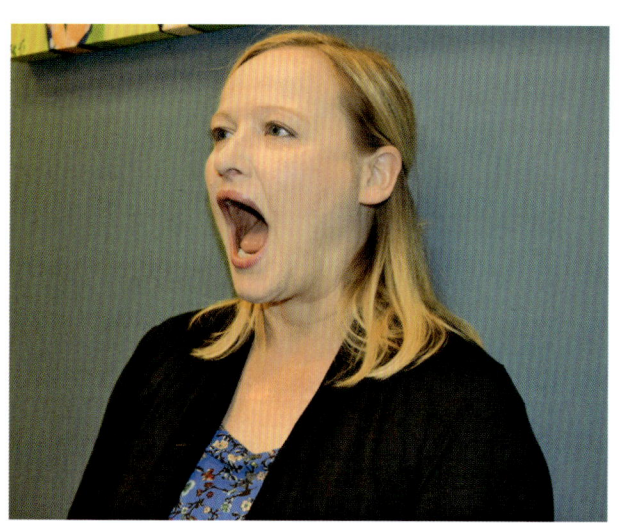

图4-17 下颌主动开合

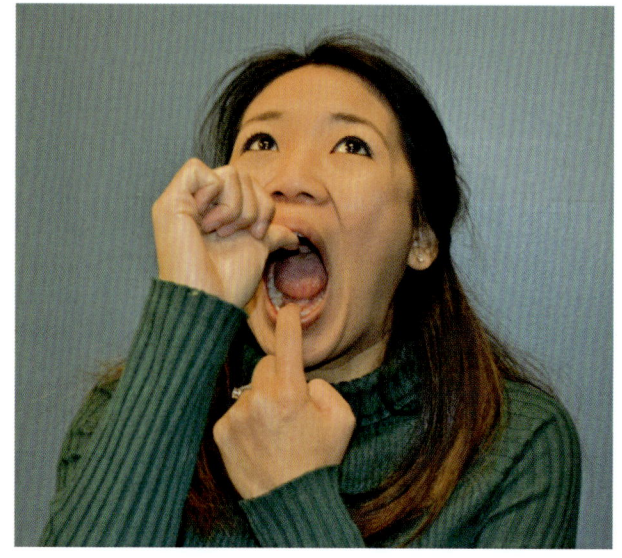

图4-18 下颌被动开合

活动性和力量。
- 用力吞咽，增强舌根和咽的收缩力度。
- 马萨科（Masako）动作，使得舌根更加靠近咽后壁。
- 摇动练习，使得上段食管括约肌打开更持久且幅度更大。
- 门德尔松（Mendelsohn）动作，可以改善咽腔的运动和上段食管括约肌的松弛。

多学科团队

头颈癌的治疗需要多个学科专家的长期跟踪随访。在多学科团队的支持下，接受头颈癌治疗的患者对其诊断、肿瘤治疗的早期和长期影响以及治疗的社会心理和情感表现有了更深入的了解。

多学科团队在治疗的早期就介入。从确诊时起患者就开始与头颈癌治疗团队的各个成员沟通，包括头颈肿瘤外科医生、肿瘤内科医生、放疗科医生、牙科医生、言语康复师、营养师和护理人员。头颈癌治疗开始前，这些成员参与治疗方案的计划、治疗相关并发症的风险评估和社会心理支持。在治疗过程中，多学科团队主要关注患者的当下状态、整个治疗过程中病情的发展以及是否需要调整治疗方案来缓解副反应。头颈癌治疗结束后，多学科团队继续参与疾病的随访、监测治疗相关副反应和改善生活质量的支持处理[27]。

在治疗吞咽困难方面，言语语言治疗师是头颈癌治疗团队不可或缺的一部分。在患者接受手术或药物治疗前，言语语言治疗师首先评估吞咽功能，分析是否存在吞咽困难的情况和治疗过程中出现吞咽功能下降的风险。在治疗前期，患者可以咨询言语语言治疗师癌症治疗可能导致的功能损伤。在癌症治疗的早期就可以开始预防性吞咽练习，使用代偿性策略和动作改善吞咽功能，以及改善饮食方案。在治疗的过程中，言语语言治疗师对吞咽功能进行持续性评估，改善饮食方案，指导代偿性策略。癌症治疗结束之后，言语语言治疗师评估急性期和远期的吞咽困难情况，并提供康复指导。

小 结

吞咽困难目前仍是头颈癌治疗后一个重要的并发症。吞咽功能受损可以发生在治疗后恢复期的早期和晚期。外科手术和内科治疗技术的不断进步使得我们对吞咽功能的保护得到不断的加强。言语语言治疗师是头颈癌治疗团队中不可或缺的部分，为吞咽困难的评估和诊断提供专业支持。通过全面的诊断和早期的干预，可以实现吞咽功能的保存、饮食的有限调整以及生活质量的维持。

参考文献

[1] Chaturvedi AK, Engels EA, Pfeiffer RM, Hernandez BY, Xiao W, Kim E, Biang B, Goodman MT, Sibug-Saber M, Cozen W, Liu L, Lynch CF, Wentzensen N, Jordan RC, Altekruse S, Anderson WF, Rosenberg RS, Gillison ML. Human papillomavirus and rising oropharyngeal cancer incidence in the United States. J Clin Oncol. 2011; 29(32): 4294–301.

[2] Aylward A, Abdelaziz S, Hunt JP, Buchmann LO, Cannon RB, Rowe K, Snyder J, Wan Y, Deshmukj V, Newman M, Fraser A, Smith K, Herget K, Lloyd S, Hitchcock Y, Hashibe M, Monroe MM. Rates of dysphagia related diagnoses in long-term survivors of head and neck cancers. Otolaryngol Head Neck Surg. 2019; 161(4): 643–51. https://doi.org/10.1177/0194599819850154.

[3] Iseli TA, Kulbersh BD, Iseli CE, Carroll WR, Rosenthal EL, Magnuson JS. Functional outcomes after transoral robotic surgery for head

and neck cancer. Otolaryngol Head Neck Surg. 2009; 141(2): 166−71.

[4] Hutcheson KA, Holsinger FC, Kupferman ME, Lewin JS. Functional outcomes after TORS for oropharyngeal cancer: a systematic review. Eur Arch Otorhinolaryngol. 2014; 272(2): 463−71.

[5] Park YM, Kim WS, Byeon HK, Lee SY, Kim SH. Oncological and functional outcomes of transoral robotic surgery for oropharyngeal cancer. Br J Oral Maxillofac Surg. 2013; 51(5): 408−12.

[6] Hirano M, Matsuoka H, Kuroiwa Y, Sato K, Tanaka S, Yoshida T. Dysphagia following various degrees of surgical resection for oral cancer. Ann Otol Rhinol Laryngol. 1992; 101(2): 138−41.

[7] Lewin JS, Hutcheson KA, Barringer DA, May AH, Roberts DB, Holsinger FC, Diaz EM Jr. Functional analysis of swallowing outcomes after supracricoid partial laryngectomy. Head Neck. 2008; 30(5): 559−66.

[8] Sullivan PA, Hartig GK. Dysphagia after total laryngectomy. Curr Opin Otolaryngol Head Neck Surg. 2001; 9(3): 139−46.

[9] Maclean J, Cotton S, Perry A. Dysphagia following a total laryngectomy: the effect on quality of life, functioning, and psychological well-being. Dysphagia. 2009; 24(3): 314−21.

[10] Kronenberger MB, Meyers AD. Dysphagia following head and neck cancer surgery. Dysphagia. 1994; 9(4): 236−44.

[11] Rancati T, Schwarz M, Allen AM, Feng F, Popovtzer A, Mittal B, Eisbruch A. Radiation dose−volume effects in the larynx and pharynx. Int J Radiat Oncol Biol Phys. 2010; 76(3): S64−9.

[12] Platteaux N, Dirix P, Dejaeger E, Nuyts S. Dysphagia in head and neck cancer patients treated with chemoradiotherapy. Dysphagia. 2010; 25(2): 139−52.

[13] Guchelaar HJ, Vermes A, Meerwaldt JH. Radiation-induced xerostomia: pathophysiology, clinical course and supportive treatment. Support Care Cancer. 1997; 5(4): 281−8.

[14] Maria OM, Eliopoulos N, Muanza T. Radiation-induced oral mucositis. Front Oncol. 2017; 7: 89.

[15] Deshpande TS, Blanchard P, Wang L, Foote RL, Zhang X, Frank SJ. Radiation-related alterations of taste function in patients with head and neck cancer: a systematic review. Curr Treat Options in Oncol. 2018; 19(12): 72.

[16] Murphy, B. A., & Gilbert, J. (2009). Dysphagia in head and neck cancer patients treated with radiation: assessment, sequelae, and rehabilitation. In Seminars in radiation oncology (19, 1, pp. 35−42). Philadelphia: WB Saunders.

[17] Sonies BC, Weiffenbach J, Atkinson JC, Brahim J, Macynski A, Fox PC. Clinical examination of motor and sensory functions of the adult oral cavity. Dysphagia. 1987; 1(4): 178−86.

[18] Palmer JB, Kuhlemeier KV, Tippett DC, Lynch C. A protocol for the videofluorographic swallowing study. Dysphagia. 1993; 8(3): 209−14.

[19] Rosenbek JC, Robbins JA, Roecker EB, Coyle JL, Wood JL. A penetration-aspiration scale. Dysphagia. 1996; 11(2): 93−8.

[20] Eisenhuber E, Schima W, Schober E, Pokieser P, Stadler A, Scharitzer M, Oschatz E. Videofluoroscopic assessment of patients with dysphagia: pharyngeal retention is a predictive factor for aspiration. Am J Roentgenol. 2002; 178(2): 393−8.

[21] Kendall KA, McKenzie S, Leonard RJ, Gonçalves MI, Walker A. Timing of events in normal swallowing: a videofluoroscopic study. Dysphagia. 2000; 15(2): 74−83.

[22] Langmore SE, Kenneth SM, Olsen N. Fiberoptic endoscopic examination of swallowing safety: a new procedure. Dysphagia. 1988; 2(4): 216−9.

[23] Wu CH, Ko JY, Hsiao TY, Hsu MM. Dysphagia after radiotherapy: endoscopic examination of swallowing in patients with nasopharyngeal carcinoma. Ann Otol Rhinol Laryngol. 2000; 109(3): 320−5.

[24] Garcia JM, Chambers E IV. Managing dysphagia through diet modifications. Am J Nurs. 2010; 110(11): 26−33.

[25] Logemann JA, et al. Effects of postural change on aspiration in head and neck surgical patients. Otolaryngol Head Neck Surg. 1994; 110(2): 222−7.

[26] Carnaby-Mann G, et al. "Pharyngocise": randomized controlled trial of preventative exercises to maintain muscle structure and swallowing function during head-and-neck chemoradiotherapy. Int J Radiat Oncol Biol Phys. 2012; 83(1): 210−9.

[27] Kelly SL, et al. Multidisciplinary clinic care improves adherence to best practice in head and neck cancer. Am J Otolaryngol. 2013; 34(1): 57−60.

第 5 章

Kelechi Nwachuku, Daniel E. Johnson, and Jennifer R. Grandis

头颈鳞癌的突变景观：通过分析循环肿瘤 DNA 进行检测和监测

The Mutational Landscape of Head and Neck Squamous Cell Carcinoma: Opportunities for Detection and Monitoring Via Analysis of Circulating Tumor DNA

引 言

头颈鳞状细胞癌（HNSCC）至少部分源于致癌信号通路中遗传变异的累积，导致细胞异常生长和存活[1-4]。过去十年中一系列的基因组研究成果为理解头颈鳞癌的突变景观提供了信息。阐明头颈鳞癌中的关键遗传变异，可能会指导针对性治疗的实施，从而改变这种致死性恶性肿瘤的预后。

尽管目前对头颈鳞癌的遗传基础有了更深的理解，但大多数头颈鳞癌病例仍然确诊时即为晚期，影响预后和生存[5]。传统筛查方法依赖于体格检查，这通常需要有经验的临床医生和专业设备。理解头颈鳞癌的突变谱系可能有助于非侵入性技术的应用，如评估血液和（或）唾液中的循环肿瘤 DNA（ctDNA）[5]。在头颈鳞癌患者中，血浆和唾液都含有可检测的包含肿瘤突变的循环 DNA 片段，这些片段在癌症的早期阶段就可以检测到，这或许可以应用于高危个体中早期检测头颈鳞癌[5]。此外，高敏感性和特异性的非侵入性方法也可能用于头颈鳞癌患者治疗后的监测[6]。本章我们将总结对当前头颈鳞癌突变谱系的研究成果，进而探究 ctDNA 作为早期检测和监测头颈鳞癌工具的潜力。

头颈鳞癌的突变谱系

大量的基因组测序研究已经深刻揭示头颈鳞癌的突变谱系[1,7-9]。这种突变要么赋予功能增益（驱动突变），或导致功能丧失，要么无明显的功能影响（沉默突变）。在本章中，我们仅限讨论已

K. Nwachuku
School of Medicine, University of California at San Francisco, San Francisco, CA, USA

D. E. Johnson · J. R. Grandis (✉)
Department of Otolaryngology – Head and Neck Surgery, University of California at San Francisco, San Francisco, CA, USA
e-mail: Jennifer.Grandis@ucsf.edu

知的会改变编码蛋白功能的基因突变。包括最常见的肿瘤抑制基因如 TP53、CDKN2A、NOTCH1 和 PTEN 的突变，以及 PIK3CA、CCND1、EGFR 和 HRAS 的致癌性改变（突变或扩增）（表 5-1）。

TP53 的缺失和（或）突变是头颈鳞癌中最常见的体细胞基因组改变，头颈鳞癌中的突变率为 72%[7]。与头颈鳞癌相关的 TP53 突变改变了 p53 的功能活性，包括感知和修复 DNA 损伤，以及在广泛 DNA 损伤响应中诱导凋亡。TP53 突变被认为在头颈鳞癌致癌的早期阶段发挥作用[10]。同样，肿瘤抑制基因 CDKN2A 的改变也与头颈鳞癌有关。CDKN2A 编码依赖于细胞周期的激酶抑制剂 p16/INK4A，其作用是阻止细胞周期从 G1 期进展到 S 期[11]。CDKN2A 可以通过多种机制在头颈鳞癌中下调或失活，包括启动子区域的低甲基化、基因缺失、拷贝数丢失和突变，其失活导致的细胞周期活性失调可促进肿瘤发生。CCND1（细胞周期编码蛋白 D1）的扩增导致该致癌基因的过度表达，并在许多头颈鳞癌患者中进一步增强 CDKN2A 功能丧失的影响[3]。另一个头颈鳞癌中常见的突变基因是抑制基因 NOTCH1，它在 15% 的肿瘤中发生突变[9, 12]，NOTCH1 蛋白是一种跨膜受体，可以在细胞生长和分化中发挥多种作用。

EGFR 基因已被认为是头颈鳞癌发展的原癌基因。EGFR 编码表皮生长因子受体，是 HER 家族受体酪氨酸激酶的细胞表面成员。通过配体结合激活后，EGFR 通过 PI3K/AKT、RAS/RAF/MEK/ERK 和 PLC/PKC 途径发出信号，以促进细胞增殖和存活，以及侵袭和转移[13]。EGFR 基因扩增常常导致其在绝大多数头颈鳞癌细胞和肿瘤中过度表达，现已证明是头颈鳞癌中致癌的关键驱动因素[13]。

头颈鳞癌中也常常存在 EGFR 下游编码细胞内信号蛋白的基因突变，特别是 PIK3CA 和 HRAS[9]。PIK3CA 编码磷脂酰肌醇-3 激酶（PI3K）的 p110α 催化亚基，在细胞增殖、迁移和存活调控中异常重要。现已发现 PIK3CA 在头颈鳞癌中既有突变也有扩增，会导致头颈鳞癌患者生存率下降[14, 15]。PI3K 信号通路受肿瘤抑制因子 PTEN 的负向调控，但很多 PTEN 的基因突变或表观遗传修饰均可能导致头颈鳞癌中 PTEN 功能或表达丧失[16]。此外，原癌基因 HRAS 的激活突变在头颈鳞癌中的发生率为 6%[7]。然而，在其他癌症中发生率很高的 KRAS 激活突变在头颈鳞癌中并未发现[7]。

一些研究较少的基因，包括 FBXW7、CASP8、FGF/FGFR、HLA-A/B、TGFBR2、FAT1、AJUBA、NSD1 和 KMT2D 等也被发现在头颈鳞癌中频繁突变（表 5-1）。FBXW7，或称 F-Box and WD Repeat Domain Containing 7，是一个肿瘤抑制基因，编码泛素蛋白连接酶复合体的一个组分[14]。有趣的是，含有 FBXW7 的复合体会靶向 NOTCH1 进行蛋白降解，而 FBXW7 的突变会终止这一过程。CASP8 编码外源性凋亡途径中的一个核心蛋白酶（caspase-8），在 9% 的头颈鳞癌中发生突变[7]，研究显示与头颈鳞癌相关的 CASP8 突变抑制死亡受体介导的凋亡，并促进 NF-κB 的激活，从而促进细胞侵袭、迁移和肿瘤生长[17, 18]。也有报道称 CASP8 突变可与 HRAS 突变在头颈鳞癌中并存[19]。成纤维细胞生长因子及其受体（FGF/FGFR）信号通路在调节细胞功能如迁移、分化、增殖和抑制凋亡中起着关键作用。FGFR1 基因突变被认为是低风险头颈鳞癌患者（低龄、HPV 阴性患者，不吸烟不饮酒）的可能驱动因素。值得注意的是，低风险头颈鳞癌患者与高风险患者存在不同的突变谱[20]。在免疫监视/识别途径中也发生了突变，特别是在 HLA-A/B 和转化生长因子 β 受体 2（TGFBR2）基因中，强调了免疫系统在头颈鳞癌致癌过程中的重要作用。涉及 WNT 信号通路的基因，特别是 FAT1 和 AJUBA，也与头颈鳞癌有关。FAT1（或称 FAT 非典型钙黏蛋白 1）是一个肿瘤抑制基因，在 29% 的头颈鳞癌中发生突变[7]。FAT1 蛋白通常作用是抑制与 WNT 信号相关的 β-连环蛋白的核转位。FAT1 的突变导致 WNT 信号过度活跃，并促进头颈鳞癌中的肿瘤形成。AJUBA 也可作为 WNT 信号的负向调控

表 5-1 头颈鳞癌中的突变基因

基 因	功 能	遗传突变的主要类型[a]	在头颈鳞癌中的遗传突变频率（%）[b]	突变的功能影响
在 HPV 阴性肿瘤中起主要作用的基因突变				
TP53（肿瘤蛋白 p53）	编码肿瘤抑制蛋白 p53	LOF, DEL	HPV+: 2% HPV−: 84%	丧失肿瘤抑制
CDKN2A（周期素依赖性激酶抑制剂 2A）	编码肿瘤抑制蛋白 p16（INK4A）和 p14（ARF）	LOF, DEL	HPV+: 0% HPV−: 57%	丧失肿瘤抑制
NOTCH1（Notch 同源物 1）	编码受体蛋白 Notch 1，参与 Notch 信号通路，已知在头颈鳞癌中作为肿瘤抑制因子	LOF	HPV+: 17% HPV−: 26%	丧失肿瘤抑制
PTEN（磷酸酶和张力蛋白同源物）	编码肿瘤抑制因子 PTEN	DEL, LOF	HPV+: 6% HPV−: 12%	丧失肿瘤抑制
CCND1（周期素 D1）	编码周期素 D1，与 CDK4 或 CDK6 形成复合物	AMP	HPV+: 3% HPV−: 31%	细胞周期调控失常，促进肿瘤形成
EGFR（表皮生长因子受体）	编码表皮生长因子受体，调节细胞增殖和存活	AMP	HPV+: 6% HPV−: 15%	促进肿瘤细胞增殖和存活
HRAS（HRas 原癌基因，GTP 酶）	编码 H-Ras，细胞分裂调节因子，指导生长和分裂	GOF	HPV+: 0% HPV−: 5%	无节制的细胞生长和分裂
FBXW7（含 F-Box 和 WD 重复域蛋白 7）	编码一个泛素蛋白连接酶复合物的组成部分	LOF	HPV+: 3% HPV−: 7%	蛋白酶体介导的蛋白降解调控失常，包括周期素 E
CASP8（胱天蛋白酶 8）	编码外在凋亡途径中的中心蛋白酶（胱天蛋白酶-8）	LOF	HPV+: 3% HPV−: 11%	丧失凋亡和肿瘤抑制
FGFR1（成纤维细胞生长因子受体 1）	编码成纤维细胞生长因子受体 1，调节细胞迁移、分化、增殖和存活	AMP	HPV+: 0% HPV−: 10%	促进肿瘤存活和生长
TGFBR2（转化生长因子 β 受体 2）	编码 TGF-β 受体类型 2	LOF	HPV+: 6% HPV−: 6%	促进肿瘤生长和增殖
FAT1（FAT 非典型钙黏蛋白 1）	编码肿瘤抑制蛋白 FAT 1	LOF, DEL	HPV+: 3% HPV−: 32%	丧失肿瘤抑制
AJUBA（Ajuba LIM 蛋白）	是 WNT 途径基因，调节有丝分裂、细胞间黏附和基因转录	LOF	HPV+: 0% HPV−: 7%	Wnt/β-catenin 信号和细胞分化调控失常
NSD1（核受体结合 SET 结构域蛋白 1）	编码组蛋白甲基转移酶	LOF	HPV+: 8% HPV−: 12%	改变染色质结构，导致基因表达模式变化
KMT2D（N-甲基转移酶 2D）	编码组蛋白甲基转移酶	LOF	HPV+: 17% HPV−: 18%	改变染色质结构，导致基因表达模式变化
FHIT（脆性组氨酸三联体二腺苷三磷酸酶）	编码 P1-P3-双（5′-腺苷）三磷酸水解酶，参与嘌呤代谢和肿瘤抑制	DEL	HPV+: 0% HPV−: 3%	丧失肿瘤抑制
CUL3（Cullin-3）	编码 Cullin-3，氧化应激途径蛋白	DEL	HPV+: 3% HPV−: 6%	氧化损伤

续表

基因	功能	遗传突变的主要类型[a]	在头颈鳞癌中的遗传突变频率（%）[b]	突变的功能影响
KEAP1（Kelch 样 ECH 相关蛋白 1）	编码 KEAP1，氧化应激途径蛋白	LOF	HPV+：0% HPV−：5%	氧化损伤
NFE2L2（核因子，红细胞 2 样 2）	编码 NRF2，氧化应激途径蛋白	AMP，GOF	HPV+：0% HPV−：14%	氧化损伤
在 HPV 阳性肿瘤中起主要作用的基因突变				
PIK3CA（磷脂酰肌醇 -4,5- 二磷酸 3 激酶催化亚单位 α）	编码 p110α 蛋白，PI3K 酶的催化亚单位，参与细胞增殖、迁移和存活	AMP，GOF	HPV+：56% HPV−：34%	促进肿瘤细胞增殖和存活
HPVE6/7（人乳头瘤病毒，E6 和 E7）	病毒致癌基因编码 E6 和 E7，分别失活 p53 和 pRb	病毒致癌基因	HPV+：100% HPV−：0%	丧失肿瘤抑制
RB1（RB 转录共抑制因子 1）	编码 RB 肿瘤抑制蛋白	LOF	HPV+：6% HPV−：4%	丧失肿瘤抑制
BRCA1/2（乳腺癌 1/2 型易感性蛋白）	编码肿瘤抑制蛋白	LOF	HPV+：3% HPV−：3%（BRCA1） HPV−：4%（BRCA2）	丧失肿瘤抑制
HLA-A/B（主要组织相容性复合体，I 类，A 和 B）	编码人类白细胞抗原（HLA）复合体，帮助身体区分自身抗原和外来抗原	LOF	HPV+：11% HPV−：7%	可能使免疫系统较难抵御癌症
ATM（ATM 丝氨酸/苏氨酸激酶）	编码 DNA 修复蛋白 ATM	DEL	HPV+：8% HPV−：5%	DNA 不稳定促进致癌
TP63（肿瘤蛋白 p63）	调节细胞增殖、分化、黏附和存活	AMP	HPV+：28% HPV−：19%	促进细胞侵袭和迁移
STAT1（信号转导及转录激活因子 1）	编码转录因子 STAT1，介导对 IFN 的免疫反应	AMP	HPV+：6% HPV−：5%	STAT1 介导的免疫反应可能丧失，促进致癌
SOX2（性别决定区 Y 盒 2）	编码在胚胎和神经干细胞中维持多能性的转录因子	AMP	HPV+：28% HPV−：21%	促进肿瘤生长和增殖
TRAF3（肿瘤坏死因子受体相关因子 3）	介导肿瘤坏死因子受体超家族的信号转导	LOF	HPV+：22% HPV−：1%	TRAF3 介导的免疫反应可能丧失，促进致癌
CYLD（CYLD 赖氨酸 63 去泛素化酶）	编码去泛素化酶，调节 NF-κB	LOF	HPV+：11% HPV−：3%	凋亡调控失常
DDX3X（DEAD 盒 螺旋酶 3，X 连锁）	编码 RNA 螺旋酶 DDX3X	DEL	HPV+：3% HPV−：5%	可能调控 DNA 翻译和细胞周期失常
E2F1（E2F 转录因子 1）	编码肿瘤抑制蛋白 E2F	AMP	HPV+：19% HPV−：2%	丧失肿瘤抑制
JAK2（Janus 激酶 2）	编码非受体型酪氨酸激酶 JAK2，介导细胞因子受体信号	AMP	HPV+：6% HPV−：7%	促进肿瘤细胞增殖和存活

注：[a] LOF，功能丧失；DEL，缺失；AMP，扩增；GOF，功能增益。
[b] 突变频率数据来源于 TCGA（The Cancer Genome Atlas）数据库分析结果。该研究对 279 例头颈鳞状细胞癌进行了基因组特征解析。

因子，与头颈鳞癌相关的 AJUBA 突变可能会上调致癌 WNT 信号通路[21]。头颈鳞癌中其他常见的突变基因包括核受体结合 SET 结构域蛋白（NSD1）和 N-甲基转移酶 2D（KMT2D），它们编码组蛋白甲基转移酶。这些基因的突变导致染色质结构的改变，进而改变基因表达模式，促进肿瘤形成[22]。

HPV 阳性与 HPV 阴性头颈鳞癌的突变谱比较

在美国和全球诊断的大多数头颈鳞癌病例都是烟草相关的 HPV 阴性（HPV−）肿瘤。然而，由 HPV 驱动的（HPV+）头颈鳞癌（特别是口咽部）的发病率正在上升，全球每年新诊断的 HPV+ 头颈鳞癌病例数量不断增加[23]。HPV+ 头颈鳞癌通常对化疗和放疗有更好的反应，总体预后也更好。值得注意的是，HPV+ 和 HPV−头颈鳞癌的突变谱上具有显著差异，这为理解 HPV+ 肿瘤治疗反应和预后更好提供了重要线索。在 HPV−头颈鳞癌中，TP53 的遗传改变发生率为 84%，但在 HPV+ 头颈鳞癌中却很少[7]。相反，HPV+ 头颈鳞癌中 p53 表达的丧失是由 HPV E6 致癌蛋白驱动的，该蛋白促进 p53 蛋白的蛋白酶体降解。同样，HPV E7 蛋白促进视网膜母细胞瘤（RB）蛋白的蛋白酶体降解。值得注意的是，尽管 HPV−头颈鳞癌的突变特征以嘌呤（A-G）和嘧啶（C-T）的核苷酸转换为特征，但 HPV+ 头颈鳞癌在 TpC 位点上以胞嘧啶到胸腺嘧啶（C>T）突变为主[7, 24, 25]。这是因为病毒诱导载脂蛋白 B mRNA 编辑酶，类似催化多肽（APOBEC）家族酶的增加，导致胞嘧啶脱氨酶介导的突变增加[25]。此外，APOBEC 被认为在 PIK3CA 中产生致癌的 E542K（c.1624G > A）和 E545K（c.1633G > A）典型突变，这一点值得注意，因为 PIK3CA 突变似乎在 HPV+ 头颈鳞癌中更常见[26]。尽管 HPV+ 和 HPV−头颈鳞癌都由 p53 表达（通过 E6 或遗传性缺失）或功能（通过突变）的丧失以及 RB 表达（通过 E7）或功能（通过 CDKN2A 改变）的丧失驱动，但作用的机制完全不同[23]。

HPV+ 头颈鳞癌肿瘤还被发现 DNA 修复途径相关的基因（BRCA1/2、ATM 和 Fanconi 贫血基因），JAK/STAT 信号（Janus 激酶 1/2 和 STAT1）；FGF 信号（FGFR2、FGFR3 和 FGFR4），以及 PIK3CA、KRAS、E2F1、HLA-A/B、KMT2C、TRAF3、CYLD 和 DDX3X（表 5-1）[27-29]的富集改变。在 22% 的 HPV+ 肿瘤中发现 TRAF3 的缺失或截断突变，在 11% 中发现 CYLD 的截断或错义突变。这些基因的突变导致 NF-κB 信号通路的组成性激活[30]。研究表明，目前在美国诊断的所有口咽鳞状细胞癌中，超过一半是 HPV+，与 HPV−口咽肿瘤相比，其表观遗传修饰不同，包括病毒和宿主的甲基化和染色质修饰[31]。在 HPV+ 头颈鳞癌中 DNA 损伤反应途径的突变增加可能是 HPV+ 病例的化疗和放射敏感性增加及总体生存率提高的原因。

尽管曾有小规模研究表明，HPV+ 与 HPV− 肿瘤相比，其总体突变负荷较低，但实际上却是相当的（在癌症相关基因中，14.4 体细胞外显子突变与 15.2 相当），这一点也可以通过 TCGA 数据分析证实[27, 32]。除了 TP53 的改变差异外，HPV−肿瘤表现出更高比例的氧化应激途径基因（KEAP1-CUL3-NFE2L2）的改变、CDKN2A 的失活、CCND1 基因的扩增、编码 RTKs 的基因以及 TERT 启动子[2, 8, 10, 33]。HPV−肿瘤也有大量的 EGFR 扩增位点，这在 HPV+ 肿瘤中未发现[2, 7, 27]。值得注意的是，FAT1 的功能缺失突变在 HPV+ 头颈鳞癌中不常见，但在 HPV−头颈鳞癌中普遍存在，分别为 3% 和 32%[7, 34]。

与早期头颈鳞癌相关的突变

头颈鳞癌的发生是通过一系列组织病理学和临床阶段发展而来的，每个阶段都伴随着特定的遗传学改变（图 5-1）[35]。这种进展从良性增生开始，到异常增生，进而原位癌（CIS），最后是侵袭性肿瘤，即头颈鳞癌。当按 HPV 状态分层时，早期头颈鳞癌的遗传学改变与晚期肿瘤是不同的。HPV 相关肿瘤的最早阶段是由 HPV 感染

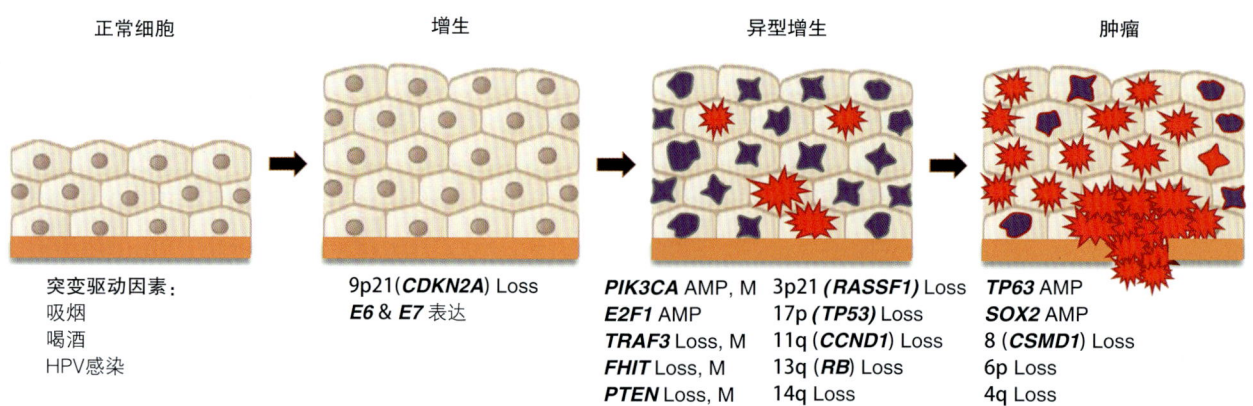

图 5-1 向侵袭性头颈鳞癌进展的各阶段相关的遗传改变。旁边列出的位点包含括号中的基因。未指定基因的位点是定义不明确的微卫星区域。AMP，扩增；M，突变；Loss，由缺失和（或）表观遗传变化导致的遗传丢失

隐窝上皮导致病毒癌基因 E6 和 E7 的表达[24]。这些癌基因通过失活 p53 和 RB 来破坏被感染细胞的细胞周期调控，启动 HPV 诱导的致癌过程[36,37]。介导 HPV+ 头颈鳞癌的确切驱动突变在很大程度上仍然未知[38]。实际上，在扁桃体中很少发现异型增生病变，而 HPV 驱动的头颈鳞癌最常在这里发展[38]。通过 PIK3CA 癌基因的突变和（或）扩增激活 PI3K 途径在 HPV+ 头颈鳞癌中相对常见，发生在 50%～60% 的肿瘤中[38]。HPV 感染后，基底层细胞的异常分化和 E2F 转录因子 1（E2F1）的上调随之而来，这通常与异型增生一起发生[24]。CIS 随后发生，与 TRAF3、脆弱组氨酸三联体基因（FHIT）和 PTEN 的失活突变或缺失相关[24,36]。最后，异常细胞通过基底膜侵袭（癌变转化），这通常伴随着 TP63、SOX2 和 PIK3CA 的增加[24,36,39]。

烟草和酒精可导致 DNA 损伤和基因组改变，促进 HPV-肿瘤的发展（图 5-1）。发展为头颈鳞癌的第一个阶段是增生，这通常伴随着 9p21 染色体的丢失——CDKN2A 的位置[24,35]。增生发展为异型增生，这通常与 3p21 和 17p 染色体的丢失相关——分别是肿瘤抑制基因 Ras 关联结构域家族成员 1（RASSF1）和 TP53 的位置[35,36]。异型增生随后发展为原位癌，这与 11q 染色体（包含 CCND1）、13q 染色体（靠近 Rb 位点）、14q（复制数目不明确的微卫星序列）的丢失相关。原位癌在侵袭通过基底膜后转变为头颈鳞癌，这与 8 号、6p 和 4q 染色体的丢失相关[35]。8 号染色体包含肿瘤抑制基因 CUB 和 CSMD1，而 6p 和 4q 染色体由定义不明确的微卫星区域组成，包括 TCTE、D6S265、D6S105（6p 染色体）、D8S262、D8S261、D8S273、D8S167 和 D8S257（8 号染色体），这些区域在侵袭性肿瘤中丢失的比率很高（大约 40%）[35,36]。在肿瘤形成过程中丢失比率很高的其他微卫星区域还包括 D3S1007、D3S1284、D3S1038、D3S1067（3p 染色体）、FABP2、D4S1613（4 号染色体）、D9S736、IFN-α、D9S171（9p21 染色体）、JNT-2、D11S873、PYGM（11q13 染色体）、D13S133、D13S170（13q21 染色体）、D14S51、D14S81（14q 染色体）、TP53 和 CHRNB-1（17p13 染色体）[35,36]。Sidransky 等人在头颈鳞癌患者的唾液 DNA 检测中测试了这 23 个微卫星标志物的集合，并将它们与健康对照组进行比较，发现 86% 的头颈鳞癌组（在肿瘤中发现微卫星改变的子集中有 96%）检测到微卫星改变，而健康对照组没有检测到微卫星改变[40]。进一步确立了这些微卫星标志物与头颈鳞癌之间的关联，类似于循环肿瘤 DNA（ctDNA），提示了检测和监测头颈鳞癌的方法。许多研究也开始关注并探究微小 RNA（miRNA）在头颈鳞癌中的作用[36,41]。

头颈鳞癌相关突变在引起肿瘤形成中的作用仍然在很大程度上未知，对这点的深层理解受到癌前病变进展到癌症的测序研究缺乏的阻碍。

TP53 是目前被认为是致病突变的最有力证据，因为它被发现在肿瘤邻近黏膜上皮和异型增生组织中的小 p53 免疫阳性灶中发生突变，导致了头颈鳞癌的点—面—肿瘤—转移进展模型。这个模型表明，口腔黏膜前体细胞中的 TP53 突变是随后致癌变化的预兆[36,38,42]。这一假设得到了在工程化小鼠模型中获得的数据支持[38,43]。研究还表明，口腔异型增生上皮病变有很高的恶性进展风险[44]。

头颈鳞癌中的循环肿瘤 DNA（ctDNA）

尽管治疗干预取得了进展，但过去几十年头颈鳞癌的预后仍然没有改善，5 年生存率约为 50%[5]。延迟诊断是这一困境的原因之一，它与更高风险（30%）的晚期肿瘤和较差预后相关[45]。通过非侵入性检测新生物标志物来监测高危个体和（或）可疑病变，有可能减少这种诊断延迟。

细胞游离 DNA（cfDNA）是从小死亡细胞脱落的核酸小片段，存在于体液中。在癌症患者中，一部分 cfDNA 变成了循环肿瘤 DNA（ctDNA），它携带肿瘤特异性的遗传和表观遗传改变，包括突变和甲基化模式，均可作为头颈鳞癌诊断的生物标志物[41]。

肿瘤检测

在头颈鳞癌患者中，肿瘤 DNA 不仅在血液中可存在，而且由于与口腔和咽部肿瘤紧邻的原因，在唾液中也可以被检测到（图 5-2）[4]。头颈鳞癌患者中 ctDNA 的存在使得这种 DNA 的分析成为一个特别有吸引力的诊断测试。此外，获取 ctDNA 相对非侵入性[46]。循环 DNA 也可以在早期疾病中检测到，并已显示出检测微小残留疾病（许多基于影像学方法的局限性，如 MRI、超声、CT 等）的潜力[46-48]。此外，尽管存在肿瘤异质性，但是对 ctDNA 的分析仍有潜力能跟踪肿瘤的动态变化，这克服了当前检测方法的另一个主要限制，特别是那些依赖于组织活检的方法[49]。研究还发现 ctDNA 水平与肿瘤的大小和阶段相关，进一步证明了它作为癌症检测和监测方式的潜力[50-55]。

由于体液中目标核酸水平可能非常低（例如，

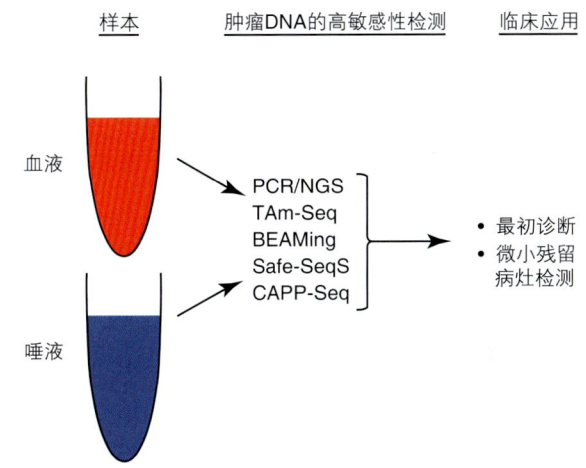

图 5-2 对血液或唾液进行分析以进行诊断或检测微小残留病变

每毫升仅 1 个突变 DNA 片段），因此需要高度敏感的技术来分析 ctDNA 中的突变[41,51]。这些技术包括"标记-扩增子深度测序"（TAm-Seq）、"珠子、乳液、扩增和磁性"（BEAMing）、"安全测序系统"（Safe-SeqS）、"癌症个性化深度测序分析"（CAPP-Seq）以及与全外显子组测序（WES）或下一代测序（NGS）相结合的 PCR 扩增（图 5-2）[41,56]。

几项研究已经应用这些方法研究了 ctDNA 在头颈鳞癌检测中的实用性[4]。Agrawal 等对 93 名头颈鳞癌患者的唾液和（或）血浆中的 DNA 进行了检测，并在 30 名患者（32%）中识别出 E7 基因[4]。在其余 63 名患者（HPV-个体）中，评估了在头颈鳞癌中常见的基因和基因区域的体细胞突变，包括 PIK3CA、FBXW7、TP53、HRAS、CDKN2A 和 NRAS。在这项研究中，通过多重 PCR 和大规模测序，63 个样本中的 58 个样本鉴定出了驱动突变。剩余的 5 个样本使用全基因组测序来检测驱动突变。总体上，最常突变的基因是 TP53，这一发现得到了其他研究的证实（63名 HPV-患者中有 86%）[5]。在 25 个 HPV+ 患者样本中，也有 12 个样本被鉴定出突变。在同一研究中，当对 47 名患者的唾液和血浆同时进行测试时，ctDNA 的检出率为 96%。当按肿瘤部位分开分析时，分别在下咽、喉、口咽和口腔肿瘤中 ctDNA 的检出率分别为 100%（$n=3$）、100%（$n=7$）、91%（$n=22$）和 100%（$n=15$）。在比较唾液和血浆检测时，Agrawal 等人表明，唾液在口腔癌中优先富集 ctDNA，100% 的口腔癌在唾液中被检测到，而其他上呼吸道肿瘤患者的唾液中检出率为 47%～70%[5]。唾液还被证明可以确定原发肿瘤的 HPV 状态，敏感度和特异度分别为 92.9% 和 100%[57]。血浆在确定肿瘤 HPV 状态方面也有类似的敏感度（96%），并且在除口腔外的肿瘤患者中富集 ctDNA，血浆样本中的检出率为 86%～100%，而口腔癌患者的血浆中检出率为 80%。此外，血浆中 ctDNA 的检测对晚期疾病更敏感，而唾液中的检测对早期癌症更敏感。值得注意的是，在晚期头颈鳞癌患者中，ctDNA 水平本身预示着生存率降低。

这些研究，以及大型头颈鳞癌基因研究[7,9,12]表明，包括 PIK3CA、NOTCH1、TP53、CDKN2A 和 HPV16 DNA 序列的小组能够检测到超过 95% 的侵袭性头颈鳞癌[4]。需要在高危队列中进行进一步研究，以确定这种方法能够在症状和体检发现以前检测到癌症。

肿瘤监测

ctDNA 分析不仅可以用于早期肿瘤检测，还可以用于早期复发识别和治疗反应监测[4,41]。越来越多的研究正在确定 ctDNA 在这一领域的应用[41]。一项研究调查了肿瘤切除术后患者血浆或唾液中的肿瘤 DNA 存在情况[4]。在纳入研究的 9 名患者中，有 3 名患者在复发前被发现存在肿瘤 DNA。相比之下，在持续显示无复发证据的 5 名患者中，中位随访 12 个月期间未检测到肿瘤 DNA[4]。这表明 ctDNA 可能作为复发的早期识别器，从而可以更早地启动治疗。

在通过评估 ctDNA 监测治疗反应方面，Binder 等人研究了通过分析头颈鳞癌患者血浆中的突变 EGFR 和 RAS 来研究西妥昔单抗耐药的治疗分子机制[58]。他们发现，在疾病进展的患者中，有相当一部分（46%）发展出 KRAS、HRAS 或 NRAS 突变，而在非进展的患者亚组中未检测到 RAS 突变。这种相关性是显著的——RAS 突变克隆与临床耐药（卡方检验 $P=0.032$），表明 RAS 突变在很大程度上解释了头颈鳞癌患者对 EGFR 靶向治疗的获得性耐药，尽管在未接受过西妥昔单抗治疗的原发性肿瘤中，RAS 突变相对罕见。这项研究表明 ctDNA 检测可以作为监测治疗反应并指导治疗决策的有效手段，有优化患者治疗策略的潜力。目前关于 ctDNA 在头颈鳞癌肿瘤监测中的应用研究较少，但随着对该方法的重要性和前景的认识加深，研究数量正在增加。

小结和未来方向

头颈鳞癌的突变谱是一个不断扩展的知识体系，具有指导疾病的检测和管理的潜力。大约 2/3 的头颈癌在晚期识别，头颈鳞癌的预后和生存率仍然较差。需要新的方法来早期检测头颈鳞癌以改善结果。循环 DNA 已经在多个头颈鳞癌队列中显示出作为非侵入性获得的生物标志物的巨大潜力。利用头颈鳞癌的突变特征在体液中识别肿瘤 DNA 已经展示了在早期阶段检测肿瘤和监测肿瘤复发及治疗反应的潜力。

尽管在理解头颈鳞癌特征性突变方面取得了巨大进展，但由于缺乏对癌前病变的突变分析研究，特别是 HPV+ 头颈鳞癌，对明确的驱动突变的识别受到限制。此外，头颈鳞癌起源于上呼吸消化道不同的解剖部位（下咽、喉、口咽、口腔），可能具有不同的分子特征，头颈鳞癌的整体突变谱可能无法揭示导致不同解剖部位肿瘤形成和进展的关键突变。此外，TCGA 队列中的大多数样本以及许多其他测序研究中的样本大都来自口腔，而咽部和喉部肿瘤在基因组上的描述较少[24]。迄今为止，ctDNA 作为头颈鳞癌管理中的生物标志物的研究也主要限于口腔癌，并且包含的病例数量相对较少。需要在更大的头颈鳞癌队列中进一步研究 ctDNA，以完全确定这种方法对于早期检测原发性和复发性疾病的价值。

致谢：本工作得到了美国国立卫生研究院资助项目 R01 DE024728（D.E.J.）、R01 DE023685 和 R35 CA231998（J.R.G.），以及美国癌症协会的支持。

参 考 文 献

[1] Li H, et al. Genomic analysis of head and neck squamous cell carcinoma cell lines and human tumors: a rational approach to preclinical model selection. Mol Cancer Res. 2014; https: //doi. org/10.1158/1541-7786. MCR-13-0396.
[2] Van Waes C, Musbahi O. Genomics and advances towards precision medicine for head and neck squamous cell carcinoma. Laryngoscope Investig Otolaryngol. 2017; 2: 310–9.
[3] Hoesli RC, et al. Genomic sequencing and precision medicine in head and neck cancers. Eur J Surg Oncol. 2017; https://doi.org/10.1016/j.ejso.2016.12.002.
[4] Papadopoulos N, et al. Detection of somatic mutations and HPV in the saliva and plasma of patients with head and neck squamous cell carcinomas. Sci Transl Med. 2015; 7: 293ra104–293ra104.
[5] Perdomo S, et al. Circulating tumor DNA detection in head and neck cancer: evaluation of two different detection approaches. Oncotarget. 2017; 8: 72621–32.
[6] van Ginkel JH, Huibers MMH, van Es RJJ, de Bree R, Willems SM. Droplet digital PCR for detection and quantification of circulating tumor DNA in plasma of head and neck cancer patients. BMC Cancer. 2017; 17: 1–8.
[7] Lawrence MS, et al. Comprehensive genomic characterization of head and neck squamous cell carcinomas. Nature. 2015; 517: 576–82.
[8] Gaykalova DA, et al. Novel insight into mutational landscape of head and neck squamous cell carcinoma. PLoS One. 2014; https://doi.org/10.1371/journal.pone.0093102.
[9] Stransky N, et al. The mutational landscape of head and neck squamous cell carcinoma. Science (80-). 2011; 333: 1157–60.
[10] Morris LGT, et al. The molecular landscape of recurrent and metastatic head and neck cancers. JAMA Oncol. 2016; 3: 244.
[11] Padhi S, et al. Role of CDKN2A/p16 expression in the prognostication of oral squamous cell carcinoma. Oral Oncol. 2017; 73: 27.
[12] Agrawal N, et al. Exome sequencing of head and neck squamous cell carcinoma reveals inactivating mutations in NOTCH1. Science (80-). 2011; https://doi.org/10.1126/science.1206923.
[13] Brand TM, Iida M, Wheeler D, L. Molecular mechanisms of resistance to the EGFR monoclonal antibody cetuximab. Cancer Biol Ther. 2011; https://doi.org/10.4161/cbt.11.9.15050.
[14] Kommineni N, Jamil K, Pingali U, Addala L, Mur N. Association of PIK3CA gene mutations with head and neck squamous cell carcinomas. Neoplasma. 2015; 62: 72.
[15] Hedberg ML, et al. Use of nonsteroidal anti-inflammatory drugs predicts improved patient survival for *PIK3CA*-altered head and neck cancer. J Exp Med. 2019; 216: 419 LP–427.
[16] Shao X, et al. Mutational analysis of the PTEN gene in head and neck squamous cell carcinoma. Int J Cancer. 1998; https://doi.org/10.1002/(SICI)1097-0215(19980831)77: 5 < 684: : AID-IJC4 > 3.0.CO; 2-R.
[17] Li C, Egloff AM, Sen M, Grandis JR, Johnson DE. Caspase-8 mutations in head and neck cancer confer resistance to death receptor-mediated apoptosis and enhance migration, invasion, and tumor growth. Mol Oncol. 2014; https://doi.org/10.1016/j.molonc.2014.03.018.
[18] Ando M, et al. Cancer-associated missense mutations of caspase-8 activate nuclear factor-κB signaling. Cancer Sci. 2013; https://doi.org/10.1111/cas.12191.
[19] Pickering CR, et al. Integrative genomic characterization of oral squamous cell carcinoma identifies frequent somatic drivers. Cancer Discov. 2013; https://doi.org/10.1158/2159-8290. CD-12-0537.
[20] Tillman BN, et al. Fibroblast growth factor family aberrations as a putative driver of head and neck squamous cell carcinoma in an epidemiologically low-risk patient as defined by targeted sequencing. Head Neck. 2016; https://doi.org/10.1002/hed.24292.
[21] Haraguchi K, et al. Ajuba negatively regulates the Wnt signaling pathway by promoting GSK-3β-mediated phosphorylation of β-catenin. Oncogene. 2007; 27: 274.
[22] Abba MC, et al. The head and neck cancer cell oncogenome: a platform for the development of precision molecular therapies. Oncotarget. 2015; https://doi.org/10.18632/oncotarget.2417.
[23] Dok R, Nuyts S. HPV positive head and neck cancers: molecular pathogenesis and evolving treatment strategies. Cancers. 2016; https: //

doi.org/10.3390/cancers8040041.

[24] Faraji, F. et al. The genome-wide molecular landscape of HPV-driven and HPV-negative head and neck squamous cell carcinoma293–325 (2018). doi: https: //doi. org/10.1007/978-3-319-78762-6_11.

[25] Hayes DN, Van Waes C, Seiwert TY. Genetic landscape of human papillomavirus-associated head and neck cancer and comparison to tobacco-related tumors. J Clin Oncol. 2015; https: //doi.org/10.1200/JCO.2015.62.1086.

[26] Henderson S, Chakravarthy A, Su X, Boshoff C, Fenton TR. APOBEC-mediated cytosine deamination links PIK3CA helical domain mutations to human papillomavirus-driven tumor development. Cell Rep. 2014; https: //doi.org/10.1016/j.celrep.2014.05.012.

[27] Seiwert TY, et al. Integrative and comparative genomic analysis of HPV-positive and HPV-negative head and neck squamous cell carcinomas. Clin Cancer Res. 2015; https: //doi. org/10.1158/1078-0432. CCR-13-3310.

[28] Shih JW, Tsai TY, Chao CH, Wu Lee YH. Candidate tumor suppressor DDX3 RNA helicase specifically represses cap-dependent translation by acting as an eIF4E inhibitory protein. Oncogene. 2008; https: //doi.org/10.1038/sj.onc.1210687.

[29] Zhang J, et al. Attenuated TRAF3 fosters activation of alternative NF-κB and reduced expression of antiviral interferon, TP53, and RB to promote HPV-positive head and neck cancers. Cancer Res. 2018; https: //doi.org/10.1158/0008-5472. CAN-17-0642.

[30] Hajek M, et al. TRAF3/CYLD mutations identify a distinct subset of human papillomavirus-associated head and neck squamous cell carcinoma. Cancer. 2017; https: //doi.org/10.1002/cncr.30570.

[31] Harbison RA, et al. The mutational landscape of recurrent versus nonrecurrent human papillomavirus–related oropharyngeal cancer. JCI Insight. 2018; https: //doi.org/10.1172/jci. insight.99327.

[32] Hayes DN, Grandis JR, El-Naggar AK. The Cancer Genome Atlas: integrated analysis of genome alterations in squamous cell carcinoma of the head and neck. J Clin Oncol. 2013; 31: 6009.

[33] Cho J, Johnson DE, Grandis JR. Therapeutic implications of the genetic landscape of head and neck cancer. Semin Radiat Oncol. 2018; https: //doi.org/10.1016/j.semradonc.2017.08.005.

[34] Kim KT, Kim BS, Kim JH. Association between FAT1 mutation and overall survival in patients with human papillomavirus-negative head and neck squamous cell carcinoma. Head Neck. 2016; https: //doi.org/10.1002/hed.24372.

[35] Califano J, et al. Genetic progression model for head and neck cancer: implications for field cancerization. Cancer Res. 1996; 56: 2488.

[36] Leemans CR, Braakhuis BJM, Brakenhoff RH. The molecular biology of head and neck cancer. Nat Rev Cancer. 2011; https: //doi.org/10.1038/nrc2982.

[37] Zur Hausen H. Papillomaviruses and cancer: from basic studies to clinical. Papillomaviruses and cancer: from basic studies to clinical application. Nat Rev Cancer. 2002; 2(5): 342–50. https: //doi.org/10.1038/nrc798.

[38] Leemans CR, Snijders PJF, Brakenhoff RH. The molecular landscape of head and neck cancer. Nat Rev Cancer. 2018; https: //doi.org/10.1038/nrc.2018.11.

[39] Nekulova M, Holcakova J, Coates P, Vojtesek B. The role of P63 in cancer, stem cells and cancer stem cells. Cell Mol Biol Lett. 2011; https: //doi.org/10.2478/s11658-011-0009-9.

[40] Spafford MF, et al. Detection of head and neck squamous cell carcinoma among exfoliated oral mucosal cells by microsatellite analysis. Clin Cancer Res. 2001; 7: 607–12.

[41] van Ginkel JH, Slieker FJB, de Bree R, van Es RJJ, Willems SM. Cell-free nucleic acids in body fluids as biomarkers for the prediction and early detection of recurrent head and neck cancer: a systematic review of the literature. Oral Oncol. 2017; 75: 8–15.

[42] Wood HM, et al. The genomic road to invasion-examining the similarities and differences in the genomes of associated oral pre-cancer and cancer samples. Genome Med. 2017; https: //doi.org/10.1186/s13073-017-0442-0.

[43] Lim X, et al. Interfollicular epidermal stem cells self-renew via autocrine Wnt signaling. Science (80-). 2013; https: //doi.org/10.1126/science.1239730.

[44] Torres-Rendon A, Stewart R, Craig GT, Wells M, Speight PM. DNA ploidy analysis by image cytometry helps to identify oral epithelial dysplasias with a high risk of malignant progression. Oral Oncol. 2009; https: //doi.org/10.1016/j.oraloncology.2008.07.006.

[45] Gómez I, Seoane J, Varela-Centelles P, Diz P, Takkouche B. Is diagnostic delay related to advanced-stage oral cancer? A meta-analysis. Eur J Oral Sci. 2009; https: //doi. org/10.1111/j.1600-0722.2009.00672. x.

[46] Han X, Wang J, Sun Y. Circulating tumor DNA as biomarkers for cancer detection. Genom Proteom Bioinform. 2017; https: //doi.org/10.1016/j.gpb.2016.12.004.

[47] Shaw JA, et al. Genomic analysis of circulating cell-free DNA infers breast cancer dormancy. Genome Res. 2012; https: //doi.org/10.1101/gr.123497.111.

[48] Chaudhuri AA, Binkley MS, Osmundson EC, Alizadeh AA, Diehn M. Predicting radiotherapy responses and treatment outcomes through analysis of circulating tumor DNA. Semin Radiat Oncol. 2015; https: //doi.org/10.1016/j.semradonc.2015.05.001.

[49] Ignatiadis M, Lee M, Jeffrey SS. Circulating tumor cells and circulating tumor DNA: challenges and opportunities on the path to clinical utility. Clin Cancer Res. 2015; https: //doi. org/10.1158/1078-0432. CCR-14-1190.

[50] Forshew T, et al. Noninvasive identification and monitoring of cancer mutations by targeted deep sequencing of plasma DNA. Sci Transl Med. 2012; https: //doi.org/10.1126/scitranslmed.3003726.

[51] Bettegowda C, et al. Detection of circulating tumor DNA in early- and late-stage human malignancies. Sci Transl Med. 2014; https: //doi.org/10.1126/scitranslmed.3007094.

[52] Diehl F, et al. Circulating mutant DNA to assess tumor dynamics. Nat Med. 2008; https: //doi. org/10.1038/nm.1789.

[53] Newman AM, et al. An ultrasensitive method for quantitating circulating tumor DNA with broad patient coverage. Nat Med. 2014; https://doi.org/10.1038/nm.3519.

[54] Sausen M, et al. Clinical implications of genomic alterations in the tumour and circulation of pancreatic cancer patients. Nat Commun. 2015; https://doi.org/10.1038/ncomms8686.

[55] Beaver JA, et al. Detection of cancer DNA in plasma of patients with early-stage breast cancer. Clin Cancer Res. 2014; https://doi.org/10.1158/1078-0432. CCR-13-2933.

[56] Heitzer E, Ulz P, Geigl JB. Circulating tumor DNA as a liquid biopsy for cancer. Clin Chem. 2015; https://doi.org/10.1373/clinchem.2014.222679.

[57] Chai RC, et al. A pilot study to compare the detection of HPV-16 biomarkers in salivary oral rinses with tumour p16INK4a expression in head and neck squamous cell carcinoma patients. BMC Cancer. 2016; https://doi.org/10.1186/s12885-016-2217-1.

[58] Braig F, et al. Liquid biopsy monitoring uncovers acquired RAS-mediated resistance to cetuximab in a substantial proportion of patients with head and neck squamous cell carcinoma. Oncotarget. 2016; https://doi.org/10.18632/oncotarget.8943.

第 6 章

Taichiro Nonaka and David T. W. Wong

头颈癌循环生物标志物

Circulating Biomarkers in Head and Neck Cancer

引 言

头颈癌在 2018 年被列为全球第七大常见癌症，新增病例约为 88 万例，死亡约 45 万例[1]。鳞状细胞癌（SCC）是最主要的组织学类型，主要发生在口咽黏膜。尽管手术和治疗选择有所改进，但总体生存率多年来基本保持不变。目前，现有的筛查技术，如影像学和蛋白质标志物，尚不足以在早期检测头颈癌。组织活检是标准的诊断方法，但它无法提供有关肿瘤异质性和演变的信息[2]。液体活检因其可以以微创的方式提供实时信息，被认为是一种理想的癌症检测方法[3]。循环肿瘤 DNA（ctDNA）、循环肿瘤细胞（CTC）和外泌体 miRNA 是新兴的生物标志物，可应用于癌症检测、治疗计划和疗效监测[4]。值得注意的是，ctDNA 和外泌体 miRNA 存在于包括唾液在内的多种体液中，被视为极具前景的肿瘤标志物[5]。在本章中，我们总结了目前现有的循环生物标志物（ctDNA、CTC 和外泌体 miRNA）及它们在早期检测和治疗头颈癌中的潜在临床应用。

循环肿瘤 DNA 和循环肿瘤细胞

早期检测

循环肿瘤 DNA（ctDNA）是指来源于在血液中自由循环的癌症细胞的游离 DNA。癌症患者的 ctDNA 浓度高于健康人[6]。ctDNA 主要来源于凋亡或坏死的肿瘤细胞，并包含肿瘤的突变信息（图 6-1）。1994 年，Vasioukhin 和 Sorenson 等首次证实了在血浆游离 DNA 中检测到肿瘤特异性 RAS 突变的存在[7, 8]。其他多项研究表明，在肺癌[9]、乳腺癌[10, 11]和结直肠癌[12, 13]中，血浆 ctDNA 与相应肿瘤样本之间在突变特征上高度一致。

最近的一项原理验证研究表明，ctDNA 在头颈癌是一种极具前景的生物标志物[14]。在一项包含 93 名头颈鳞状细胞癌（HNSCC）患者（包括 20 例早期癌症患者）的队列研究中，对

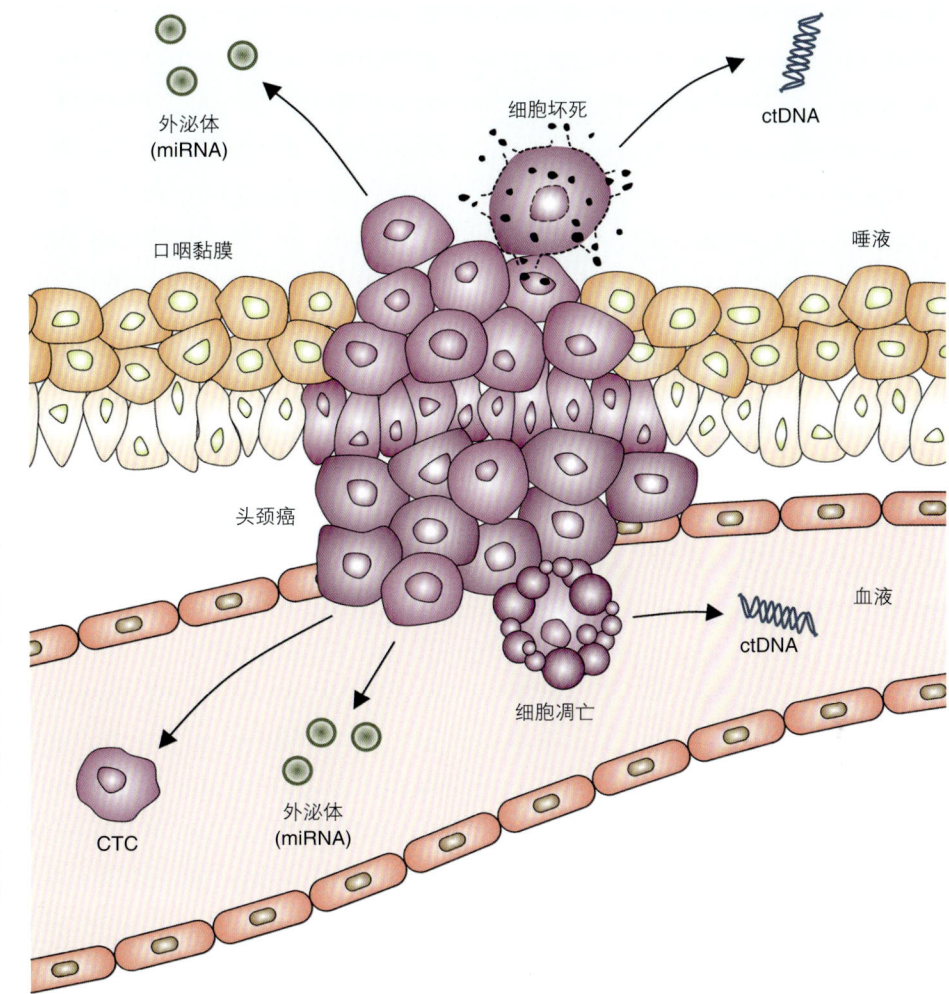

图 6-1 头颈癌中的循环生物标志物。循环肿瘤 DNA（ctDNA）、循环肿瘤细胞（CTC）和外泌体 miRNA 是存在于血浆和（或）唾液中的互补生物标志物。凋亡的肿瘤细胞将 ctDNA 释放到血液中，而坏死的肿瘤细胞将 ctDNA 释放到唾液中。肿瘤细胞将外泌体 miRNA 释放到血液和唾液中。原发肿瘤和转移性病灶将 CTC 释放到血液中（经允许引自参考文献［3］。版权：2018，SAGE Publications）

患者血浆和唾液样本进行体细胞突变（*TP53*、*PIK3CA*、*NOTCH1*、*FBXW7*、*CDKN2A*、*NRAS* 和 *HRAS*）和人乳头瘤病毒（HPV16 和 18）的检测（表 6-1）。研究发现，对于口咽癌、下咽癌和喉癌，血浆 ctDNA 比唾液 ctDNA 的灵敏度更高（86%~100% vs 47%~70%）。然而，在口腔癌中，唾液 ctDNA 比血浆 ctDNA 的灵敏度更高（100% vs 80%），表明口腔癌来源的 DNA 更容易在唾液中检测到，这主要是由于肿瘤与唾液的近距离接触。重要的是，当同时检测血浆和唾液时，无论肿瘤位置或分期如何，ctDNA 的总体检测率达 96%。这些发现表明，为了获得高灵敏度的结果，应根据肿瘤类型选择合适的体液进行组合检测。*TP53* 是口腔癌患者血浆中检测到的最常见的 ctDNA（85%），在其他部位的肿瘤（口咽癌 100%，下咽癌 100%，喉癌 86%）中也是如此。相比之下，HPV16 DNA 的检测频率略低，可能是因为 *TP53* 突变和 HPV 阳性通常是相互排斥的[15]。癌症基因组图谱网络在 243 个 HPV 阴性样本中显示了高达 86% 的 *TP53* 突变率，而在 36 个 HPV 阳性病例中仅有一个（2.8%）存在非同义 *TP53* 突变，这与该数据一致[16]。

对于病毒为病因的癌症（如鼻咽癌），检测与癌症相关的病毒 DNA 可能是一种识别早期疾病的有效策略。Chan 等人对无症状志愿者的血浆 Epstein-Barr 病毒（EBV）DNA 进行了筛查，发现 1 318 名参与者中有 69 人（5.2%）携带病毒 DNA，其中 3 人被确诊为鼻咽癌[17]。他们在一项包含 20 174 名参与者的前瞻性队列中进一步验证了该结果，结果显示 309 名持续 EBV 阳性的参与者中有 34 人（11%）发展为鼻咽癌[18]。在人群中筛查血浆中的病毒 DNA 是检测早期癌

表 6-1　头颈鳞状细胞癌中唾液和血浆 ctDNA 生物标志物特征概述

		ctDNA	阳性率（%）（检出数/样本数）		
			唾　液	血　浆	唾液或血浆[a]
部位	口腔	TP53	100（36/36）	85（11/13）	100（13/13）
		PIK3CA	100（2/2）	50（1/2）	100（2/2）
		NOTCH1	100（3/3）	NA	NA
		CDKN2A	100（2/2）	NA	NA
		易位	100（2/2）[b]	NA	NA
		HPV16 DNA	100（1/1）	NA	NA
		（总计）	100（46/46）	80（12/15）	100（15/15）
	口咽	TP53	80（4/5）	100（1/1）	100（1/1）
		PIK3CA	25（2/8）[b]	100（5/5）	100（5/5）
		FBXW7	67（2/3）	100（3/3）	100（3/3）
		HPV16 DNA	41（7/17）	92（11/12）	92（11/12）
		NRAS	0（0/1）	0（0/1）	0（0/1）
		（总计）	47（16/34）[b]	91（20/22）	91（20/22）
	喉	TP53	70（7/10）	86（6/7）	100（7/7）
	下咽	TP53	67（2/3）	100（3/3）	100（3/3）
分期	早期（Ⅰ+Ⅱ）	TP53	100（16/16）	75（6/8）	100（8/8）
		HPV16 DNA	100（2/2）	100（1/1）	100（1/1）
		PIK3CA	100（1/1）	0（0/1）	100（1/1）
		NOTCH1	100（1/1）	NA	NA
		（总计）	100（20/20）	70（7/10）	100（10/10）
	晚期（Ⅲ+Ⅳ）	TP53	87（33/38）	94（15/16）	100（16/16）
		PIK3CA	33（3/9）b	100（6/6）	100（6/6）
		FBXW7	67（2/3）	100（3/3）	100（3/3）
		HPV16 DNA	38（6/16）	91（10/11）	91（10/11）
		NOTCH1	100（2/2）	NA	NA
		CDKN2A	100（2/2）	NA	NA
		易位	100（2/2）	NA	NA
		NRAS	0（0/1）	0（0/1）	0（0/1）
		（总计）	70（51/73）[b]	92（34/37）	95（35/37）
HPV	HPV16	HPV16 DNA	40（12/30）	86（18/21）	86（18/21）
总计			76（71/93）[b]	87（41/47）	96（45/47）

注：经允许引自参考文献［3］。版权：2018，SAGE Publications。
所有生物标志物数据和检出率均来自 Wang 等人（2015）发表的安全测序系统（Safe-SeqS）和数字聚合酶链式反应的结果。
NA，不适用。
[a] "唾液或血浆"中的检出率仅在患者的唾液和血浆数据都可用时计算。
[b] 一名唾液中 PIK3CA 阴性但人乳头瘤病毒（HPV）阳性的患者被计入总数。

症的极具前景的方法。

一些原发和转移性肿瘤将 CTC 释放到血液中（图 6-1）。CTC 能够提供完整的细胞信息，且 CTC 水平的升高具有诊断特征。在多项研究中，CTC 已被尝试用于原发性肿瘤和转移复发的诊断[19]。Nichols 等人和 He 等人报告称，在被诊断为头颈癌的患者中，分别在 15 例中的 6 例（40.0%）和 9 例中的 3 例（33.3%）中检测到了 CTC[20, 21]。Buglione 和他的团队报告称，相比于早期肿瘤，CTC 在晚期肿瘤中更为常见[22]。此外，Jatana 等人和 Gröbe 等人报告称，CTC 数量的增加与较差的预后相关，CTC 的存在与局部复发相关[23, 24]。然而，在癌症的早期检测方面，CTC 的敏感性似乎远低于 ctDNA。Bettegowda 等人报告称，在早期膀胱癌、乳腺癌和结直肠癌中未检测到 CTC，而 ctDNA 在 81% 的这些癌症中被检测到[11]。这些发现表明，CTC 的存在提示肿瘤分期较晚，代表了一种预后标志，而不是早期诊断标志（图 6-2a）。

治疗选择

循环肿瘤细胞（CTC）可用于检测药物靶点的存在。西妥昔单抗（Cetuximab）是一种靶向表皮生长因子受体（EGFR）胞外结构域的单克隆抗体，已被批准用于晚期头颈鳞状细胞癌（HNSCC）的治疗[25, 26]。检测 CTC 表面的 EGFR 表达可为抗 EGFR 治疗提供重要信息（图 6-2a）。例如，与传统化疗相比，西妥昔单抗治疗 HNSCC 更能显著减少 EGFR 阳性 CTC[27]。

EGFR 下游信号分子参与了 HNSCC 对西妥昔单抗的耐药性。在西妥昔单抗治疗前筛查 *RAS* 突变尤为重要，因为携带活性 *RAS* 突变的肿瘤对 EGFR 靶向治疗无反应。Braig 等人研究了接受西妥昔单抗治疗的 20 名 HNSCC 患者液体活检队列中的血浆 ctDNA，发现 20 名患者中有 6 名（30%）获得了 *KRAS*、*NRAS* 或 *HRAS* 突变[28]。在 ctDNA 或 CTC 中检测到 *RAS* 突变可能有助于定制抗 EGFR 治疗，因为这些突变与治疗效果和疾病进展显著相关。更重要的是，应在治疗过程中监测突变负荷，以可靠地预测西妥昔单抗反应的丧失。因此，CTC 可用于突变监测，以指导治疗决策。

在肿瘤微环境中，肿瘤细胞可以表达程序性死亡配体 1（PD-L1），其可下调效应 T 细胞的活性，从而保护肿瘤免受免疫攻击[29]。检测 CTC 表面表达的 PD-L1 可以预测对抗 PD-L1 免疫治疗的反应（图 6-2a）[30]。在乳腺癌中，Mazel 等人报告称在 16 名患者中有 11 名（68.8%）检测到 PD-L1 阳性 CTC，表明其在治疗计划中的用途[31]。在其他肿瘤类型中，如肺癌[32]、膀胱癌[33]、前列腺癌和结直肠癌[34]，也有报道称 CTC 上 PD-L1 表达与较差的生存率显著相关。在头颈癌中，Strati 等人发现，在 94 名患者中，24 人（25.5%）的 CD45$^-$EpCAM$^+$CTC 在疗前表达 PD-L1，34 名患者中 8 人（23.5%）在化疗后表达 PD-L1，54 名患者中 12 人（22.2%）在治疗结束时表达 PD-L1[35]。Oliveira-Costa 等人研究了来自口腔鳞状细胞癌（OSCC）的 CD45$^-$细胞角蛋白（CK）$^+$CTC 中的 PD-L1 表达，发现了 PD-L1 的转录和蛋白质表达，表明其在监测患者治疗反应中的用途[36]。此外，Kulasinghe 等人从一名喉癌患者中分离出 CD45$^-$EpCAM$^+$CK$^+$CTC，并通过免疫细胞化学法检测到 PD-L1 的高表达[37]。

尽管有证据表明检测 CTC 水平有助于治疗方案的选择，但由于 CTC 数量极低，检测 CTC 仍具有挑战性。据估计，每 7.5 mL 血液中仅存在 1~2 个 CTC，使其研究变得困难[21]。目前，CellSearch[38] 是美国食品药物监督管理局（FDA）批准的唯一 CTC 分离平台。CellSearch 是一个基于 EpCAM 上皮标志物表达的标准化半自动系统，能够对 CTC 进行阳性选择。针对 HNSCC 患者中小部分 CTC 的治疗靶标测试正在研究中，但其临床实用性尚未确定。

治疗反应监测

与影像学相比，ctDNA 在实时监测治疗反应方面具有优势[39]。在预测治疗反应方面，

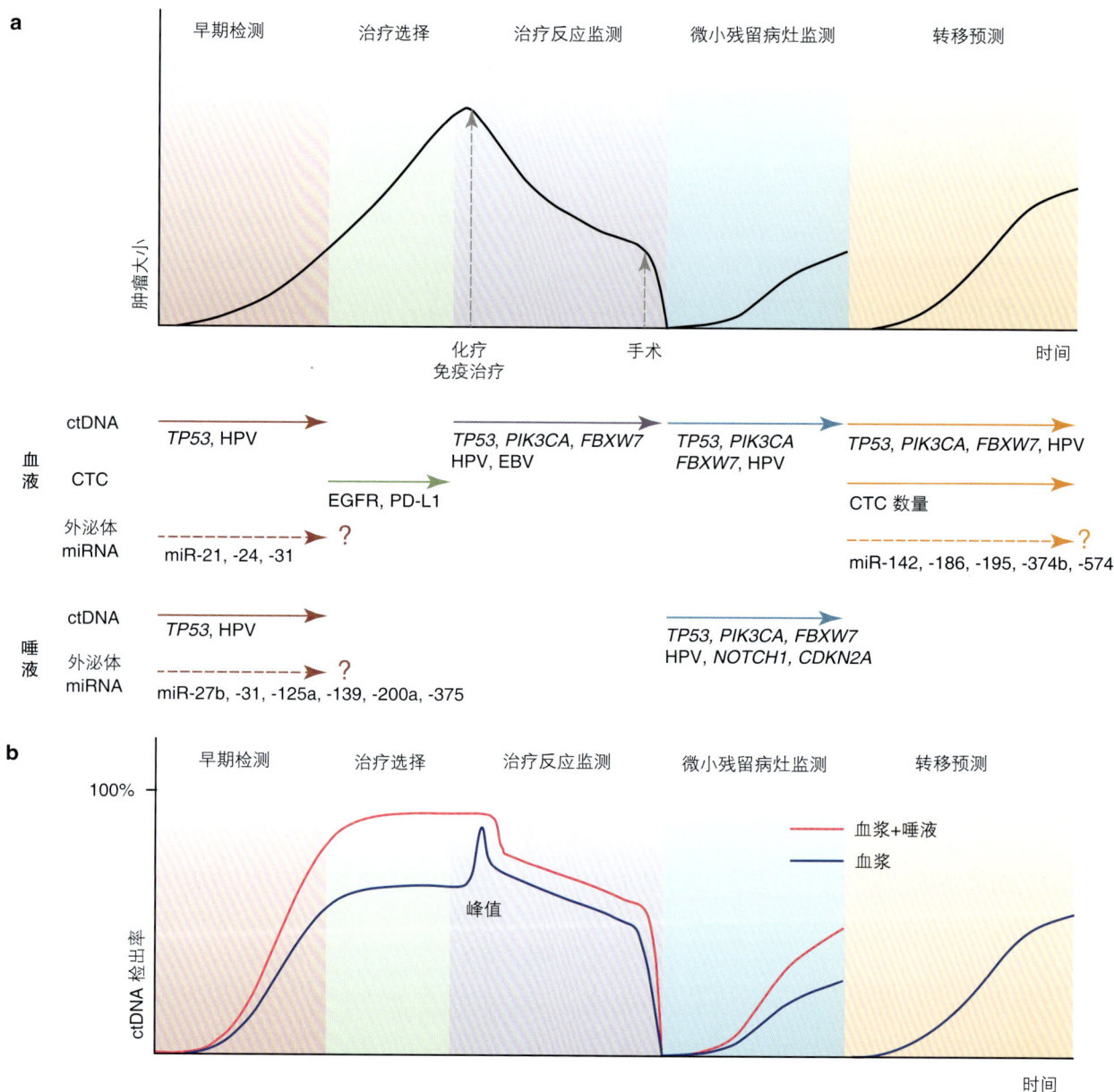

图 6-2　循环生物标志物在头颈癌治疗中的潜在临床应用。a. 头颈癌患者在接受化疗（或免疫疗法）和手术过程中的疾病管理和肿瘤大小的时间示意图。血浆 ctDNA 分析可用于早期检测、治疗反应监测、微小残留病灶（MRD）监测和转移预测。CTC 分析可以协助靶向治疗的选择。外泌体 miRNA 目前在临床应用中提供的信息有限。唾液 ctDNA 分析可以提供补充信息。b. 联合使用血浆和唾液 ctDNA 相比单独使用血浆 ctDNA 具有更高的癌症检测灵敏度。ctDNA 水平的峰值反映了系统性治疗引起的肿瘤细胞短暂死亡（经允许引自参考文献［3］。版权：2018，SAGE Publications）

ctDNA 比 CTC 或其他癌症抗原（如 CA15-3）更敏感（图 6-2a）[40]。通过检测不同突变的早期动态变化，可以在全身治疗的情况下预测治疗反应，从而实现早期的治疗干预。

一项检测鼻咽癌化疗期间 EBV 清除率的研究表明，血浆 EBV DNA 的中位半衰期为 3.99 天（范围为 1.85～28.29 天）[41]。另一项研究报告称，结直肠癌术后血浆 ctDNA（APC、KRAS、TP53 和 PIK3CA）的半衰期为 114 分钟，这表明 ctDNA 是监测肿瘤大小快速变化的最理想生物标志物，因其快速动态变化[12]。上述研究表明，化疗或手术期间癌症患者的肿瘤动态可以通过 ctDNA 测量进行可靠监测（图 6-2a）。目前，一项评估 ctDNA 作为 HNSCC 治疗反应生物标志物的临床试验正在进行中，结果尚待公布（ClinicalTrials.gov 标识符：NCT03540563）。

微小残留病灶（MRD）监测

已有研究表明，ctDNA 水平可用于手术后微小残留病灶（MRD）的监测[42]。理论上，ctDNA 的检测可能是评估 MRD 的最佳方法，因为基于 PCR 的方法具有高灵敏度，且能够有效地进行检测（图 6-2a）。Diehl 等人成功检测到结直肠癌患者游离 DNA 中低至 0.01% 的突变，并发现 MRD 患者在术后一年内复发[12]。另一项对 230 名结直肠癌患者的前瞻性研究显示，术后 ctDNA 阴性患者的无复发生存率为 90%，而 ctDNA 阳性患者为 0%[43]。对 55 名乳腺癌患者的研究表明，术后 ctDNA 检测可以准确预测无复发生存率[44]。鉴别 MRD 阳性患者能否改善癌症患者的生存状况尚有待证实，但根据 ctDNA 水平将患者分为高风险和低风险组，可以更早进行治疗干预。

转移预测

使用 ctDNA 作为替代标志物的想法是基于其与原发性肿瘤和继发性肿瘤具有共同的突变特征[11, 40]。许多研究表明，ctDNA 是一种敏感的检测转移的标志物，能够反映包括头颈癌在内的多种癌症的肿瘤负荷[11, 40, 45]。

CTC 计数的预后价值也已通过大型临床试验在各种肿瘤类型中得到证实[46-48]。且越来越多的证据表明，CTC 检测与头颈癌患者的低生存率相关[23, 24, 49, 50]。此外，CTC 数量与头颈癌区域性转移的高发病率相关[51]。然而，由于个体之间 CTC 数量的高度差异，难以确定与不良预后相关的 CTC 阈值。尽管 CTC 分析的临床价值仍存在争议，但有证据表明，术后或系统治疗后的 CTC 数量可以预测治疗效果和转移风险（图 6-2a）[52]。

CTC 数量少，检测难度大。CellSearch 方法选择表达 EpCAM 的肿瘤细胞；因此，上皮间质转化过程中 EpCAM 的下调可能导致 CTC 无法被检测到。事实上，在转移性乳腺癌患者中，只有 1/3 的 CTC 是 EpCAM 阳性[53]。结合使用不同技术和标志物可以克服这一局限性。考虑到这一点，我们建议联合使用 ctDNA 和 CTC，这可能是评估头颈癌转移风险的理想策略。

循环外体 miRNA

外泌体是源自内吞作用的纳米级细胞外囊泡，携带多种细胞成分（如 DNA、RNA 和蛋白质），在细胞间的分子信息交换中发挥重要作用[54]。鉴于外泌体的成分，外泌体有可能被用作癌症生物标志物。外泌体包含的成分中，miRNA 被认为是癌症诊断的关键标志物，因为它们可调控癌基因和抑癌基因[55]。由于血浆和肿瘤中 miRNA 谱之间的相关性，一组外泌体 miRNA 形成了肿瘤生物标志物[56, 57]。这推动了使用 miRNA 特征作为诊断工具的研究[58-60]，包括头颈部恶性肿瘤。Summerer 等人进行的一项研究表明，循环 miR-142、miR-186、miR-195、miR-374b 和 miR-574 的高表达是头颈癌的预后生物标志物[61]。同样，在头颈癌患者的血浆中检测到 miR-21 和 miR-24 水平升高[62, 63]。此外，miR-31 在头颈癌患者血浆中也呈现高表达，并在肿瘤切除后降低，表明其可能来源于肿瘤[63]。肿瘤抑制性 miR-486 的下调与口腔鳞癌（OSCC）的复发高度相关，提示 miR-486 可用于监测 OSCC 术后复发的生物标志物[64]。这些发现提供了大量证据，证明外泌体 miRNA 可以作为诊断癌症有价值的工具（图 6-2a）。

miRNA 数据库 miRandola 提供了一个大型的细胞外非编码 RNA 目录，这些 RNA 在多种疾病中被发现，目前包含 1 002 种 miRNA，共 3 283 个条目（http：//mirandola.iit.cnr.it/）[65]。尽管经

过广泛研究，但外泌体 miRNA 的可靠性由于研究方法不一致而受到影响，导致结果不一致[66]。此外，尚未确认免疫细胞是否对循环 miRNA 水平有显著贡献。系统性或局部炎症可能会扰乱 miRNA 的表达及其可重复性，即使在同一个体中也会如此[67]。由此，对于外泌体 miRNA 在头颈癌诊断中的表现尚无共识，且需要更多的研究进一步表征外泌体 miRNA。需要在大规模临床试验中采用标准化的协议进行验证，以证明外泌体 miRNA 在临床环境中的价值。

唾液诊断

在过去十年中，唾液研究人员开发了唾液诊断方法，以检测口腔和全身性疾病[68]。蛋白质组学研究表明，唾液中的某些成分来源于与血液的生理相互作用，显示出唾液蛋白质组中有 20%～30% 反映了血浆的成分[69, 70]。这种血液和唾液之间的关系揭示了另一种诊断全身性疾病的资源。唾液在临床诊断中具有独特的优势。唾液可以无创采集，不会给引起患者不适。唾液不会凝结，因此比血液更容易处理和加工。由于唾液包含多种成分并与血液有紧密的生理联系，因此可以被视为口腔和全身健康的一面"镜子"，使其成为一种极具吸引力的疾病诊断生物液体。

唾液 ctDNA

基因组分析显示，约 70% 的唾液游离 DNA 来自宿主，其余 30% 来自微生物[71]。研究发现，唾液 ctDNA 作为早期口腔癌的生物标志物比血浆 ctDNA 更为敏感（表 6-1）。一项原理验证研究表明，在早期口腔癌患者的唾液中检测到 $TP53$ ctDNA，其灵敏度为 100%[14]。即使在其他部位癌症（如口咽癌、下咽癌和喉癌）患者中，也有 67%～80% 的患者在唾液中检测到 $TP53$ ctDNA，使其成为检测头颈癌的潜在生物标志物（图 6-2a）。

Qureishi 等人研究了在口咽鳞状细胞癌（OPSCC）患者的唾液中通过 PCR 检测 HPV DNA 的准确性，结果表明诊断准确性令人满意，阳性预测值为 96%[72]。与手术活检的 p16 相关免疫组化（IHC）相比，唾液检测的灵敏度和特异度分别为 72% 和 90%。在一项前瞻性研究中，Martin-Gomez 等人确认了漱口水是获取 OPSCC 患者 HPV DNA 的可靠且非侵入性来源[73]。在 171 例病例中，漱口水与肿瘤标本在 HPV16 方面的一致率为 74%。其他 HPV 类型（如 HPV 18、31、33 和 35）显示出更高的一致率（> 94%），证明了在唾液中检测 HPV 的可行性（图 6-2a）。口腔 HPV 检测的另一个可能意义在于在 HPV 阳性 OPSCC 治疗后的疾病监测。Ahn 等人通过一项回顾性研究表明，治疗后唾液 HPV 阳性状态与较高的复发风险相关（风险比为 10.7；95% CI：2.36～48.50）（$P = 0.002$）[74]。Rettig 等人也得出了类似结果，评估了唾液中 HPV DNA 的预测价值[75]。在 124 名 HPV 阳性 OPSCC 的前瞻性队列中，治疗前 54% 的患者漱口水样本中存在 HPV DNA，而治疗后仅有 5%。重要的是，6 例中有 5 例（83%）漱口水样本中持续存在 HPV DNA 的患者出现了复发，提示唾液可能是一个潜在的监测工具。唾液富含来源于口咽腔肿瘤细胞的肿瘤或 HPV 特异性 DNA，同时分析血浆和唾液可以使筛查头颈癌的效果最大化（图 6-2b）。

唾液 miRNA

循环的游离 miRNA 在唾液中出乎意料地稳定[76]。与外源性 miRNA 相比，唾液中的内源性 miRNA 降解速率较慢。唾液 miRNA 的分析显示它们被包裹在外泌体中，使其能够抵抗核糖核酸酶（RNase）的破坏[77, 78]。一些研究表明，唾液 miRNA 可以作为头颈癌的潜在生物标志物。Park 等人报告称，与健康个体相比，口腔癌患者唾液中的 miR-125a 和 miR-200a 显著减少[76]。同样地，与健康对照组相比，从口腔癌患者唾液中收集的 miR-139 和 miR-375 的表达水平也有所下降[79,80]。此外，在口腔癌患者唾液中观察到 miR-27b 和 miR-31 的表达水平增加[81,82]。重要的是，miR-139 和 miR-31 的表达水平在病变切除后恢复到基线水平，提示其作为预后生物标志物的潜力[79,81]。尽管某些唾液 miRNA 可能作为头颈癌的推测性生物标志物，但需要进一步研究以验证这些发现并阐明相关分子机制。

唾液外泌体

唾液外泌体是由唾液腺和（或）口腔上皮细胞分泌的纳米级细胞外囊泡（EV）。它们被磷脂双层包裹，包含反映其来源细胞的独特蛋白质载体（图 6-3）。常见的检测到的蛋白质包括四跨膜蛋白、热激蛋白、水通道、主要组织相容性复合物（MHC）以及 Rab GTPases 和 ESCRT[83,84]。其他外泌体中的蛋白质包括信号传导、细胞骨架、代谢和载体蛋白。对哺乳动物 EV 的全面分析生成了在不同类型的从细胞、组织或体液中分离出的 EV 中发现的成分（蛋白质、核酸和脂质）目录。这些数据库可在 Vesiclepedia（http://www.microvesicles.org）[85] 和 ExoCarta（http://www.exocarta.org）[86] 上公开获取。

肿瘤来源的外泌体的纳米结构为外泌体的表征增加了另一层复杂性[87]。使用原子力显微镜（AFM）和场发射扫描电子显微镜（FESEM）进行纳米结构分析显示健康供体的唾液外泌体具有三叶结构，表明其弹性机械性质[88,89]。未施加压力时，唾液外泌体具有球形形态，由于其致密的脂质膜中嵌入的蛋白质，其表面呈现异质性。口腔癌患者单个囊泡水平的唾液外泌体表征显示出不规则形态和聚集[90]。研究还表明，口腔癌患者唾液外泌体的尺寸增大（98.3 ± 4.6 nm），而健康个体的外泌体尺寸为 67.4 ± 2.9 nm（$P < 0.05$）。这些形态异常表明某些唾液外泌体由直接释放到唾液中的肿瘤来源外泌体组成。此外，高分辨率 AFM 在口腔癌唾液中识别出多泡体（MVB）（图 6-4）[90]。MVB 中的膜破裂表明了外泌体释放的位点以及核酸的丝状延伸。这些研究的图像表明唾液外泌体是口腔癌的潜在指示物。

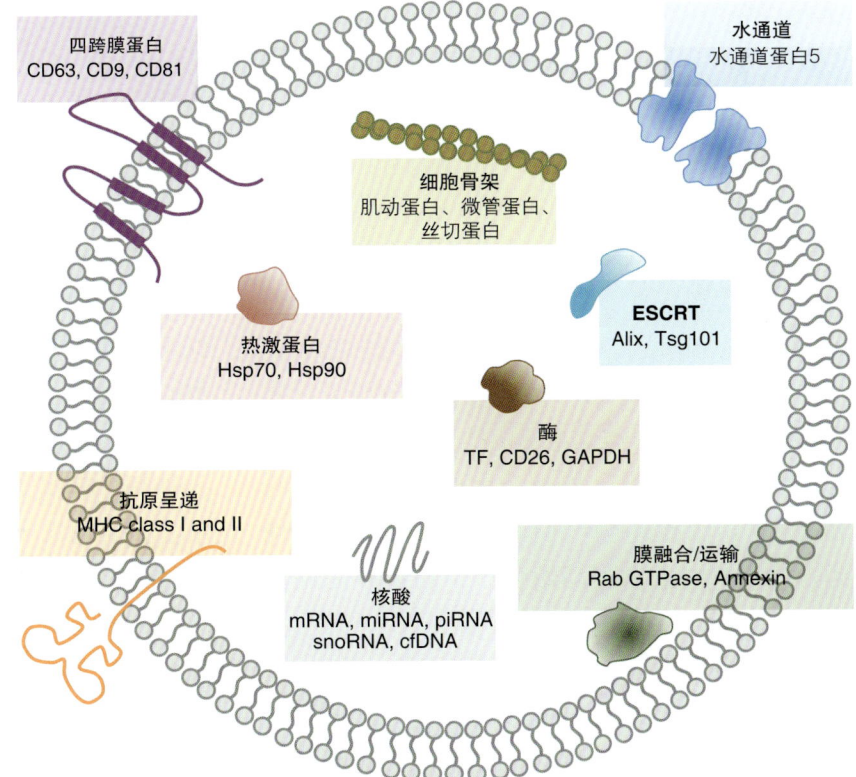

图 6-3 唾液外泌体的结构和成分。外泌体被磷脂双层包围。大多数唾液外泌体的膜蛋白标志物包括四跨膜蛋白、水通道和主要组织相容性复合物（MHC）Ⅰ类。囊泡内的内容物包括核酸（RNA 和 DNA）和各种胞质蛋白，如酶、热激蛋白、细胞骨架、内体分拣复合体（ESCRT）相关蛋白以及原始亲本细胞的膜融合 / 转运相关蛋白（经允许引自参考文献 [68]。版权：2017，Elsevier Inc.）

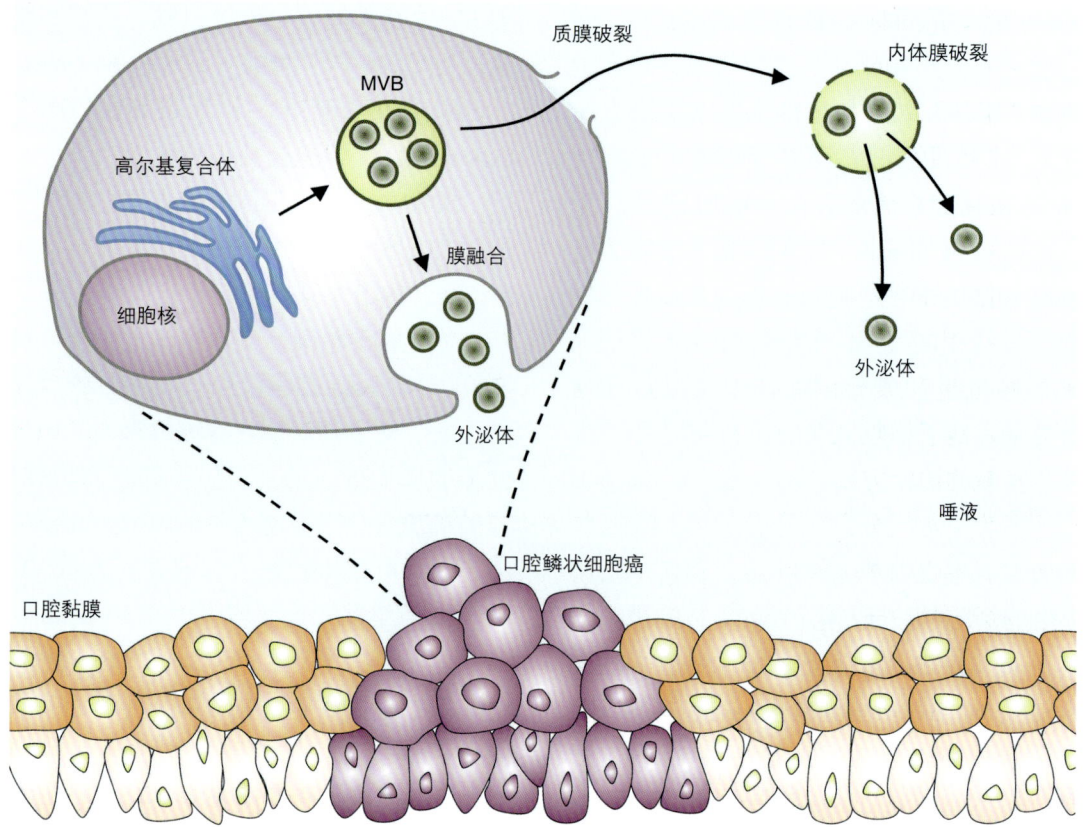

图6-4 口腔鳞状细胞癌（OSCC）中的外泌体生成及其直接释放到唾液中。外泌体通过反面高尔基网生成并积聚在多泡体（MVB）中。外泌体通过两种不同的机制释放到唾液中；通过膜融合的持续释放或通过膜破裂的异常释放（经允许引自参考文献［68］。版权：2017，Elsevier Inc.）

小结与未来展望

越来越多的证据表明，循环生物标志物在患者分层和疾病状态监测方面的临床应用潜力。活跃释放于血浆和唾液中的ctDNA优先用于头颈癌的早期检测，而来自转移性病灶的循环肿瘤细胞（CTC）则可用于预测不良预后。对CTC表面分子（如EGFR、PD-L1）表达的分析可以提供规划免疫治疗所需的重要信息。其他循环生物标志物，如外泌体miRNA，也可以提供额外的信息层次。因此，靶向具有独立释放机制的多种生物标志物可能会提高癌症诊断的特异度和灵敏度。

一个关键问题是循环生物标志物（ctDNA、CTC和外泌体miRNA）在多大程度上能代表整个肿瘤。就此而言，生物标志物的评估应涵盖所有肿瘤特征的包容性。CTC无法代表异质性肿瘤，这在一定程度上降低了它们的临床相关性，尽管CTC被认为具有完整的细胞信息。外泌体则被认为能够代表肿瘤的较大部分，因为它们被认为源自整个肿瘤，反映了肿瘤的异质性特征。然而，外泌体miRNA是通过反面高尔基网选择性组装的，仅能代表细胞miRNA的一部分。需要使用标准化方案进行大规模患者队列研究，以确定每种方法（单独或组合）是否可以改善总体生存率。

同时分析多种体液中的循环生物标志物是提供补充信息的理想策略，并且是将液体活检应用于个性化医疗的重要里程碑。利用唾液是无创的，且其包含的信息丰富，因此，唾液诊断有望实现精准医学计划的目标。

唾液外泌体学（saliva-exosomics）是指通过使用先进的"组学"技术研究唾液外泌体的下一代唾液组学，旨在更好地描述其特定功能和生物标志物[68]。在癌症患者中，唾液中含有一组源自癌变病灶的独特外泌体（图6-5）。这可能是由唾液腺对癌源性外泌体的加工和选择所致。然而，即使在具有相同类型和分期的肿瘤患者中，唾液外泌体的数量和成分也存在很大差异，因此，需要更深入地了解唾液外泌体，以建立生物标志物并开发新的治疗方法。

在临床环境中常规分离和分析循环生物标志物极具挑战性。建立简单、快速且经济的技术来分析循环生物标志物对于即刻应用至关重要。当前的技术（如ddPCR、下一代测序）存在成本高、处理时间长和数据操作复杂等缺点。我们开发了一种新型的唾液活检技术，称为电场诱导释放与测量（EFIRM），该技术可以直接检测极少量的ctDNA和RNA，仅需40 μL唾液[91-93]。将这种电化学传感技术和其他出色的组件（如快速生物标志物分离技术）相结合，将有助于有效检测循环生物标志物，推动开发用于常规临床使用的即时检测设备。

致谢：本研究得到了美国国立卫生研究院的资助，项目编号为：UH2/UH3 CA206126、U01 CA233370和 U01 DE017790（D.T.W.W.）；DE027759 和 DE029272（T.N.）。

利益冲突声明：D.T.W.W. 是 Liquid Diagnostics、葛兰素史克公司、箭牌公司和高露洁棕榄公司的顾问。

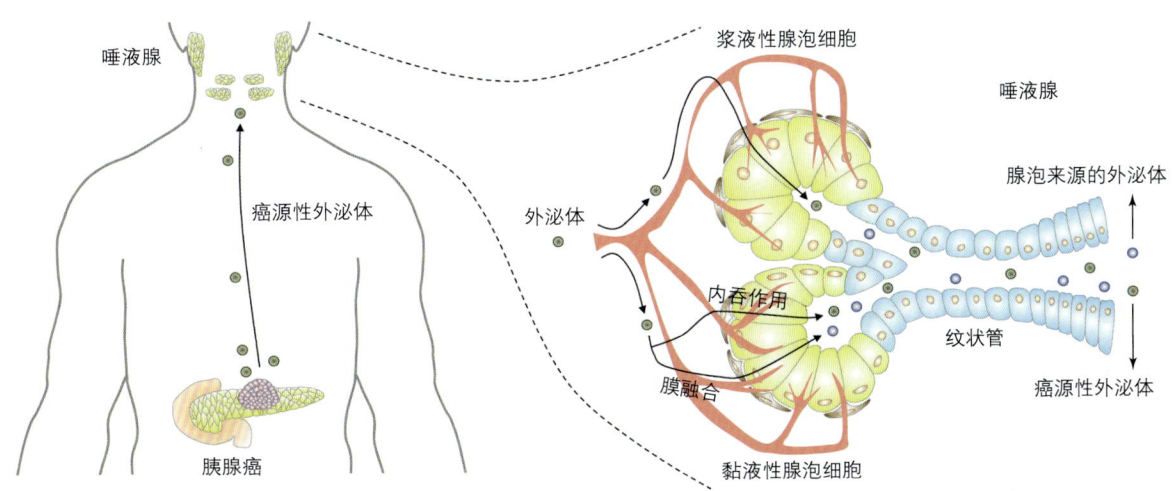

图6-5 外泌体介导的癌症衍生产物从远端肿瘤传输至唾液腺组织的示意图。癌源性外泌体进入循环系统并到达唾液腺。唾液腺腺泡细胞通过内吞作用或膜融合吸收外泌体。两种不同的唾液外泌体被释放到唾液中。癌源性外泌体通过内吞作用后在对侧腔膜外泌的方式释放，而腺泡来源的外泌体通过多泡体（MVB）与质膜的融合释放。这两种唾液外泌体均携带癌症衍生的产物（经允许引自参考文献[68]。版权：2017，Elsevier Inc.）

参考文献

[1] Bray F, Ferlay J, Soerjomataram I, Siegel RL, Torre LA, Jemal A. Global cancer statistics 2018: GLOBOCAN estimates of incidence and mortality worldwide for 36 cancers in 185 countries. CA Cancer J Clin. 2018; 68: 394-424.

[2] Gerlinger M, Rowan AJ, Horswell S, Math M, Larkin J, Endesfelder D, Gronroos E, Martinez P, Matthews N, Stewart A, Tarpey P, Varela I, Phillimore B, Begum S, McDonald NQ, Butler A, Jones D, Raine K, Latimer C, Santos CR, Nohadani M, Eklund AC, Spencer-Dene B, Clark G, Pickering L, Stamp G, Gore M, Szallasi Z, Downward J, Futreal PA, Swanton C. Intratumor heterogeneity and branched

evolution revealed by multiregion sequencing. N Engl J Med. 2012; 366: 883–92.
[3] Nonaka T, Wong DTW. Liquid biopsy in head and neck cancer: promises and challenges. J Dent Res. 2018; 97: 701–8.
[4] Siravegna G, Marsoni S, Siena S, Bardelli A. Integrating liquid biopsies into the management of cancer. Nat Rev Clin Oncol. 2017; 14: 531–48.
[5] Weber JA, Baxter DH, Zhang S, Huang DY, Huang KH, Lee MJ, Galas DJ, Wang K. The microRNA spectrum in 12 body fluids. Clin Chem. 2010; 56: 1733–41.
[6] Leon SA, Shapiro B, Sklaroff DM, Yaros MJ. Free DNA in the serum of cancer patients and the effect of therapy. Cancer Res. 1977; 37: 646–50.
[7] Sorenson GD, Pribish DM, Valone FH, Memoli VA, Bzik DJ, Yao SL. Soluble normal and mutated DNA sequences from single-copy genes in human blood. Cancer Epidemiol Biomark Prev. 1994; 3: 67–71.
[8] Vasioukhin V, Anker P, Maurice P, Lyautey J, Lederrey C, Stroun M. Point mutations of the N-ras gene in the blood plasma DNA of patients with myelodysplastic syndrome or acute myelogenous leukaemia. Br J Haematol. 1994; 86: 774–9.
[9] Newman AM, Bratman SV, To J, Wynne JF, Eclov NC, Modlin LA, Liu CL, Neal JW, Wakelee HA, Merritt RE, Shrager JB, Loo BW Jr, Alizadeh AA, Diehn M. An ultrasensitive method for quantitating circulating tumor DNA with broad patient coverage. Nat Med. 2014; 20: 548–54.
[10] Beaver JA, Jelovac D, Balukrishna S, Cochran R, Croessmann S, Zabransky DJ, Wong HY, Toro PV, Cidado J, Blair BG, Chu D, Burns T, Higgins MJ, Stearns V, Jacobs L, Habibi M, Lange J, Hurley PJ, Lauring J, VanDenBerg D, Kessler J, Jeter S, Samuels ML, Maar D, Cope L, Cimino-Mathews A, Argani P, Wolff AC, Park BH. Detection of cancer DNA in plasma of patients with early-stage breast cancer. Clin Cancer Res. 2014; 20: 2643–50.
[11] Bettegowda C, Sausen M, Leary RJ, Kinde I, Wang Y, Agrawal N, Bartlett BR, Wang H, Luber B, Alani RM, Antonarakis ES, Azad NS, Bardelli A, Brem H, Cameron JL, Lee CC, Fecher LA, Gallia GL, Gibbs P, Le D, Giuntoli RL, Goggins M, Hogarty MD, Holdhoff M, Hong SM, Jiao Y, Juhl HH, Kim JJ, Siravegna G, Laheru DA, Lauricella C, Lim M, Lipson EJ, Marie SK, Netto GJ, Oliner KS, Olivi A, Olsson L, Riggins GJ, Sartore-Bianchi A, Schmidt K, Shih M, Oba-Shinjo SM, Siena S, Theodorescu D, Tie J, Harkins TT, Veronese S, Wang TL, Weingart JD, Wolfgang CL, Wood LD, Xing D, Hruban RH, Wu J, Allen PJ, Schmidt CM, Choti MA, Velculescu VE, Kinzler KW, Vogelstein B, Papadopoulos N, Diaz LA Jr. Detection of circulating tumor DNA in early- and late-stage human malignancies. Sci Transl Med. 2014; 6: 224ra24.
[12] Diehl F, Schmidt K, Choti MA, Romans K, Goodman S, Li M, Thornton K, Agrawal N, Sokoll L, Szabo SA, Kinzler KW, Vogelstein B, Diaz LA Jr. Circulating mutant DNA to assess tumor dynamics. Nat Med. 2008; 14: 985–90.
[13] Thierry AR, Mouliere F, El Messaoudi S, Mollevi C, Lopez-Crapez E, Rolet F, Gillet B, Gongora C, Dechelotte P, Robert B, Del Rio M, Lamy PJ, Bibeau F, Nouaille M, Loriot V, Jarrousse AS, Molina F, Mathonnet M, Pezet D, Ychou M. Clinical validation of the detection of KRAS and BRAF mutations from circulating tumor DNA. Nat Med. 2014; 20: 430–5.
[14] Wang Y, Springer S, Mulvey CL, Silliman N, Schaefer J, Sausen M, James N, Rettig EM, Guo T, Pickering CR, Bishop JA, Chung CH, Califano JA, Eisele DW, Fakhry C, Gourin CG, Ha PK, Kang H, Kiess A, Koch WM, Myers JN, Quon H, Richmon JD, Sidransky D, Tufano RP, Westra WH, Bettegowda C, Diaz LA Jr, Papadopoulos N, Kinzler KW, Vogelstein B, Agrawal N. Detection of somatic mutations and HPV in the saliva and plasma of patients with head and neck squamous cell carcinomas. Sci Transl Med. 2015; 7: 293ra104.
[15] Leemans CR, Braakhuis BJ, Brakenhoff RH. The molecular biology of head and neck cancer. Nat Rev Cancer. 2011; 11: 9–22.
[16] The Cancer Genome Atlas Network. Comprehensive genomic characterization of head and neck squamous cell carcinomas. Nature. 2015; 517: 576–82.
[17] Chan KC, Hung EC, Woo JK, Chan PK, Leung SF, Lai FP, Cheng AS, Yeung SW, Chan YW, Tsui TK, Kwok JS, King AD, Chan AT, van Hasselt AC, Lo YM. Early detection of nasopharyngeal carcinoma by plasma Epstein-Barr virus DNA analysis in a surveillance program. Cancer. 2013; 119: 1838–44.
[18] Chan KCA, Woo JKS, King A, Zee BCY, Lam WKJ, Chan SL, Chu SWI, Mak C, Tse IOL, Leung SYM, Chan G, Hui EP, Ma BBY, Chiu RWK, Leung SF, van Hasselt AC, Chan ATC, Lo YMD. Analysis of plasma Epstein-Barr virus DNA to screen for nasopharyngeal cancer. N Engl J Med. 2017; 377: 513–22.
[19] Alix-Panabieres C, Pantel K. Clinical applications of circulating tumor cells and circulating tumor DNA as liquid biopsy. Cancer Discov. 2016; 6: 479–91.
[20] He S, Li P, Long T, Zhang N, Fang J, Yu Z. Detection of circulating tumour cells with the CellSearch system in patients with advanced-stage head and neck cancer: preliminary results. J Laryngol Otol. 2013; 127: 788–93.
[21] Nichols AC, Lowes LE, Szeto CC, Basmaji J, Dhaliwal S, Chapeskie C, Todorovic B, Read N, Venkatesan V, Hammond A, Palma DA, Winquist E, Ernst S, Fung K, Franklin JH, Yoo J, Koropatnick J, Mymryk JS, Barrett JW, Allan AL. Detection of circulating tumor cells in advanced head and neck cancer using the CellSearch system. Head Neck. 2012; 34: 1440–4.
[22] Buglione M, Grisanti S, Almici C, Mangoni M, Polli C, Consoli F, Verardi R, Costa L, Paiar F, Pasinetti N, Bolzoni A, Marini M, Simoncini E, Nicolai P, Biti G, Magrini SM. Circulating tumour cells in locally advanced head and neck cancer: preliminary report about their possible role in predicting response to non-surgical treatment and survival. Eur J Cancer. 2012; 48: 3019–26.
[23] Grobe A, Blessmann M, Hanken H, Friedrich RE, Schon G, Wikner J, Effenberger KE, Kluwe L, Heiland M, Pantel K, Riethdorf S. Prognostic relevance of circulating tumor cells in blood and disseminated tumor cells in bone marrow of patients with squamous cell carcinoma of the oral cavity. Clin Cancer Res. 2014; 20: 425–33.
[24] Jatana KR, Lang JC, Chalmers JJ. Identification of circulating tumor cells: a prognostic marker in squamous cell carcinoma of the head

and neck? Future Oncol. 2011; 7: 481−4.

[25] Bonner JA, Harari PM, Giralt J, Azarnia N, Shin DM, Cohen RB, Jones CU, Sur R, Raben D, Jassem J, Ove R, Kies MS, Baselga J, Youssoufian H, Amellal N, Rowinsky EK, Ang KK. Radiotherapy plus cetuximab for squamous-cell carcinoma of the head and neck. N Engl J Med. 2006; 354: 567−78.

[26] Vermorken JB, Mesia R, Rivera F, Remenar E, Kawecki A, Rottey S, Erfan J, Zabolotnyy D, Kienzer HR, Cupissol D, Peyrade F, Benasso M, Vynnychenko I, De Raucourt D, Bokemeyer C, Schueler A, Amellal N, Hitt R. Platinum-based chemotherapy plus cetuximab in head and neck cancer. N Engl J Med. 2008; 359: 1116−27.

[27] Tinhofer I, Hristozova T, Stromberger C, Keilhoiz U, Budach V. Monitoring of circulating tumor cells and their expression of EGFR/phospho-EGFR during combined radiotherapy regimens in locally advanced squamous cell carcinoma of the head and neck. Int J Radiat Oncol Biol Phys. 2012; 83: e685−90.

[28] Braig F, Voigtlaender M, Schieferdecker A, Busch CJ, Laban S, Grob T, Kriegs M, Knecht R, Bokemeyer C, Binder M. Liquid biopsy monitoring uncovers acquired RAS-mediated resistance to cetuximab in a substantial proportion of patients with head and neck squamous cell carcinoma. Oncotarget. 2016; 7: 42988−95.

[29] Baumeister SH, Freeman GJ, Dranoff G, Sharpe AH. Coinhibitory pathways in immunotherapy for Cancer. Annu Rev Immunol. 2016; 34: 539−73.

[30] Butt AQ, Mills KH. Immunosuppressive networks and checkpoints controlling antitumor immunity and their blockade in the development of cancer immunotherapeutics and vaccines. Oncogene. 2014; 33: 4623−31.

[31] Mazel M, Jacot W, Pantel K, Bartkowiak K, Topart D, Cayrefourcq L, Rossille D, Maudelonde T, Fest T, Alix-Panabieres C. Frequent expression of PD-L1 on circulating breast cancer cells. Mol Oncol. 2015; 9: 1773−82.

[32] Boffa DJ, Graf RP, Salazar MC, Hoag J, Lu D, Krupa R, Louw J, Dugan L, Wang Y, Landers M, Suraneni M, Greene SB, Magana M, Makani S, Bazhenova L, Dittamore RV, Nieva J. Cellular expression of PD-L1 in the peripheral blood of lung cancer patients is associated with worse survival. Cancer Epidemiol Biomark Prev. 2017; 26: 1139−45.

[33] Anantharaman A, Friedlander T, Lu D, Krupa R, Premasekharan G, Hough J, Edwards M, Paz R, Lindquist K, Graf R, Jendrisak A, Louw J, Dugan L, Baird S, Wang Y, Dittamore R, Paris PL. Programmed death-ligand 1 (PD-L1) characterization of circulating tumor cells (CTCs) in muscle invasive and metastatic bladder cancer patients. BMC Cancer. 2016; 16: 744.

[34] Satelli A, Batth IS, Brownlee Z, Rojas C, Meng QH, Kopetz S, Li S. Potential role of nuclear PD-L1 expression in cell-surface vimentin positive circulating tumor cells as a prognostic marker in cancer patients. Sci Rep. 2016; 6: 28910.

[35] Strati A, Koutsodontis G, Papaxoinis G, Angelidis I, Zavridou M, Economopoulou P, Kotsantis I, Avgeris M, Mazel M, Perisanidis C, Sasaki C, Alix-Panabieres C, Lianidou E, Psyrri A. Prognostic significance of PD-L1 expression on circulating tumor cells in patients with head and neck squamous cell carcinoma. Ann Oncol. 2017; 28: 1923−33.

[36] Oliveira-Costa JP, de Carvalho AF, da Silveira da GG, Amaya P, Wu Y, Park KJ, Gigliola MP, Lustberg M, Buim ME, Ferreira EN, Kowalski LP, Chalmers JJ, Soares FA, Carraro DM, Ribeiro-Silva A. Gene expression patterns through oral squamous cell carcinoma development: PD-L1 expression in primary tumor and circulating tumor cells. Oncotarget. 2015; 6: 20902−20.

[37] Kulasinghe A, Perry C, Kenny L, Warkiani ME, Nelson C, Punyadeera C. PD-L1 expressing circulating tumour cells in head and neck cancers. BMC Cancer. 2017; 17: 333.

[38] Riethdorf S, Fritsche H, Muller V, Rau T, Schindlbeck C, Rack B, Janni W, Coith C, Beck K, Janicke F, Jackson S, Gornet T, Cristofanilli M, Pantel K. Detection of circulating tumor cells in peripheral blood of patients with metastatic breast cancer: a validation study of the CellSearch system. Clin Cancer Res. 2007; 13: 920−8.

[39] Haber DA, Velculescu VE. Blood-based analyses of cancer: circulating tumor cells and circulating tumor DNA. Cancer Discov. 2014; 4: 650−61.

[40] Dawson SJ, Tsui DW, Murtaza M, Biggs H, Rueda OM, Chin SF, Dunning MJ, Gale D, Forshew T, Mahler-Araujo B, Rajan S, Humphray S, Becq J, Halsall D, Wallis M, Bentley D, Caldas C, Rosenfeld N. Analysis of circulating tumor DNA to monitor metastatic breast cancer. N Engl J Med. 2013; 368: 1199−209.

[41] Wang WY, Twu CW, Chen HH, Jan JS, Jiang RS, Chao JY, Liang KL, Chen KW, Wu CT, Lin JC. Plasma EBV DNA clearance rate as a novel prognostic marker for metastatic/recurrent nasopharyngeal carcinoma. Clin Cancer Res. 2010; 16: 1016−24.

[42] Reinert T, Scholer LV, Thomsen R, Tobiasen H, Vang S, Nordentoft I, Lamy P, Kannerup AS, Mortensen FV, Stribolt K, Hamilton-Dutoit S, Nielsen HJ, Laurberg S, Pallisgaard N, Pedersen JS, Orntoft TF, Andersen CL. Analysis of circulating tumour DNA to monitor disease burden following colorectal cancer surgery. Gut. 2016; 65: 625−34.

[43] Tie J, Wang Y, Tomasetti C, Li L, Springer S, Kinde I, Silliman N, Tacey M, Wong HL, Christie M, Kosmider S, Skinner I, Wong R, Steel M, Tran B, Desai J, Jones I, Haydon A, Hayes T, Price TJ, Strausberg RL, Diaz LA Jr, Papadopoulos N, Kinzler KW, Vogelstein B, Gibbs P. Circulating tumor DNA analysis detects minimal residual disease and predicts recurrence in patients with stage II colon cancer. Sci Transl Med. 2016; 8: 346ra92.

[44] Garcia-Murillas I, Schiavon G, Weigelt B, Ng C, Hrebien S, Cutts RJ, Cheang M, Osin P, Nerurkar A, Kozarewa I, Garrido JA, Dowsett M, Reis-Filho JS, Smith IE, Turner NC. Mutation tracking in circulating tumor DNA predicts relapse in early breast cancer. Sci Transl Med. 2015; 7: 302ra133.

[45] Lebofsky R, Decraene C, Bernard V, Kamal M, Blin A, Leroy Q, Rio Frio T, Pierron G, Callens C, Bieche I, Saliou A, Madic J, Rouleau E, Bidard FC, Lantz O, Stern MH, Le Tourneau C, Pierga JY. Circulating tumor DNA as a non-invasive substitute to metastasis biopsy for tumor genotyping and personalized medicine in a prospective trial across all tumor types. Mol Oncol. 2015; 9: 783−90.

[46] Groot Koerkamp B, Rahbari NN, Buchler MW, Koch M, Weitz J. Circulating tumor cells and prognosis of patients with resectable colorectal liver metastases or widespread metastatic colorectal cancer: a meta-analysis. Ann Surg Oncol. 2013; 20: 2156–65.

[47] Ma X, Xiao Z, Li X, Wang F, Zhang J, Zhou R, Wang J, Liu L. Prognostic role of circulating tumor cells and disseminated tumor cells in patients with prostate cancer: a systematic review and meta-analysis. Tumour Biol. 2014; 35: 5551–60.

[48] Wang S, Zheng G, Cheng B, Chen F, Wang Z, Chen Y, Wang Y, Xiong B. Circulating tumor cells (CTCs) detected by RT-PCR and its prognostic role in gastric cancer: a meta-analysis of published literature. PLoS One. 2014; 9: e99259.

[49] Jatana KR, Balasubramanian P, Lang JC, Yang L, Jatana CA, White E, Agrawal A, Ozer E, Schuller DE, Teknos TN, Chalmers JJ. Significance of circulating tumor cells in patients with squamous cell carcinoma of the head and neck: initial results. Arch Otolaryngol Head Neck Surg. 2010; 136: 1274–9.

[50] Kulasinghe A, Perry C, Jovanovic L, Nelson C, Punyadeera C. Circulating tumour cells in metastatic head and neck cancers. Int J Cancer. 2015; 136: 2515–23.

[51] Hristozova T, Konschak R, Stromberger C, Fusi A, Liu Z, Weichert W, Stenzinger A, Budach V, Keilholz U, Tinhofer I. The presence of circulating tumor cells (CTCs) correlates with lymph node metastasis in nonresectable squamous cell carcinoma of the head and neck region (SCCHN). Ann Oncol. 2011; 22: 1878–85.

[52] Toss A, Mu Z, Fernandez S. Cristofanilli M. CTC enumeration and characterization: moving toward personalized medicine. Ann Transl Med. 2014; 2: 108.

[53] de Albuquerque A, Kaul S, Breier G, Krabisch P, Fersis N. Multimarker analysis of circulating tumor cells in peripheral blood of metastatic breast cancer patients: a step forward in personalized medicine. Breast Care (Basel). 2012; 7: 7–12.

[54] Simons M, Raposo G. Exosomes — vesicular carriers for intercellular communication. Curr Opin Cell Biol. 2009; 21: 575–81.

[55] Chen X, Liang H, Zhang J, Zen K, Zhang CY. Secreted microRNAs: a new form of intercellular communication. Trends Cell Biol. 2012; 22: 125–32.

[56] Mitchell PS, Parkin RK, Kroh EM, Fritz BR, Wyman SK, Pogosova-Agadjanyan EL, Peterson A, Noteboom J, O'Briant KC, Allen A, Lin DW, Urban N, Drescher CW, Knudsen BS, Stirewalt DL, Gentleman R, Vessella RL, Nelson PS, Martin DB, Tewari M. Circulating microRNAs as stable blood-based markers for cancer detection. Proc Natl Acad Sci U S A. 2008; 105: 10513–8.

[57] Rosenfeld N, Aharonov R, Meiri E, Rosenwald S, Spector Y, Zepeniuk M, Benjamin H, Shabes N, Tabak S, Levy A, Lebanony D, Goren Y, Silberschein E, Targan N, Ben-Ari A, Gilad S, Sion-Vardy N, Tobar A, Feinmesser M, Kharenko O, Nativ O, Nass D, Perelman M, Yosepovich A, Shalmon B, Polak-Charcon S, Fridman E, Avniel A, Bentwich I, Bentwich Z, Cohen D, Chajut A, Barshack I. MicroRNAs accurately identify cancer tissue origin. Nat Biotechnol. 2008; 26: 462–9.

[58] Rabinowits G, Gercel-Taylor C, Day JM, Taylor DD, Kloecker GH. Exosomal microRNA: a diagnostic marker for lung cancer. Clin Lung Cancer. 2009; 10: 42–6.

[59] Skog J, Wurdinger T, van Rijn S, Meijer DH, Gainche L, Sena-Esteves M, Curry WT Jr, Carter BS, Krichevsky AM, Breakefield XO. Glioblastoma microvesicles transport RNA and proteins that promote tumour growth and provide diagnostic biomarkers. Nat Cell Biol. 2008; 10: 1470–6.

[60] Taylor DD, Gercel-Taylor C. MicroRNA signatures of tumor-derived exosomes as diagnostic biomarkers of ovarian cancer. Gynecol Oncol. 2008; 110: 13–21.

[61] Summerer I, Unger K, Braselmann H, Schuettrumpf L, Maihoefer C, Baumeister P, Kirchner T, Niyazi M, Sage E, Specht HM, Multhoff G, Moertl S, Belka C, Zitzelsberger H. Circulating microRNAs as prognostic therapy biomarkers in head and neck cancer patients. Br J Cancer. 2015; 113: 76–82.

[62] Hsu CM, Lin PM, Wang YM, Chen ZJ, Lin SF, Yang MY. Circulating miRNA is a novel marker for head and neck squamous cell carcinoma. Tumour Biol. 2012; 33: 1933–42.

[63] Liu CJ, Kao SY, Tu HF, Tsai MM, Chang KW, Lin SC. Increase of microRNA miR-31 level in plasma could be a potential marker of oral cancer. Oral Dis. 2010; 16: 360–4.

[64] Yan Y, Wang X, Veno MT, Bakholdt V, Sorensen JA, Krogdahl A, Sun Z, Gao S, Kjems J. Circulating miRNAs as biomarkers for oral squamous cell carcinoma recurrence in operated patients. Oncotarget. 2017; 8: 8206–14.

[65] Russo F, Di Bella S, Vannini F, Berti G, Scoyni F, Cook HV, Santos A, Nigita G, Bonnici V, Lagana A, Geraci F, Pulvirenti A, Giugno R, De Masi F, Belling K, Jensen LJ, Brunak S, Pellegrini M, Ferro A. miRandola 2017: a curated knowledge base of non-invasive biomarkers. Nucleic Acids Res. 2018; 46: D354–D9.

[66] Ono S, Lam S, Nagahara M, Hoon DS. Circulating microRNA biomarkers as liquid biopsy for cancer patients: Pros and Cons of current assays. J Clin Med. 2015; 4: 1890–907.

[67] Pritchard CC, Kroh E, Wood B, Arroyo JD, Dougherty KJ, Miyaji MM, Tait JF, Tewari M. Blood cell origin of circulating microRNAs: a cautionary note for cancer biomarker studies. Cancer Prev Res (Phila). 2012; 5: 492–7.

[68] Nonaka T, Wong DTW. Saliva-Exosomics in cancer: molecular characterization of cancer-derived exosomes in saliva. Enzyme. 2017; 42: 125–51.

[69] Bandhakavi S, Stone MD, Onsongo G, Van Riper SK. Griffin TJ. A dynamic range compression and three-dimensional peptide fractionation analysis platform expands proteome coverage and the diagnostic potential of whole saliva. J Proteome Res. 2009; 8: 5590–600.

[70] Yan W, Apweiler R, Balgley BM, Boontheung P, Bundy JL, Cargile BJ, Cole S, Fang X, Gonzalez-Begne M, Griffin TJ, Hagen F, Hu S, Wolinsky LE, Lee CS, Malamud D, Melvin JE, Menon R, Mueller M, Qiao R, Rhodus NL, Sevinsky JR, States D, Stephenson JL, Than

S, Yates JR, Yu W, Xie H, Xie Y, Omenn GS, Loo JA, Wong DT. Systematic comparison of the human saliva and plasma proteomes. Proteomics Clin Appl. 2009; 3: 116–34.

[71] Rylander-Rudqvist T, Hakansson N, Tybring G, Wolk A. Quality and quantity of saliva DNA obtained from the self-administered oragene method — a pilot study on the cohort of Swedish men. Cancer Epidemiol Biomark Prev. 2006; 15: 1742–5.

[72] Qureishi A, Ali M, Fraser L, Shah KA, Moller H, Winter S. Saliva testing for human papilloma virus in oropharyngeal squamous cell carcinoma: a diagnostic accuracy study. Clin Otolaryngol. 2018; 43: 151–7.

[73] Martin-Gomez L, Giuliano AR, Fulp WJ, Caudell J, Echevarria M, Sirak B, Abrahamsen M, Isaacs-Soriano KA, Hernandez-Prera JC, Wenig BM, Vorwald K, McMullen CP, Wadsworth JT, Slebos RJ, Chung CH. Human papillomavirus genotype detection in oral gargle samples among men with newly diagnosed oropharyngeal squamous cell carcinoma. JAMA Otolaryngol Head Neck Surg. 2019; 145: 460.

[74] Ahn SM, Chan JY, Zhang Z, Wang H, Khan Z, Bishop JA, Westra W, Koch WM, Califano JA. Saliva and plasma quantitative polymerase chain reaction-based detection and surveillance of human papillomavirus-related head and neck cancer. JAMA Otolaryngol Head Neck Surg. 2014; 140: 846–54.

[75] Rettig EM, Wentz A, Posner MR, Gross ND, Haddad RI, Gillison ML, Fakhry C, Quon H, Sikora AG, Stott WJ, Lorch JH, Gourin CG, Guo Y, Xiao W, Miles BA, Richmon JD, Andersen PE, Misiukiewicz KJ, Chung CH, Gerber JE, Rajan SD, D'Souza G. Prognostic implication of persistent human papillomavirus type 16 DNA detection in oral rinses for human papillomavirus-related oropharyngeal carcinoma. JAMA Oncol. 2015; 1: 907–15.

[76] Park NJ, Zhou H, Elashoff D, Henson BS, Kastratovic DA, Abemayor E, Wong DT. Salivary microRNA: discovery, characterization, and clinical utility for oral cancer detection. Clin Cancer Res. 2009; 15: 5473–7.

[77] Gallo A, Tandon M, Alevizos I, Illei GG. The majority of microRNAs detectable in serum and saliva is concentrated in exosomes. PLoS One. 2012; 7: e30679.

[78] Michael A, Bajracharya SD, Yuen PS, Zhou H, Star RA, Illei GG, Alevizos I. Exosomes from human saliva as a source of microRNA biomarkers. Oral Dis. 2010; 16: 34–8.

[79] Duz MB, Karatas OF, Guzel E, Turgut NF, Yilmaz M, Creighton CJ, Ozen M. Identification of miR-139-5p as a saliva biomarker for tongue squamous cell carcinoma: a pilot study. Cell Oncol (Dordr). 2016; 39: 187–93.

[80] Wiklund ED, Gao S, Hulf T, Sibbritt T, Nair S, Costea DE, Villadsen SB, Bakholdt V, Bramsen JB, Sorensen JA, Krogdahl A, Clark SJ, Kjems J. MicroRNA alterations and associated aberrant DNA methylation patterns across multiple sample types in oral squamous cell carcinoma. PLoS One. 2011; 6: e27840.

[81] Liu CJ, Lin SC, Yang CC, Cheng HW, Chang KW. Exploiting salivary miR-31 as a clinical biomarker of oral squamous cell carcinoma. Head Neck. 2012; 34: 219–24.

[82] Momen-Heravi F, Trachtenberg AJ, Kuo WP, Cheng YS. Genomewide study of salivary microRNAs for detection of oral cancer. J Dent Res. 2014; 93: 86S–93S.

[83] Gonzalez-Begne M, Lu B, Han X, Hagen FK, Hand AR, Melvin JE, Yates JR. Proteomic analysis of human parotid gland exosomes by multidimensional protein identification technology (MudPIT). J Proteome Res. 2009; 8: 1304–14.

[84] Ogawa Y, Miura Y, Harazono A, Kanai-Azuma M, Akimoto Y, Kawakami H, Yamaguchi T, Toda T, Endo T, Tsubuki M, Yanoshita R. Proteomic analysis of two types of exosomes in human whole saliva. Biol Pharm Bull. 2011; 34: 13–23.

[85] Kalra H, Simpson RJ, Ji H, Aikawa E, Altevogt P, Askenase P, Bond VC, Borras FE, Breakefield X, Budnik V, Buzas E, Camussi G, Clayton A, Cocucci E, Falcon-Perez JM, Gabrielsson S, Gho YS, Gupta D, Harsha HC, Hendrix A, Hill AF, Inal JM, Jenster G, Kramer-Albers EM, Lim SK, Llorente A, Lotvall J, Marcilla A, Mincheva-Nilsson L, Nazarenko I, Nieuwland R, Nolte-'t Hoen EN, Pandey A, Patel T, Piper MG, Pluchino S, Prasad TS, Rajendran L, Raposo G, Record M, Reid GE, Sanchez-Madrid F, Schiffelers RM, Siljander P, Stensballe A, Stoorvogel W, Taylor D, Thery C, Valadi H, van Balkom BW, Vazquez J, Vidal M, Wauben MH, Yanez-Mo M, Zoeller M, Mathivanan S. Vesiclepedia: a compendium for extracellular vesicles with continuous community annotation. PLoS Biol. 2012; 10: e1001450.

[86] Simpson RJ, Kalra H, Mathivanan S. ExoCarta as a resource for exosomal research. J Extracell Vesicles. 2012: 1.

[87] Cheng J, Nonaka T, Wong DTW. Salivary exosomes as nanocarriers for cancer biomarker delivery. Materials (Basel). 2019; 12: 654.

[88] Palanisamy V, Sharma S, Deshpande A, Zhou H, Gimzewski J, Wong DT. Nanostructural and transcriptomic analyses of human saliva derived exosomes. PLoS One. 2010; 5: e8577.

[89] Sharma S, Rasool HI, Palanisamy V, Mathisen C, Schmidt M, Wong DT, Gimzewski JK. Structural-mechanical characterization of nanoparticle exosomes in human saliva, using correlative AFM, FESEM, and force spectroscopy. ACS Nano. 2010; 4: 1921–6.

[90] Sharma S, Gillespie BM, Palanisamy V, Gimzewski JK. Quantitative nanostructural and single-molecule force spectroscopy biomolecular analysis of human-saliva-derived exosomes. Langmuir. 2011; 27: 14394–400.

[91] Pu D, Liang H, Wei F, Akin D, Feng Z, Yan Q, Li Y, Zhen Y, Xu L, Dong G, Wan H, Dong J, Qiu X, Qin C, Zhu D, Wang X, Sun T, Zhang W, Li C, Tang X, Qiao Y, Wong DT, Zhou Q. Evaluation of a novel saliva-based epidermal growth factor receptor mutation detection for lung cancer: a pilot study. Thorac Cancer. 2016; 7: 428–36.

[92] Tu M, Wei F, Yang J, Wong D. Detection of exosomal biomarker by electric field-induced release and measurement (EFIRM). J Vis Exp. 2015: 52439.

[93] Wei F, Lin CC, Joon A, Feng Z, Troche G, Lira ME, Chia D, Mao M, Ho CL, Su WC, Wong DT. Noninvasive saliva-based EGFR gene mutation detection in patients with lung cancer. Am J Respir Crit Care Med. 2014; 190: 1117–26.

第 7 章

Zhong Chen, Ramya Viswanathan, Ethan L. Morgan, Jun Jeon, and Carter Van Waes

头颈癌中的促炎信号通路和基因组特征

Proinflammatory Signaling Pathways and Genomic Signatures in Head and Neck Cancers

引 言

炎症和免疫反应的失调已被观察到并被认为在癌症的发病机制和治疗抵抗中起着重要作用，包括头颈癌（HNC）。在头颈癌中，头颈鳞状细胞癌（HNSCC）是最主要的病理类型，占大约90%，并且是研究最广泛的。HNSCC和其他病理亚型的头颈癌异常表达一系列细胞因子、趋化因子和可溶性因子，这些因子促进肿瘤细胞的生长、生存、迁移，以及肿瘤微环境（TME）中的炎症和血管生成反应，从而促进肿瘤发生。在这些因子中，肿瘤细胞表达的白细胞介素-1（IL-1）和免疫细胞及其他细胞在TME中表达的肿瘤坏死因子（TNF）诱导NF-κB的激活，NF-κB是调节细胞因子表达、肿瘤恶性生物学表型及免疫失调反应的一组转录因子。对HNSCC和其他头颈癌的信号通路和基因组改变的剖析显示，许多这些通路汇聚于NF-κB以及其他调节多基因和恶性表型特征的转录因子，从而识别出感兴趣的通路。蛋白质泛素化和蛋白酶体在调节NF-κB中起关键作用，并且是基因组或其他改变的目标之一，因此可能是潜在的治疗靶点。癌症基因组图谱（TCGA）和细胞系库及患者来源的异种移植模型的基因组特征已识别出影响这些通路的几个关键、反复出现的改变，这些改变可以启用机制和临床前研究以识别新的治疗靶点。功能基因组学使用RNAi、CRISPR和药物库可以与这些发现整合，以识别代表治疗关键靶点的驱动因子和介质。在本章中，我们总结了HNSCC的发现历史和当前进展，重点关注促炎信号通路和基因组特征。主题包括：① 促炎细胞因子、趋化因子和生长因子的网络，重点关注它们在HNSCC发病机制中的作用、共表达模式、临床相关性和治疗潜力；② NF-κB信号传导及其与其他通路的交叉以及相关的当前生物标志物识别和药物开发；③ 通过泛素化调节炎症信号传导，与基因组改变和转录组表达的关联，以及药物发现的最新进展；④ 促炎和其他信号分子的基因组特征和转录组景观，包括HNSCC TCGA和Pan TCGA项目的概述、人类细胞系的高通量特征描述，以及全基因组基因活动和功能分析。尖端实验技术的进步，如高通量测序、单

Z. Chen (✉) · R. Viswanathan · E. L. Morgan · J. Jeon · C. Van Waes (✉)
Tumor Biology Section, Head and Neck Surgery Branch, National Institute on Deafness and Other Communication Disorders, National Institutes of Health, Bethesda, MD, USA
e-mail: chenz@nidcd.nih.gov; vanwaesc@nidcd.nih.gov

细胞亚群分析、多重染色和成像，加上大数据采集、计算管道和生物信息学能力，使我们能够以前所未有的规模和深度精确理解和构建 HNSCC 的分子图谱。癌症的全面特征描述显著影响了如何以分子亚型将 HNSCC 分类，并改变了我们对患者诊断、预后和治疗的临床实践。

促炎细胞因子、趋化因子和生长因子的网络

恶性细胞和基质细胞分泌的细胞因子、趋化因子及其他可溶性因子在 TME 中发挥着关键作用，促进细胞生长、生存、炎症、迁移、血管生成、治疗抵抗及其他复杂的相互作用[1-4]（图7-1）。这些因子通过局部和全身环境中的促炎信号传导，影响头颈癌的表型。本节总结了这些因子在头颈癌发展、预后和治疗反应中的作用，这可能有助于研究人员阐明可能与现有靶向和免疫疗法协同作用的潜在靶点。

白细胞介素、趋化因子和生长因子在头颈癌发病机制中的作用

能够传递炎症信号的可溶性因子包括多种不同类别的信号分子，这些分子是由 TME 中的免疫细胞、基质细胞和上皮细胞分泌和使用的小型蛋白质，用于调节免疫和炎症反应。由于同一信号分子的受体可能位于 TME 的不同区域，理解它们在肿瘤和免疫细胞群体中的平行和重叠的下

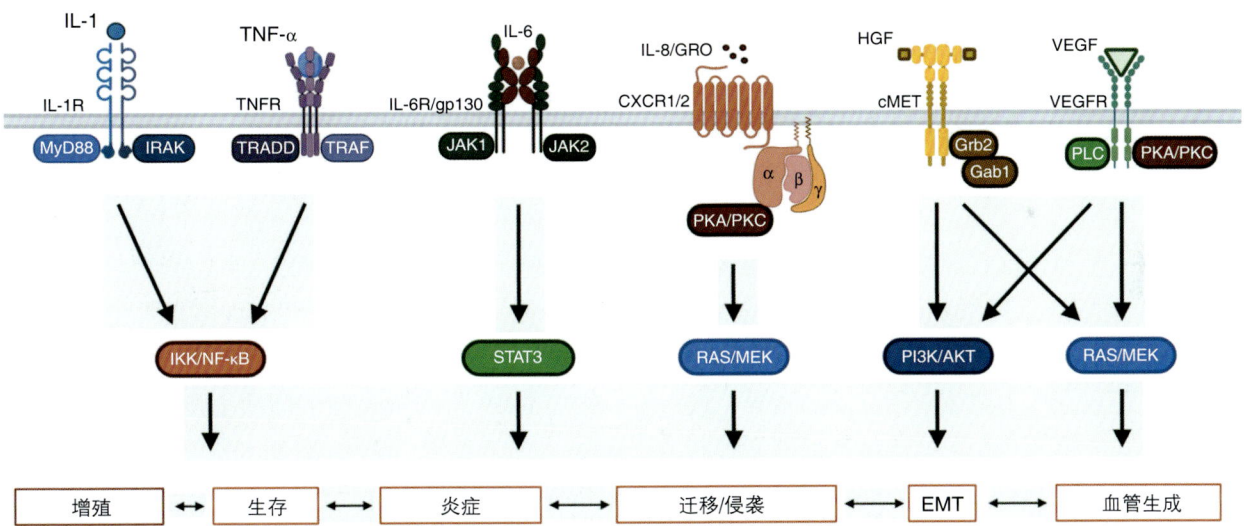

图 7-1　头颈鳞状细胞癌（HNSCC）中促炎和促血管生成的细胞因子、趋化因子和生长因子的网络。这些因子由肿瘤微环境中的癌细胞、炎症细胞或基质细胞产生。它们的受体具有独特的细胞外结构域用于配体结合，以及细胞内结构域用于信号传导。具体来说，白细胞介素-1α 或白细胞介素-1β 与白细胞介素-1 受体（IL-1R1）的细胞外免疫球蛋白结构域结合，通过 MyD88 和 IRAK 传导细胞内信号，激活 IKK 和 NF-κB 通路。肿瘤坏死因子 α（TNF-α）与三聚体 TNF 受体（TNFR）结合，通过 TRADD 和 TRAF 介导的受体死亡域（DD）传导信号。白细胞介素-6 受体（IL-6R）的多聚结构由与 gp130 复合的 IL-6R 链组成，通过 JAK1/2 介导信号传导并激活 STAT3 通路。白细胞介素-8（IL-8）或 GRO 与 CXCR1/2 结合，这些是七跨膜 G 蛋白偶联受体（Gα、Gβ、Gγ），通过蛋白激酶 A 和蛋白激酶 C（PKA/C）介导信号传导以激活 RAS/MEK 通路。肝细胞生长因子（HGF）与 c-MET 结合，通过适配蛋白 Gab1 和 Grb2 介导下游信号，激活 PI3K/AKT 和 RAS/MEK 通路。血管内皮生长因子（VEGF）与 VEGFR 结合，形成受体二聚体，然后激活磷脂酶 C（PLC）和 PKA/C，通过 RAS/MEK 和 PI3K/AKT 通路介导信号传导。这些信号通路的激活共同促进了 HNSCC 的肿瘤发生，包括增强细胞增殖、生存、炎症、迁移、侵袭、上皮-间质转化（EMT）和血管生成（图由 BioRender.com 制作）

游效应对于多靶点治疗具有重要意义。值得注意的是炎症和生长介质相关的蛋白家族，包括白细胞介素（IL）细胞因子、肿瘤坏死因子（TNF）、趋化因子和生长因子受体酪氨酸激酶家族的成员（图7-1）。在TME中，这些因子、通路和介质通过促进癌细胞增殖、生存、迁移、炎症、抗肿瘤免疫和血管生成，在癌症发病机制和根除之间的平衡中发挥关键作用[5]。

IL-1家族是癌症免疫和炎症的关键调节剂，能够直接或间接促进肿瘤的炎症反应、转移和血管生成。IL-1α/β及其通过1型IL-1受体（IL-1R）的相互作用在癌症中的作用已被广泛研究[6]。IL-1信号通过IL-1R辅佐蛋白和适配蛋白MyD88的募集至受体复合物而启动，这导致下游的促炎效应通路的激活，例如IKK和NF-κB通路[7]。已知内皮细胞中的IL-1R可以触发NF-κB非依赖性通路分子，例如MYD88-ARNO-ARF6级联反应，以破坏炎症性疾病模型中的血管稳定性，这在肿瘤发生中也可能具有重要意义[8]。IL-1可能由HNSCC细胞和招募至TME的免疫细胞表达。我们的早期研究表明，IL-1-IL1R-IKK-NF-κB信号轴异常活跃，并在两个鳞状细胞癌（SCC）小鼠模型中对肿瘤发生和转移有贡献[9-12]，这与患者血清和肿瘤样本中的水平增加一致。TNF-α和TNF相关的凋亡诱导配体（TRAIL）是另一类细胞因子家族，可以在压力或放射治疗下被诱导，或由T淋巴细胞产生，并在不同情境下促进癌细胞的生存或死亡[13-17]。TNF结合TNF家族受体，可以诱导IKK-NF-κB和促生存基因，或通过胱天蛋白酶介导的细胞死亡[18]。我们证明，NF-κB和IL-1及TNF下游的其他转录共因子反应元件普遍存在，并调节包括IL-6、IL-8、IL-8同源生长调节基因-α（GRO-α），粒细胞-巨噬细胞集落刺激因子（GM-CSF）和血管内皮生长因子（VEGF）在内的多种促炎和促血管生成的细胞因子的表达。大量研究证实这些细胞因子和生长因子与癌症密切相关。从生物学上看，IL-6能够通过各种下游途径启动其活动[19-21]，并被认为促进增殖、EMT和促肿瘤炎症反应[11,20,21]。

几种被归类为趋化因子的细胞因子与肿瘤细胞恶性生物学行为相关[22]。对于GRO-α和IL-8等因子，其下游机制及其对HNSCC表型的促进作用已被阐明[23,24]。GRO-α或CXCL1主要通过G蛋白偶联受体CXCR2发挥作用，调节肿瘤的生存和扩散，其作用机制涉及PI3K/AKT/mTOR、RAS/RAF/MEK/ERK和NF-κB通路[10,24-27]。IL-8或CXCL8是一种与CXCR1和CXCR2结合的白细胞介素。证据表明，IL-8的表达在HNSCC中增加的同时，还受IL-1α、表皮生长因子受体（EGFR）拮抗剂和肝细胞生长因子（HGF）等其他因素的影响[17,25,26,28]。从机制上看，IL-8的效应在一定程度上依赖于CXCR1/2介导的NOD1/RIP2和NF-κB信号通路[23]。

主要因其在刺激生长和血管生成中的作用而知名的因子，如VEGF、HGF和GM-CSF，也在各种HNSCC细胞系和模型中被观察到[9,12,14,25,26,28-30]。VEGF是促进肿瘤生长的最著名的血管生成因子之一[31]。HNSCC细胞表达VEGF受体（VEGFR）1、2和3，这些受体各自有不同的VEGF家族配体偏好和亲和力，并激活不同的下游信号通路，最终促成血管生成[32,33]。HGF是一种生长因子，调节许多正常生理过程，如组织生长、重塑、迁移、再生和分化。活化形式的HGF与细胞表面的间质上皮转化因子受体（c-Met）结合，激活诸如Src、MAPK和PI3K等细胞内信号级联反应，以增加细胞生存和运动性[34]。c-MET在许多HNSCC病例中过度表达，虽然罕见但其运动域中的突变可以增加肿瘤转移潜力，干扰放射治疗的疗效，并加重肿瘤复发情况[35]。GM-CSF是一种响应免疫激活和炎症信号的生长因子，虽然传统上与调节免疫细胞活动有关，但证据表明它也由TME中的非免疫细胞分泌，以促进癌症发病机制[36]。GM-CSF通过CD116（也称为GM-CSF受体，GMCSFR）发挥作用，它与JAK2激活密切相关，并且下游激活STAT5和MAPK以调节细胞增殖[37,38]。在各种人 HNSCC 肿瘤细胞系中都注意到了 GM-CSF 及其受体的增加表达[39]，并且研究显示在体外和体内 HNSCC 模型中 GM-CSF 能够刺激肿瘤的增殖和迁移[40]。

促炎因子的共同表达与临床相关性

研究表明，HNSCC 的许多促炎介质会共同调节，这对于评估疾病预后和治疗反应具有重要的临床意义。早期对患者血清以及各种人类 HNSCC 细胞系和肿瘤样本的研究显示，关键促炎分子如 IL-1α、IL-6、IL-8、GRO-α、GM-CSF 和 VEGF 的表达增加[14, 15]，这一结果在多个不同的实验室中得到了重复验证[41-44]。因此，某些促炎分子是共同表达和相互调节的，并且评估了将这些标志物作为一个总体进行纵向分析的预后价值。

某些明显的促炎因子模式在 HNSCC 的不同阶段差异明显。在细胞系和小鼠模型中，HNSCC 的恶性阶段与炎症细胞因子特征从癌前病变的转变开始密切相关[45, 46]。有趣的是，存在癌前口腔病变的患者的唾液样本显示出 TNF-α 和 IL-6 水平的增加[47]。最后，与非转移性细胞或正常角质形成细胞相比，一项体外研究中的转移性或复发性病变显示出 IL-6、IL-6R、TGF-β 和 VEGF 的表达增加，而促炎 TNF-α 仅由 Ⅳ 期、转移性或复发来源的细胞系分泌[48]。相应地，HNSCC 对 TNF-α 的耐药性是通过激活 NF-κB 和 BCL-2 及凋亡抑制蛋白（IAP）家族的促生存基因[49, 50]以及失活 TP53/TP63/TP73 肿瘤抑制因子家族实现的[51, 52]。

在临床上，对 HNSCC 患者的平均血清浓度进行分析，结果显示，患者的 IL-6、IL-8、HGF、VEGF 和 GRO-α 水平与匹配的对照组相比有所增加[53]。随后对接受化放疗的 Ⅲ/Ⅳ 期口咽鳞状细胞癌患者进行的为期三年的前瞻性血清研究表明，IL-6、IL-8、VEGF、HGF 和（或）GRO-α 水平的增加预示着特异性病因生存率的降低，而较高的基线 VEGF 水平与生存率的增加相关[13]。最近的研究显示，正在接受化放疗的新确诊、可治愈的 HNSCC 患者在治疗后 7 周时，其 IL-1β、IL-6 和 IL-10 水平相比于治疗前显著增加[54]。

基于细胞因子和趋化因子的治疗方案及其潜力

迄今为止讨论的许多促炎因子与 HNSCC 的发病机制密切相关，已经探索了几种策略来抑制这些因子在 HNSCC 中经常引发的致癌途径和反应。IL-1 信号在 HNSCC 细胞中起到使肿瘤细胞对 EGFR 抑制剂厄洛替尼产生耐药的作用[55]。然而，IL-1 也被证明可以增强自然杀伤细胞（NK）和 T 细胞介导的细胞毒性[56, 57]，这是西妥昔单抗促进抗肿瘤活性的机制[58]。因此，IL-1 在癌症中的对立作用使得针对 IL-1 进行治疗的合理性变得复杂。Espinosa-Cotton 等人的一项最新研究表明，重组 IL-1α 在免疫健全的小鼠中诱导了 T 细胞依赖的抗肿瘤活性，并且在接受西妥昔单抗治疗的复发/转移（R/M）HNSCC 患者中，血清 IL-1α 水平升高与良好的无进展生存期（PFS）相关[59]。这表明将 IL-1 与免疫疗法（如抗 PD1 免疫检查点疗法）联合治疗的潜力，但这尚未得到充分研究证实。

研究表明，IL-6 的表达在许多由炎症驱动的状态下会增加，并通过 IL-6 介导的正反馈回路增强 STAT3（信号转导及转录激活因子 3）的活化，从而进一步增加 HNSCC 患者的生存期和治疗抵抗[20, 60-62]。此外，肿瘤浸润性免疫细胞通过 STAT3 在肿瘤和免疫细胞中的活化效应被证明会下调抗肿瘤免疫[63-66]。这些发现显示了靶向 IL-6/STAT3 通路在 HNSCC 中的潜力。靶向 IL-6/JAK/STAT3 通路在各种炎症状态下的人体安全性和耐受性已经得到很好的验证，并且其在包括 HNSCC 在内的实体肿瘤治疗中的应用，正在临床前和临床进行活跃的研究[67]。具体而言，AZD9150，即一种 STAT3 反义寡核苷酸，在一项针对晚期淋巴瘤和非小细胞肺癌的 Ⅰ 期试验中显示出安全且有效的抗肿瘤效果，在研究的患者中实现了 44% 的疾病稳定或部分响应率。值得注意的是，一项临床前研究显示，STAT3 反应元件在 FOS 启动子上的诱饵寡核苷酸通过抑制 STAT3 与 DNA 结合抑制了 HNSCC 肿瘤生长[68]，该研究后来进入了 0 期研究，显示在 HNSCC 肿瘤中 STAT3 依赖性基因表达的减少，而且对患者没有显著毒性影响[69]。最后，结合免疫检查点疗法（ICT）和 IL-6/JAK/STAT3 通路抑制剂在各种癌症[70-72]（包括 HNSCC）中的治疗作用已被研究。目前正在进行的 durvalumab（抗 PD-L1）与 AZD9150 或 AZD5069（抗 CXCR2）用于晚期实体瘤和 R/M HNSCC 的 1b/2 期（SCORES）研究显示，与其他联合或单药治疗组相比，durvalumab 与 AZD9150 的结合组具有更高的抗肿瘤活性[73]。

最近，人们对靶向趋化因子的疗法越来越感兴趣，这些疗法旨在提高免疫检查点疗法的效果。趋化因子如 IL-8 的表达与免疫检查点疗法效果不佳相关，因为 IL-8 可以招募髓源性抑制细胞（MDSC）[74, 75]。一项涉及 1 344 名晚期癌症患者（包括鳞状细胞癌）的大型回顾性分析显示，在四个不同的Ⅲ期临床试验中，血浆中高水平的 IL-8 和肿瘤中性粒细胞浸润与免疫检查点疗法，包括 nivolumab（抗 PD1）和（或）ipilimumab（抗 CTLA4）、everolimus（mTOR 抑制剂），或 docetaxel 的疗效降低相关[74]。单细胞 RNA 测序研究显示，髓系细胞中的高 IL-8 表达与抗原呈递机制的下调有关，而抗原呈递机制对基于 T 细胞的肿瘤细胞毒性至关重要[76]。既往研究表明，MDSC 在肿瘤微环境（TME）中抑制 T 细胞功能，通过使用 SX-682 阻断 CXCR1/2 减少 MDSC 的招募，在小鼠口腔癌模型中增强了 NK 细胞和 T 细胞的免疫治疗效果[77, 78]。

总之，研究表明，促炎细胞因子、生长因子和趋化因子对头颈癌的发病机制具有直接和间接的影响。靶向该系列因子在确定头颈癌的生长、转移、预后和治疗反应监测方面具有潜在的应用价值。对这些因子如何影响致癌信号通路的机制阐明，使得能够与现有治疗方式协同的联合疗法成为可能，而那些增强免疫细胞毒性或减少免疫抑制的因子在补充免疫检查点疗法以治疗 HNSCC 方面显示出不错的潜力。

NF-κB 通路及其与其他信号的交互作用在头颈癌中作用的研究

NF-κB 是一组调节多种细胞过程的蛋白家族，包括细胞生长、凋亡、炎症和免疫反应[79]，并在多种癌症类型的肿瘤发生中发挥关键作用，包括头颈癌、肺癌、乳腺癌、前列腺癌、结肠癌、胃肠道癌、肝癌、胰腺癌和血液系统恶性肿瘤[80-85]。该家族由五个亚基组成，它们在 N 端具有保守的 REL 同源域（RHD）-RELA（p65）、RELB、c-REL、NF-κB1（p105/p50）和 NF-κB2（p100/p52）[79]。RHD 通过 N 端与 DNA 结合，并通过 C 端与 IκB 相互作用。RHD 对于 NF-κB 成员之间的二聚体形成也至关重要，如 RELA/p50、RELB/p52、c-REL/p50、RELA/RELA 和 RELA/c-REL[86, 87]。RELA、c-REL 和 RELB 作为成熟蛋白参与合成，而 p50 和 p52 则分别作为其前体蛋白复合物 p105 和 p100 的一部分参与合成。p105 和 p100 的 C 端含有 IκB 样锚蛋白重复序列，这些序列被磷酸化、泛素化，并被蛋白酶体部分降解，从而分别释放出作用后的单位 p50 和 p52[87, 88]。此外，RELA、c-REL 和 RELB 含有转录激活域（TAD），可以转录激活其靶基因，而缺乏这些 TAD 的 p50 和 p52 则依赖于与其他蛋白的相互作用来抑制或激活转录[89]。

经典和非经典 NF-κB 信号通路

在没有任何刺激的情况下，NF-κB 二聚体留在细胞质中，其核定位信号（NLS）被 IκB 抑制剂隔离。它们的激活通过 IκB 激酶（IKK）介导和通过经典与替代信号通路进行[79, 89, 90]（图 7-2）。

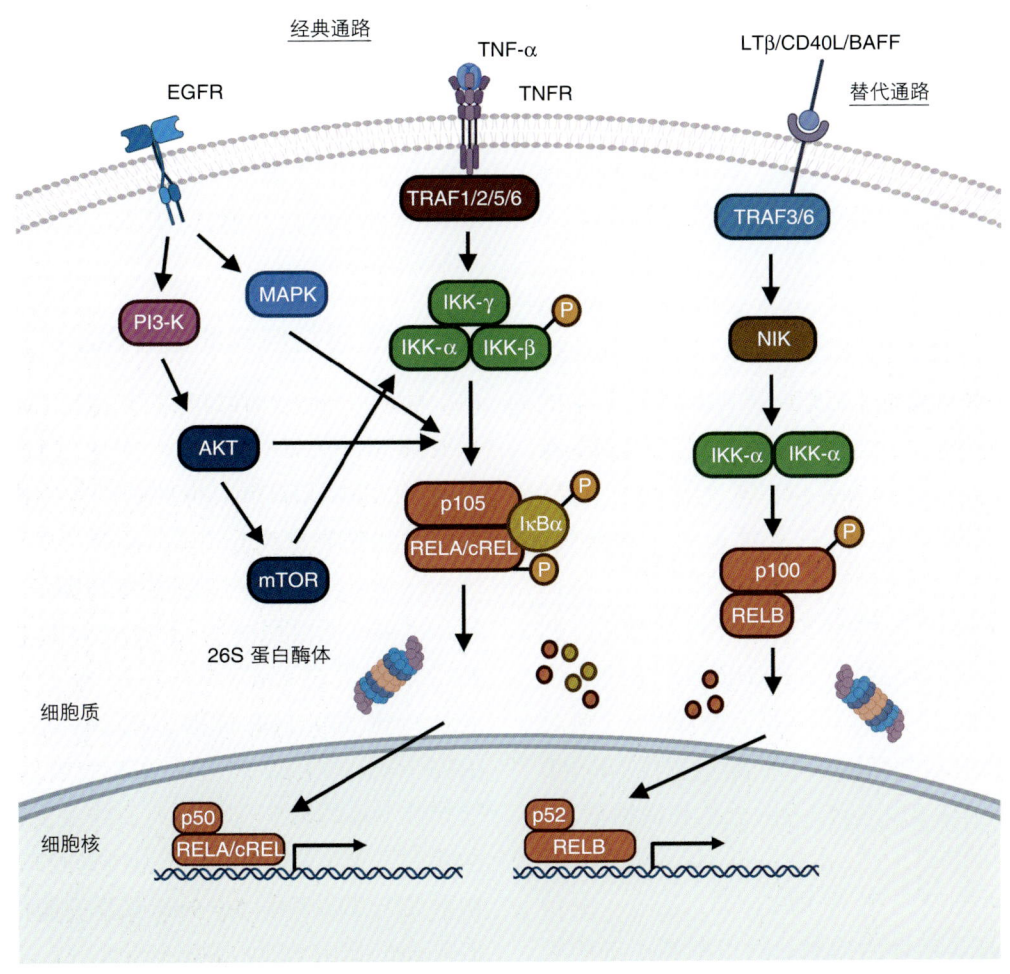

图7-2 经典和替代NF-κB信号通路。NF-κB蛋白用红色表示。经典通路（中间显示）在TNF-α等信号与其受体TNFR结合时被诱导，并由TRAF1/2/5/6介导。这导致IKK-β的磷酸化，IKK-β与IKK-α和调节蛋白IKK-γ（绿色显示）组成复合体，IKK-γ磷酸化IκB并使其被26S蛋白酶体泛素化和降解。IκB的降解和p105的蛋白酶体部分加工生成p50，导致RELA/p50或c-REL/p50二聚体的核转移并激活其靶基因。在替代通路中（右侧显示），LTβ/CD40L/BAFF与其相应受体结合，通过TRAF3/6信号传导激活NIK并激活IKK-α/IKK-α复合体。这导致p100的磷酸化和部分处理以产生p52，而后p52与RELB一起进入细胞核并调节其靶基因。其他与NF-κB信号通路交互的通路包括但不限于EGFR通路和MAPK通路（左侧显示）（图由BioRender.com制作）

经典通路在促炎细胞因子（如TNF-α或IL1）或细菌细胞壁脂多糖（LPS）与TNF受体（TNFR）或Toll样受体（TLR）结合时被激活。这个复合物磷酸化IκB，导致IκB被泛素化并被蛋白酶体降解[91]，从而暴露RELA/p50或c-REL/p50异二聚体的NLS，导致其核转位并激活靶基因（图7-2）。此外，IKK-β和其他激酶在丝氨酸536上磷酸化RELA，而蛋白激酶A则在丝氨酸276上磷酸化RELA[92]。这些磷酸化过程对于NF-κB信号传导具有重要作用，其异常激活在HNSCC患者的恶性组织中常见[93,94]。转移性细胞系依赖于IκBα与NF-κB，以及促炎细胞因子的持续激活增加[9,16,49,95]。在同系小鼠中建立的鳞状细胞癌的基因表达谱分析显示，在转移细胞中差异表达的早期响应基因与NF-κB通路激活有关[96]。当使用显性负性IκBα突变体使NF-κB失活，并通过cDNA微阵列研究小鼠SCC转化和进展的基因表达变化时，发现NF-κB调节了转移细胞中60%以上的差异表达基因。此过程还抑制了肿瘤细胞的恶性表型特征，如增殖、迁移、细胞存活、血管生成和肿瘤进展的增加，表明 NF-κB 是恶性 SCC 的关键介导者[97]。

非经典 NF-κB 通路由不同的 TNF 家族细胞因子和其他因素如 CD40、BAFF 和淋巴毒素-β（LTβ）通过 TNFR 相关因子（TRAF）3/6 和 NF-κB 诱导激酶（NIK）调节（图 7-2）。TRAF3 通过与 NIK 结合，负向调节替代 NF-κB 通路，导致 NIK 的持续泛素介导的蛋白酶体降解，从而在未刺激的细胞中保持 NIK 的稳态水平较低[78]。相反，当受体配体结合时，TRAF3 被泛素化并被蛋白酶体降解和 NIK 积累[78]。这导致 IKK-α/IKK-α 复合物的激活，通过磷酸化、泛素化和降解介导 p100 到 p52 的加工[87]，从而导致 RELB/p52 复合物的核转位和转录激活。此外，在 HNSCC TCGA 项目的 HPV 阳性肿瘤中发现了 TRAF3 缺失[98]，而我们在 TRAF3 缺乏的 HPV 阳性肿瘤和细胞系中展示了替代 NF-κB 通路成分（包括 RELB/p52）的表达和活性增加。相反，在内源性 TRAF3 水平低的 HPV 阳性细胞系中过表达 TRAF3 导致 RELB/p52 表达、定位和 NF-κB 报告活性的抑制。这也抑制了细胞生长、迁移和集落形成，并增加了肿瘤抑制蛋白的表达，表明 TRAF3 总体上在 HPV 阳性 HNSCC 细胞中作为肿瘤抑制因子起作用[99]。TRAF3 的缺失还削弱了其在 HPV 阳性 HNSCC 中的其他抗病毒信号传导作用，这可能是从表型到整合型 HPV 感染进展的一种可能方式[100]。

为了证实 HPV 阳性肿瘤预后较好的现象，并了解 NF-κB 亚基在口腔癌肿瘤发生中的角色，Mishra 等人研究了 NF-κB 不同亚基的 DNA 结合活性和表达模式，并将其与 HPV 感染的存在关联起来。从正常、癌前病变和口腔癌患者收集的组织显示，NF-κB 在口腔癌组织中持续激活，NF-κB 成员上调。NF-κB 亚基的表达随着病变严重程度的增加而增加，其中 p50 显示最高的 DNA 结合活性[101]。Gupta 等人在一系列舌癌组织和细胞系中获得了相似的结果；他们的研究表明，在 HPV 阳性和 HPV 阴性肿瘤中，p50 和 c-REL 与病变严重程度增加有关，而在 HPV 阳性 TSCC 中，RELA 与分化良好的肿瘤及较好的预后相关[102]。我们展示了经典通路成分 c-REL 在 HNSCC 中与 RELA 具有不同的作用。在 TNF-α 诱导下，c-REL 结合 TP53 家族成员 ΔNTP63，并取代 TP73，从而削弱其肿瘤抑制功能[52]。

NF-κB 通路与其他信号通路的交互作用

NF-κB 信号通路的微妙平衡也依赖于其他交互通路，例如在 HNSCC 中经常失调的 EGFR 介导的 PI3K/AKT/mTOR 通路[103]（图 7-2）。该通路由包括表皮生长因子（EGF）和转化生长因子-α（TGF-α）在内的多个配体激活，这些配体导致 I 类磷脂酰肌醇 3-激酶（PI3K）、AKT 和雷帕霉素靶蛋白（mTOR）的激活[104]。AKT、其底物 GSK 和 mTOR 能够形成一个复合体以影响 IKK-α 的磷酸化，并作为 IKK 复合体的一部分，这导致 IκB 的磷酸化和经典通路及促存活基因的激活[105-108]（图 7-2）。在 HNSCC 中，恶性表型通常与 EGFR 和 NF-κB 通路的激活有关。我们先前的研究表明，IKK-α 和 IKK-β 的过表达促进了 EGFR 通路及 NF-κB 通路关键分子的表达和激活，抑制这两条通路可能可以更好地抑制 NF-κB 通路的激活和 HNSCC 细胞的增殖[109]。

丝裂原活化蛋白激酶（MAPK）是一类丝氨酸/苏氨酸激酶，能够通过激活 IKK 来活化 NF-κB 通路[84]（图 7-2）。在激酶介导的磷酸化级联反应中，MAPK 3 激酶（MAP 3K）激活 MAPK 激酶（MKK），随后进一步激活 MAP 激酶（MAPK）。IKK 蛋白由一种叫作 TGF-β 激活激酶 1（TAK1）的 MAP 3K 活化，这进一步导致 NF-κB 通路的激活[110]。TNF-α 和 IL-1 通过另一种 MAP 3K，即 MEKK3，诱导 NF-κB 的激活。MAP 激酶还调节活化蛋白-1（AP-1）家族的一组转录因子，该家族包括几个亚家族如 Jun（c-Jun、JunB 和 JunD）和 Fos（c-Fos、FosB、Fra1 和 Fra2）[111]，这些亚家族形成二聚体并调节细胞生长、分化和凋亡等多个关键过程[112]。在多种癌症，包括口腔癌中，已经观察到 AP-1 成员，尤其是c-Fos、c-Jun和JunB，具有较高的DNA结合活性和差异表达[113,114]。在口腔癌组织中发现了c-Fos/c-Jun二聚体，而其癌前病变的对应部分则主要含有c-Jun同源二聚体[114]。同时，关键点还包括舌癌组织和癌细胞系中AP-1的高表达和DNA结合活性，当c-Fos与Fos相关抗原2（Fra-2）结合时更为明显，而在分化较差和HPV阴性的癌症中c-Jun加入了复合体[115]。

CK2（酪蛋白激酶2或Ⅱ）是另一种在HNSCC患者中高表达的蛋白激酶，与疾病的严重程度和预后相关[116,117]。CK2磷酸化IKK-β并促进NF-κB的异常激活[118]。此外，敲低CK2的特定亚基（CK2α）差异性地调节NF-κB信号通路及其下游分子和促凋亡基因如TP53和TP63，从而促进HNSCC细胞的恶性表型[119]。CK2抑制剂CX-4945抑制了包括NF-κB通路和BCL-xL表达在内的促存活介质，并增强了促凋亡的TP53和p21报告基因活性在人体HNSCC细胞系和异种移植模型中的表达，尽管在异种移植中仅显示出适度的抗肿瘤活性。当加入MEK抑制剂PD-0325901（PD-901）时，异种移植实验中的反应更佳，这表明MEK-ERK-AP-1通路对CK2抑制剂存在一定的耐药性，而MEK抑制剂PD-901在对CX-4945耐药的HNSCC细胞效果显著[120]。

当前与NF-κB通路相关的生物标志物和药物研发

人类HNSCC和小鼠同系SCC的转录组和蛋白质组研究显示，60%的差异表达基因与NF-κB通路相关，对这些基因的编辑导致肿瘤发生的改变，这表明NF-κB及其相关通路可能是HNSCC预后的潜在生物标志物[121]。大多数HNSCC病例中都观察到了NF-κB的持续激活，并且在恶性HNSCC患者中观察到磷酸化RELA的核定位增加。因此，核磷酸化RELA的强度可能成为预测恶性HNSCC风险和患者生存的蛋白质组学标志物[121]。HNSCC患者细胞系和肿瘤中由NF-κB调节的升高的促炎细胞因子及其基因也可以用作HNSCC恶性预测的生物标志物[13]。

由于NF-κB的激活依赖于IKK介导的磷酸化、泛素化和IκB的蛋白酶体降解，因此研究了蛋白酶体和IKK抑制剂。虽然发现蛋白酶体抑制剂在淋巴瘤和骨髓瘤中最为活跃，但在HNSCC和其他癌症中，与其他疗法联合使用时，它们仅诱导部分抗肿瘤活性，甚至与EGFR抑制剂有拮抗作用[122]。在一项针对HNSCC患者使用蛋白酶体抑制剂的研究中，Allen等人对来自HNSCC患者及其匹配的非癌性上皮组织的不同NF-κB亚基［包括磷酸化RELA（pRELA）、pERK1/2和pSTAT3］进行了免疫组化染色。癌组织中NF-κB包括pRELA染色增加，而在匹配的非恶性组织中，染色仅限于基底层。该模式与细胞增殖标志物核Ki67（肿瘤细胞增殖蛋白）染色相对应。此外，当比较治疗前肿瘤活检中蛋白质的存在和定位时，100%的活检中均显示包括pRELA和RELB在内的五种NF-κB蛋白、pSTAT3和pERK1/2的核共染。在某些肿瘤中，蛋白酶体抑制剂仅抑制了NF-κB和RELA，而非RELB亚基或STAT3。这些结果支持以下结论：HNSCC组织中NF-κB的核激活增加，且蛋白酶体抑制剂对替代性NF-κB和其他促存活通路的效果有限[123]。在更大规模的研究中，Gaykalova等人对100例HNSCC和13例对照进行了免疫组化，发现HPV阴性肿瘤的STAT3和NF-κB总体染色较HPV阳性肿瘤增加，尤其是STAT3和NF-κB的核激活在HPV阴性肿瘤中也高于HPV阳性肿瘤。这表明HPV阴性HNSCC具有NF-κB和STAT3通路共同激活的特征。此结果也与基因表达分析所得的转录因子（TF）特征相一致，分析显示HPV阳性和HPV阴性HNSCC在TF特征上显著不同，HPV阴性肿瘤中STAT、NF-κB和AP-1的直接靶标表达增加[124]。总体而言，由于免疫和血液毒性，发现蛋白酶体尤其是IKK抑制剂的活性有限且具有狭窄的治疗窗口，这表明靶向驱动癌基因及其对NF-κB的汇聚通路可能为HNSCC治疗提供更具体的靶点。

PI3K/mTOR 通路被认为是一个治疗靶点之一[103]。在 HNSCC 中，PI3K 的催化亚基（PI3KCA）的表达异常或突变很常见[98]。正如上文所述，PI3K-AKT 信号传导涉及通过 IKK 的 NF-κB 易位激活，以及 RELA 和 c-REL 亚基的磷酸化和辅因子 CBP/p300[125]。后者辅因子可能反向调节促存活转录因子 NF-κB 或肿瘤抑制因子 TP53 的易位激活[126]。HNSCC 中，激活的 PI3K-AKT、突变的 TP53 或 TGF-β 受体（TGFβR）的差异性显示了对 PI3K/mTOR 靶向药物的敏感性差异。PI3K/mTOR 抑制剂 PF-04691502（PF-502）能抑制促存活信号，并增强 HNSCC 的 TP53 表达，但对过表达突变型 TP53/TGFβR2 的 HNSCC 无效。这还增加了凋亡，因此，无论单独使用还是与放疗结合，均显示出显著的治疗效果。这表明，PI3K/mTOR 抑制剂 PF502 在 PI3K-AKT 通路上的作用受 TP53 性质的影响，在未来的 PI3K-mTOR 抑制剂临床试验中应考虑这些调节方面的影响[127]。

随后，在 HNSCC 的临床前模型中，测试 ATP 竞争性双重 PI3K/mTOR 抑制剂 PF-05212384 在体外和小鼠模型中增强 HNSCC 细胞对放射的敏感性。与正常人成纤维细胞相比，PF-05212384（PF-384）有效抑制了肿瘤细胞 PI3K 和 mTOR，在体外显著增强了肿瘤细胞对放射的敏感性。这也反映在 γH2AX 反应的延迟上，γH2AX 是 DNA 损伤的指标，暴露 24 小时后，细胞周期阻滞出现在暴露于 PF-05212384 的细胞中。随后，PF-384 抑制了裸鼠中 UM-SCC1 异种移植肿瘤的再生长，结果显示，PI3K/mTOR 通路可能是增强 HNSCC 细胞对放疗敏感性的良好候选信号通路，PF-384 可能作为 HNSCC 的潜在放射增敏剂[128]。然而，HNSCC 通常包含与 mTOR 通路共同激活的其他通路如 MEK/ERK/AP-1，这些可能使治疗产生抗性。因此，测试 PF-384 于一组不同 PI3KCA 表达和突变状态的 HNSCC 细胞系，显示出对不同 HNSCC 细胞系的可变活性。虽然 PF-384 在抑制 PI3K/mTOR 的直接靶点方面有效，但其对共同激活的 ERK 的作用不足以抑制小鼠中的肿瘤生长，这表明其他通路如 MEK/ERK 对 PF-384 的抗性发挥作用。当加入 MEK 抑制剂 PD-0325901（PD-901）进行治疗时，增强了 PF-384 的抗肿瘤效果[129]。

在一个机会窗试验中，经典异构调节的 PI3K-mTOR 通路抑制剂雷帕霉素被用于治疗晚期 HNSCC 患者，该治疗持续了 21 天。结果显示，接受雷帕霉素治疗的 16 名患者中有 14 名在临床上显示肿瘤体积缩小。此外，4 名患者（25%）达到了 RECIST 标准，即肿瘤缩小 30%，其中包括 1 例完全缓解，这表明抑制 mTOR 通路是 HNSCC 的一种有前景的治疗靶点[130]。mTOR 通路的另一个上游调节因子 EGFR 也成为 HNSCC 治疗的靶点。西妥昔单抗是一种针对 EGFR 的抗体，已成为 HNSCC 患者的获批治疗方案，但其价格极高且对生存期的总体影响有限[131]。两种 EGFR 酪氨酸激酶小分子抑制剂吉非替尼和厄洛替尼也已获得 FDA 批准用于抑制 EGFR 信号传导。在一项利用吉非替尼联合每周紫杉醇和放疗的剂量递增试验中，吉非替尼仅在研究的七个肿瘤中的一个中显示了 EGFR 及其下游信号的抑制。与单独使用紫杉醇和放疗相比，加入吉非替尼并未改善局部晚期 HNSCC 的预后[132]。随后，对一组 HNSCC 细胞系和肿瘤进行了吉非替尼治疗，并分析了 EGFR 及其下游信号分子的蛋白质组反应，结果表明，吉非替尼的敏感性与肿瘤中磷酸化 AKT（p-AKT）和磷酸化 STAT3（p-STAT3）的抑制直接相关，但仅在一位患者的肿瘤中得到验证。这表明 p-AKT 和 p-STAT3 可能成为预测针对少见 EGFR 驱动肿瘤发生的 HNSCC 患者的治疗敏感性的生物标志物[133]。

Soleimani 等人根据功能及其对 NF-κB 活性的影响总结了当前抑制大肠癌的 NF-κB 抑制剂。抑制剂如姜黄素，也表现出对 HNSCC 的临床活性，其通过抑制 NF-κB 的活化从而抑制细胞增殖[83]。在有癌前病变口腔病变的患者中进行的一项临床试验显示，姜黄素的临床反应稍高于安慰剂[134]，但姜黄素的溶解度和生物利用度有限。

其他对大肠癌具有临床活性的抑制剂通过调节调亡、炎症、转移、耐药性和放射抗性而发挥作用。然而，它们似乎具有一些共同特点，如消除或降低 NF-κB 信号传导、使 NF-κB 亚基失活或抑制 NF-κB 信号通路成分的磷酸化[83]。

总之，NF-κB 信号通路是大多数 HNSCC 中异常激活的关键通路。如上所述，其各种成分不仅可以用作预测疾病严重程度和患者生存的生物标志物，还可以被视为潜在的治疗候选通路。然而，NF-κB 信号通路与其他多个通路存在交叉，因此在不引起其他通路补偿性反应的情况下抑制该通路的成分仍然是一个挑战。在临床前模型中，靶向 NF-κB 及相关通路的化疗药物与放疗相联合应用似乎是更有效的治疗选择。

通过泛素化和蛋白酶体调节炎症信号传导

作为癌症特征之一，慢性炎症是恶性肿瘤的重要驱动因素[135]。因此，为了防止可能导致恶性转化的慢性炎症，炎症信号通路受到严格调控，以确保仅对炎症刺激产生适当的响应。蛋白质泛素化是许多信号通路的关键调节器，在激活和终止这些信号通路中发挥着重要作用。因此，泛素系统的缺陷可能导致炎症信号的异常激活或无法终止，进而导致慢性炎症状态[136, 137]。在这里，我们将讨论泛素系统如何调节炎症信号传导，以及该系统在 HNSCC 中作为潜在治疗靶点的可能性。

泛素系统

泛素是一种小型、高度保守、广泛表达的蛋白质，存在于从酵母到人类的所有真核生物中[136, 137]。泛素通过与蛋白质底物结合，通过逐步的酶级联反应，调节从蛋白质降解到信号传导调节的多种细胞功能[136-138]。此过程需要三类酶：E1 泛素激活酶、E2 泛素结合酶和 E3 泛素连接酶（图 7-3）。人类基因组编码了 8 种 E1 蛋白（只有 2 种参与泛素化）、大约 50 种 E2 蛋白和超过 700 种 E3 蛋白，显示了泛素系统的复杂

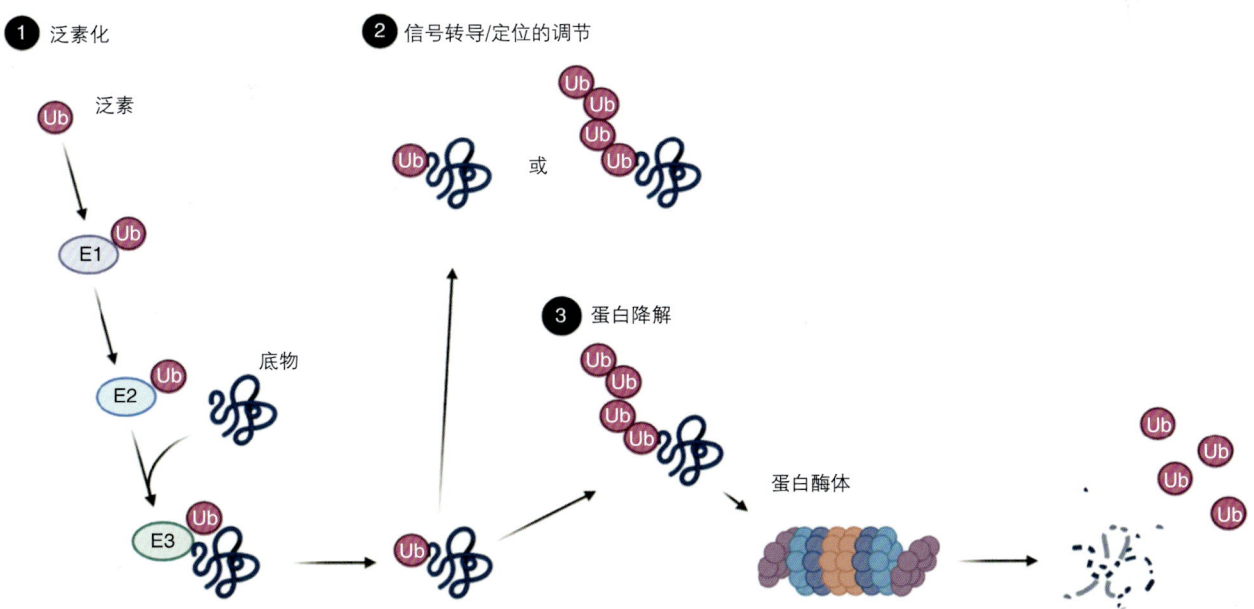

图 7-3 泛素酶级联反应和泛素-蛋白酶体系统（USP）。① 泛素酶级联反应的简化图示。向蛋白质底物添加泛素可能导致多种结果，包括：② 调节信号传导或蛋白质定位；或③ 蛋白酶体降解（图使用 BioRender.com 创建）

性[136]。E3连接酶催化泛素向蛋白质底物的转移，从而为泛素系统提供特异性[137]。此外，泛素可以通过去泛素化酶（DUB）移除，已被分类的去泛素化酶约有100种，分为7个不同的家族[138]。泛素包含76个氨基酸，其中包括7个赖氨酸残基-位于氨基酸位置的6（K6）、K11、K27、K33、K48和K63；泛素的C端可以连接到另一个泛素的这七个赖氨酸中的任何一个上，形成具有不同连接方式的多聚泛素链[137]。此外，泛素可以直接附着在另一个泛素的N端甲硫氨酸上，形成线性多聚泛素链[137]。多聚泛素链可以是线性的或分支的；除了赖氨酸连接的类型，因为这会导致不同的生物功能。例如，K11和K48多聚泛素链主要与靶向蛋白质进行降解相关，而K63多聚泛素链形成信号蛋白之间的连接，与细胞外信号传递到下游功能（如转录激活）相关[136]。

泛素介导的炎症信号调节

泛素化是炎症信号调节的关键因素，包括NF-κB、STAT3和AP-1通路，这些通路可能通过配体-受体相互作用被激活[139]，并在HNSCC中表现出异常激活。细胞因子TNF-α与TNFR1结合后，一个由TRADD、TRAF2、RIP1和cIAP1/2组成的复合物被招募到受体上。这导致E2蛋白UBC13与E3连接酶cIAP1/2对RIP1进行K63多聚泛素化[140]；这条多聚泛素链作为TAB1和TAB2的结合平台，通过其泛素结合域（UBD）进行结合[141]。这引发了TAK1的招募、自动磷酸化和激活[142]。TAK1进一步磷酸化IKK-α，随后诱导IκBα在丝氨酸32和36位置的磷酸化，导致其K48多聚泛素化、蛋白酶体降解，并继而激活NF-κB[143]。IκBα的泛素化由E3连接酶Skp1-Cullin1-F-box蛋白（SCF）$^{β-TrCP}$介导，其中β-TrCP亚基为E3连接酶提供特异性。IκBα的降解导致NF-κB亚基RELA的释放，显露其核定位序列，促进NF-κB转录激活[143]。此外，激活的TAK1还可以诱导MAPK信号通路；TAK1以依赖泛素的方式磷酸化MKK6，导致JNK/p38的激活[142]。除了TNF-α，其他细胞因子也可以通过泛素化介导促炎信号通路。IL-1α/β可以通过E3连接酶TRAF6激活NF-κB和JNK/p38信号[144]，并且其他细胞因子如IL-6和TNF-α可以直接或间接诱导STAT3激活[145]。

由IKK-γ（NEMO）、IKK-α和IKK-β组成的三聚体IKK复合物可以结合在RIP1上的K63多聚泛素链，将这些成分带到TAK1的附近，从而允许IKK复合物的磷酸化和激活[141]。除了K63多聚泛素化介导的NF-κB激活外，线性泛素化也是NF-κB激活所必需的[146,147]。线性多聚泛素化由E3连接酶线性泛素链组装复合物（LUBAC）介导[146]。LUBAC介导的泛素化对于经典的NF-κB通路和潜在的JNK介导的AP-1活性都是必需的[147]。此外，LUBAC与NEMO结合并泛素化它，这些功能对于NF-κB的激活是至关重要的。

与此同时，去泛素化酶也可以调节炎症信号，其主要是通过终止信号传导过程并防止慢性炎症的发生[148]。A20（也称为TNF诱导蛋白3，TNFAIP3）是卵巢肿瘤（OTU）家族的去泛素化酶之一，在炎症信号中有明确的作用。不寻常的是，A20还可以发挥E3连接酶的功能[149]。A20可以通过三种主要机制终止炎症信号：① A20的去泛素化功能移除RIP1和NEMO上的K63多聚泛素链；② 作为E3连接酶，A20对RIP和UBC13进行K48多聚泛素化，促进其蛋白酶体降解；③ A20干扰TRAF2/5和cIAP1/2与UBC13的相互作用，阻止其作为E3连接酶的功能[150]。另一个参与炎症信号的去泛素化酶是CYLD，属于USP家族成员[151]。CYLD移除RIP1、TRAF2、TRAF6和NEMO上的K63多聚泛素链，并去除RIP1上的M1线性多聚泛素化[152]。因此，A20和CYLD都对NF-κB和AP-1信号起负调控作用。其他去泛素化酶也能调节炎症信号：Cezanne（OTUD7BOTU家族成员）和USP21（USP家族成员），都可以移除RIP1上的K63连接的多聚泛素链[153,154]。相反，OTU家族成员OTUB1可以稳定cIAP1/2和

UBC13，增强炎症信号[155, 156]。此外，USP11 已被证明可以去泛素化并稳定 IκBα，促进 NF-κB 的核转位[157]。

HNSCC 中的泛素系统：基因组和转录组表达数据

拷贝数变异和 mRNA 表达

目前已经发表了几项全基因组研究，研究了 HNSCC 中的基因组和转录组变异[98, 158]。这些研究中有几项集中于炎症信号通路，包括 NF-κB[99, 100]。有趣的是，这些研究均强调了 HNSCC 中泛素系统变异的普遍性[159]。在对 HNSCC TCGA 数据集进行编码时，观察到编码 E3 连接酶 cIAP1/2 的 BIRC2/3（位于染色体 11q22）频繁发生扩增和过表达[98]。cIAP1/2 是 TNF-α 信号的重要介质，促进 RIP1 的 K63 介导的多聚泛素化和 TRAF3 的 K48 介导的多聚泛素化及随后的蛋白酶体降解。TCGA 研究的一个关键发现是位于染色体 14q32.32 的 TRAF3 基因在 HPV 阳性的 HNSCC 中经常被删除，并偶尔发生突变[98]。TRAF3 是一个 E3 连接酶，作为经典和替代 NF-κB 途径的负调控因子[160]。进一步研究表明，这些突变或 TRAF3 的缺失导致 NF-κB 信号增强，并促进了 HPV 阳性 HNSCC 的进展[99, 100, 160]。

体细胞突变

突变分析发现，SCF 家族 E3 连接酶 FBXW7（SCF^{FBXW7}）是 HNSCC 中最常见的突变基因之一[161]。该 E3 连接酶促进 AP-1 组分 c-Jun 和 NF-κB2 的降解，从而抑制 AP-1 和 NF-κB 信号通路[162, 163]。最普遍的 FBXW7 突变是所谓的"热点"突变（R505 > R479 > R465），发生在底物结合域；这些突变抑制 SCF^{FBXW7} 与其底物的相互作用，导致底物的稳定性增加[164]。因此，这些突变可能在 HNSCC 中促进 AP-1 和 NF-κB 信号。HNSCC 中其他常见突变出现在 CUL3 和 KEAP1 上，分别为 E3 连接酶和 CUL3 特异性适配蛋白。CUL3-KEAP1 复合物通过促进 IKK-β 的蛋白酶体降解来抑制 NF-κB 信号[165]。CUL3 或 KEAP1 的突变或缺失可能导致通过 NF-κB 的炎症信号增加。此外，在非肿瘤性 RPE 细胞中已经证明 CUL3 的失活与 TP53 的失活同时存在会导致由 NF-κB 和 AP-1 信号驱动的致癌表型[166]。有趣的是，HNSCC 中 CUL3 的突变显著与 TP53 的突变共同出现[98]，这表明 CUL3-KEAP1 E3 连接酶可能与丢失、突变或降解的 TP53 在 HNSCC 中协同作用，以促进炎症信号。此外，去泛素化酶 CYLD 在 HPV 阳性 HNSCC 中也常见突变，这种表型促进 NF-κB 信号[100]。

靶向 HNSCC 中泛素系统

上述研究已经鉴定出几个在 HNSCC 中失调的泛素系统成分，这些成分可能是有吸引力的治疗靶点。在过去的 20 年中，泛素系统作为癌症治疗的潜在靶点得到了广泛关注[167]。目前，已有多种途径被探索；由于 E3 连接酶和去泛素化酶是包含明确活性位点的酶，使用小分子抑制剂靶向这些酶具有很大潜力。然而，靶向抑制蛋白酶体是迄今为止最成功的策略，已经有几种抑制剂获得了 FDA 的批准[168]。

蛋白酶体抑制剂

泛素系统中最早被靶向抑制的成分之一是蛋白酶体，其抑制导致肿瘤抑制因子（如 TP53 和 p27）的积累。此外，抑制蛋白酶体显著抑制炎症反应；IκBα 的积累导致 NF-κB 信号传导和随后的促炎细胞因子释放的抑制[168]。因此，蛋白酶体抑制可以产生多重效果，抑制细胞增殖并促进细胞凋亡。

蛋白酶体抑制剂已在多种癌症中进行试验，包括多发性骨髓瘤（MM）和多种不同的淋巴瘤[168]。硼替佐米是一种可逆抑制剂，可与蛋白酶体的催化位点结合，目前已被 FDA 批准用于治疗多发性骨髓瘤和套细胞淋巴瘤（MCL）。后续研究表明，硼替佐米在多发性骨髓瘤和套细胞淋巴瘤中的疗效可能是由于多种机制，包括抑制增殖、诱导凋亡以及抑制 NF-κB 依赖的细胞因子分泌[169]。然而，硼替佐米的问题在于许多患者出现的内在耐药性[169]。因此，开发了第二代蛋白酶体抑制剂以克服这些问题。卡非佐米是一种不可逆的蛋白酶体抑制剂，目前已被FDA批准用于以前接受过治疗的多发性骨髓瘤患者，这些患者可能曾接受过硼替佐米的治疗[170]。

蛋白酶体抑制剂已被测试为抑制HNSCC中NF-κB信号的潜在治疗选择。早期研究显示，硼替佐米治疗抑制了小鼠和人类鳞状细胞癌中的NF-κB信号[123]。然而，尽管NF-κB被抑制，其他炎症通路（如AP-1和STAT3）未受影响，反应也不一致[171,172]。进一步的组合研究表明，硼替佐米与组蛋白去乙酰化酶（HDAC）抑制剂或顺铂联合使用，极大增强了凋亡诱导和抗肿瘤反应，但也增加了治疗毒性[173]。因此，抑制蛋白酶体在HNSCC中抑制炎症信号具有潜力，与硼替佐米或卡非佐米等下一代蛋白酶体抑制剂的联合疗法值得进一步研究。

■ **IAP拮抗剂**

近年来，泛素系统的另一个备受关注的靶点是E3连接酶cIAP1/2。如前所述，cIAP1/2在HNSCC中通常被扩增或过表达[174,175]。这些蛋白质的双重功能对于其作为癌症治疗靶点的潜力至关重要；抑制cIAP可以抑制下游炎症信号，并通过外源性途径诱导凋亡[175]。

靶向cIAP的化合物（IAP拮抗剂）模拟了天然IAP拮抗剂——凋亡酶的第二线粒体衍生激活因子（SMAC），因此也被称为SMAC模拟物。在线粒体释放后，SMAC被切割并二聚化。SMAC的N端域包含一个四氨基酸序列（AVPI；丙氨酸、缬氨酸、脯氨酸、异亮氨酸），它可以与IAP的BIR3和BIR2域结合[175]。IAP拮抗剂模拟这一序列，允许其与IAP结合。一旦结合，cIAP1/2会发生构象改变和自我泛素化，并被蛋白酶体降解[175]。此外，SMAC模拟物还靶向XIAP，从而导致半胱氨酸蛋白酶激活并引发细胞凋亡[176]。目前开发的IAP拮抗剂根据其能结合多少个BIR结构域，分为单效价或双效价。这些拮抗剂的主要作用机制是诱导TNF-α依赖性凋亡；尽管抑制了经典的NF-κB信号传导，但cIAP的耗竭会导致NIK的稳定，从而驱动替代性NF-κB信号通路[176]。这导致TNF-α自分泌生产和诱导凋亡。与此一致的是，添加死亡配体（如TNF-α和TRAIL）可增强IAP拮抗剂诱导的凋亡[177,178]。

目前，有几种IAP拮抗剂正在进行临床试验：其中四种是单效价抑制剂（Debio-1143、GDC-0917、LCL-161和GDC-0152），两种是双效价抑制剂（birinapant和HGS-1029），还有一种不基于AVPI肽（ASTX-660）。所有这些抑制剂都处于针对实体瘤的早期临床试验阶段[179]。此外，birinapant和HGS-1029正在用于淋巴瘤的研究[180]。目前，已经在卵巢癌和黑色素瘤的Ⅰ期试验中显示了临床疗效[181,182]。此外，与标准化疗（顺铂、紫杉醇）、放射疗法或免疫检查点抑制剂的联合疗法也正在进行测试[183,184]（图7-4）。

在HNSCC中，多种IAP拮抗剂在体外已被证明具有益处，并能提高HNSCC癌细胞对标准化疗药物、TNF-α和TRAIL靶向药物的敏感性[177,183]。此外，birinapant、Debio-143和LCL161可以提高HNSCC细胞对放射治疗的敏感性[177,184,185]。有趣的是，含有FADD扩增的HNSCC细胞系对IAP拮抗剂表现出更高的敏感性，并且对与放射治疗的联合疗法更加敏感，从而增强了TNF-α依赖的凋亡[177]。此外，某些IAP拮抗剂在HPV阳性的HNSCC中更为有效[185]。最近研究显示，使用IAP拮抗剂ASTX660在HNSCC中具有前景，促进了HNSCC细胞系中TNF-α和TRAIL诱导的细胞死亡，以及在临床前模型中辐射诱导的免疫源性死亡[186,187]。这些数据显示，当了解肿瘤的遗传基础或HPV状态时，IAP拮抗剂可能是最为有效的，使其在精准医学中成为一个具有吸引力的靶点。

总之，通过泛素系统抑制炎症信号传导在HNSCC中正成为一个有吸引力的治疗靶点。使用蛋白酶体抑制剂和IAP拮抗剂可以同时靶向多个致癌通路，包括抑制增殖和诱导凋亡。

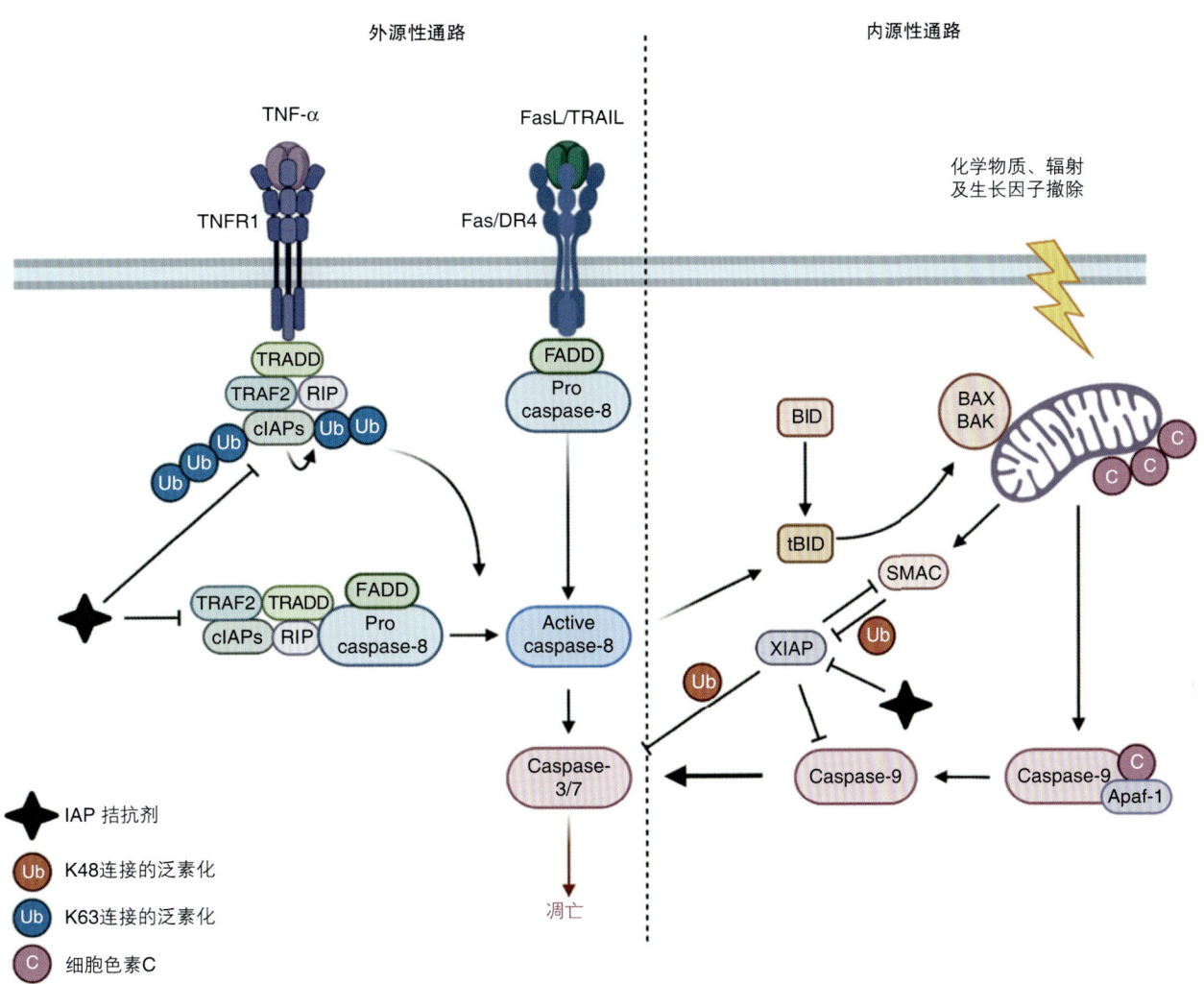

图 7-4 外源性和内源性凋亡通路。外源性凋亡通路是通过配体（TNF、FASL 或 TRAIL）与细胞死亡受体（分别为 TNFR、FAS 或 DR4）结合诱导的。TNFR1 的死亡域招募 TNF 受体相关死亡域（TRADD）蛋白，这是一个适配分子，允许 TRAF2 和 c-IAP1 及 c-IAP2 与受体复合物结合。c-IAP1/2 诱导 K63 连接的 RIP1 泛素化，随后通过 NF-κB 和 AP-1 进行下游信号传导。在没有 cIAP 情况下，RIP1 无法被泛素化，而是与适配分子 Fas 相关的死亡域（FADD）和 caspase-8 形成胞质复合物，通过 caspase-3/7 激活诱导凋亡。由于 cIAP 介导的 RIP1 泛素化防止了这些死亡诱导复合物的形成，因此可以使用 SMAC 模拟物通过降解 c-IAP 来驱动细胞死亡。内源性凋亡通路可以通过细胞毒性损伤激活，包括细胞色素 C 和 SMAC 从线粒体释放到胞质中。caspase-8 诱导 BH3 相互作用死亡域激动剂（BID）切割为截短的 BID（tBID），也可以导致线粒体通透性增加。细胞色素 C 释放到胞质中，导致 caspase-9 的激活，进而激活 caspase-3 和 caspase-7；释放的细胞色素 C 与凋亡酶激活因子（Apaf1）结合，诱导凋亡小体形成，激活 caspase-9，通过 caspase-3/7 激活诱导凋亡。此外，SMAC 从线粒体释放，可以直接抑制另一种 IAP 蛋白 XIAP。因此，SMAC 模拟物可以抑制 XIAP 以促进凋亡（图由 BioRender.com 制作）

促炎和其他信号分子的基因组特征和转录组图谱

癌症是一种复杂的遗传疾病，由具有积累基因组改变和功能缺陷的失控增殖细胞引发。最显著的遗传改变是体细胞突变，这可以通过有丝分裂的细胞谱系在表型正常的细胞中获得[188]。突变的内在机制包括固有的遗传缺陷、复制错误和（或）细胞分裂期间 DNA 修复的缺陷[188]。突变的外在机制则通过外源性诱变剂的影响介导，例如烟草烟雾和酒精中的致癌物，以及感染致癌病毒，如人乳头瘤病毒（HPV）。这些是可以增加体细胞突变率并诱导基因组不稳定性和染色体改变的强效诱导剂和促进剂[189]，尤其是在HNSCC以及来自肺、食管、宫颈和膀胱的鳞状细胞癌（SCC）中[190]。在癌细胞生长的数年或数十年中，这些遗传改变的积累可能导致异质性基因组改变的发展，这很难在临床上进行表征、分类和用于患者诊断和预后，特别是当医学实践仅基于传统病理学和组织学方法时。为了解决这些问题并理解人类癌症最全面的分子图谱，癌症基因组图谱（TCGA）和其他大型协作项目已经建立，使用尖端的基因组特征技术和大型综合数据集对主要癌症类型进行了多重深入研究。

TCGA 项目概述及 HNSCC 个体生物标志物论文

TCGA项目于2006年启动，由美国国家癌症研究所（NCI）和国家人类基因组研究所（NHGRI）资助，隶属于美国国立卫生研究院（NIH）[191]。这是一个具有里程碑意义的癌症基因组学项目，其利用了多种高通量技术平台和生物信息学分析，从分子层面上对33种主要癌症类型进行了分子表征分型。2018年，TCGA研究网络完成了这段激动人心的旅程，生成了超过2 500万兆字节的基因组、表观基因组、转录组和蛋白质组数据，并发表了30多篇特定癌症类型的"标志"（Marker）论文（表7-1）。"标志"论文被定义为由TCGA特定癌症联盟组发表的独特论文，以区别于使用TCGA数据集的其他论文[192]。

Nature于2015年1月发表了聚焦于头颈部癌症的HNSCC TCGA "标志"论文[98]。其分析了279个患者样本，包括244个HPV阴性和36个HPV阳性的HNSCC，其中最终的通路总结图展示了HNSCC中最常见的癌基因和抑癌基因的改变频率（图7-5，经允许引自参考文献[98]）。这些关键分子表达在主要通路中，包括生长受体/细胞周期、细胞死亡、免疫、细胞分化和氧化应激。若干基因组的改变影响了肿瘤坏死因子受体（TNFR）组件和汇聚于NF-κB介导信号的炎症通路。11q13/22的增益编码 FADD、BIRC2/3 或 14q32 TRAF3 的缺失，调控经典和替代的 NF-κB/REL 家族转录因子及在HNSCC中细胞死亡、迁移和炎症重要的通路。大多数HNSCC中3p的缺失及3q同染色体异倍体的结果导致促有丝分裂激酶 PIK3CA 的增益或者 PIK3CA 的突变（尤其是在HPV阳性肿瘤中）是HNSCC中最常见的癌基因改变，也与NF-κB的激活有关。NOTCH 的缺失或 TP63 的3q增益被认为与 ΔNTP63 癌基因的增强激活有关，后者促进HNSCC的干性、肿瘤发生及炎症表型。

一项针对该队列的同期研究发现，基于外显子组和转录组测序数据发现35个肿瘤（12.5%）检测到了高风险HPV类型16、33或35。该研究揭示，HPV病毒基因组的整合通过癌基因扩增、抑癌基因破坏、驱动染色体重排以及改变基因表达和DNA甲基化模式来促进宿主的肿瘤发生[197]。迄今为止，HNSCC TCGA项目已完成约530个肿瘤组织的基因组分析，包括约81个HPV阳性肿瘤组织和超过40个匹配的正常组织样本。所使用的技术涵盖六种不同的"组学"平台，包括外显子测序（exome-seq）、DNA拷贝数阵列（DNA copy-number array）、DNA甲基化阵列（DNA methylation array）、mRNA测序（mRNA-seq）、miRNA测序（miRNA-seq）以及反向相位蛋白质阵列（RPPA；详见表7-1）。

TCGA 泛癌症图谱项目的三大主题包括"起源细胞""致癌过程"和"信号通路"

我们参与了TCGA泛癌症图谱项目，该项目对包括HNSCC在内，来自12种癌症类型的3 527个肿瘤样本进行了多平台分析[198]。通过对五种基因组平台和反向相位蛋白质阵列（RPPA）数据集的多平台分类和综合分析，我们发现头颈部、肺部及部分膀胱癌的鳞状细胞癌（SCC）合并为一个亚型，该亚型具有典型的 TP53 改变、3q 染色体的拷贝数增加及p63的

表 7-1 癌症组织和细胞系的开放数据集及资源，包含基因组和蛋白质组信息以及对基因和小分子干扰的敏感性

项目名称（缩写）	主要机构	描　述	总样本数 HNSCC 样本数	网　站	参考文献
癌组织					
癌症基因组图谱（TCGA）	NCI/NHGRI/NIH	一项具有里程碑意义的癌症基因组学项目，分子表征超过 20 000 个原发癌症及匹配的正常样本，涵盖 33 种癌症类型，并生成了超过 2 500 万兆字节的基因组、表观基因组、转录组和蛋白质组数据	＞11 000 癌症样本 ＞530 HNSCC 样本	http://cancergenome.nih.gov/ https://gdc.cancer.gov https://www.cbioportal.org	Hutter and Zenklusen[191] Cancer Genome Atlas Network[98]
TCGA 泛癌症图谱（PanCanAtlas）	NCI/NHGRI/NIH	独特全面、深入且相互关联的分析，涵盖 33 种癌症类型，收集了 27 篇论文，分为三大类：起源细胞模式、致癌过程和信号通路。每个类别都有一篇旗舰论文，总结了该主题的核心发现	＞11 000 癌症样本 ＞530 HNSCC 样本	https://gdc.cancer.gov/about-data/publications/pancanatlas https://www.cell.com/pb-assets/consortium/pancanceratlas/pancani3/index.html https://www.cbioportal.org	Hoadley et al.[199] Ding et al.[200] Sanchez-Vega et al.[201] Campbell et al.[190]
正常组织					
基因型-组织表达（GTEx）	NCI/NHGRI/NHLBI/NIDA/NIMH/NINDS	一项全面的资源，用于研究组织特异性基因表达和调控。样本来自成人器官和组织捐赠者或 54 个非病变组织部位的手术捐赠者。主要的分子检测包括全基因组测序（whole genome-seq）、全外显子测序（whole exome-seq）和 RNA 测序（RNA-seq），并提供开放获取的数据，包括基因表达、定量性状位点（eQTLs）和组织学图像	～1 000 名已故成人	https://gtexportal.org/home/	GTEx Consortium, Nature, 2017[193]
癌细胞系					
癌症细胞系百科全书（CCLE）	布罗德研究所和诺华生物医学研究所	对大量人类癌症模型进行详细的遗传和药理特征分析，以开发将不同药理脆弱性与基因组和蛋白质组模式联系起来的综合分析	1 775 个细胞系 71 个 HNSCC 细胞系	https://portals.broadinstitute.org/ccle https://depmap.org/portal/ccle/	Ghandi et al.[205] Barretina, et al.[204]
RNAi/shRNA/CRISPR					
癌症中 RNA 干扰对细胞存活影响的深度探究（DRIVE）	诺华生物医学研究所	一项大规模 RNAi 筛选，通过使用平均 20 个 shRNA 敲低 7 837 个基因的 mRNA，评估其对细胞生存的影响	398 个癌症细胞系 10 个 HNSCC 细胞系	https://oncologynibr.shinyapps.io/drive/	McDonald, et al.[209]

续 表

项目名称（缩写）	主要机构	描 述	总样本数 HNSCC 样本数	网 站	参考文献
Achilles 项目	布罗德研究所	使用基因组规模的基于慢病毒的混合 shRNA 或 CRISPR-Cas9 文库，系统地识别并分类数百个基因组特征化的癌症细胞系中的基因必需性，敲除单个基因并识别影响细胞存活的基因	>700 个癌症细胞系 >40 个 HNSCC 细胞系	https://depmap.org/portal/achilles/	Behan et al.[210]
癌症依赖图谱（DepMap）	布罗德研究所和桑格研究所	整合数据集，对数百个癌症细胞系的基因组信息和对基因及小分子干扰的敏感性进行分析，以定义治疗性遗传靶点的全景	1 775 个细胞系 71 个 HNSCC 细胞系	https://depmap.org/portal/	Tsherniak et al., *Cell*, 2017[194]
药物筛选					
混合物中相对抑制的谱系分析（PRISM）	布罗德研究所和哈佛大学	一种强大的方法，能够在前所未有的规模上，快速筛选数千种药物对数百种人类癌症模型的效果，以识别敏感性的预测性生物标志物和新的治疗谱系	>500 个癌症细胞系 27 个 HNSCC 细胞系	https://depmap.org/portal/prism/	Yu et al.[213] Corsello et al.[211] Corsello et al.[212]
癌症药物敏感性基因组学（GDSC）	Wellcome Sanger 研究所和麻省总医院	使用 518 种抗癌化合物（包括细胞毒性化疗和靶向治疗）对大量表征的人类癌症细胞系进行筛选。将敏感性模式的预测与广泛的基因组数据相关联，以识别遗传特征	>1 000 个癌症细胞系 44 个 HNSCC 细胞系	https://www.cancerrxgene.org	Iorio et al., *Cell*, 2016[195]
蛋白质图谱					
人类蛋白质图谱	瑞典项目，由 Knut 和 Alice Wallenberg 基金会资助	利用各种组学技术的整合，包括基于抗体的成像、基于质谱的蛋白质组学、转录组学和系统生物学，绘制细胞、组织和器官中的所有人类蛋白质图谱。它由六个独立部分组成，包括组织图谱、细胞图谱、病理图谱、血液图谱、大脑图谱和代谢图谱	>700 个用于蛋白质表达的抗体 >500 万张癌症组织免疫组织化学图像	https://www.proteinatlas.org	Uhlén et al., *Science*, 2015[196]

ΔN 亚型的主要表达，以及免疫和增殖通路基因的高表达。该研究将多平台分类和基因组及表达特征的综合分析与组织起源相关联，为后续的 TCGA 泛癌症图谱项目奠定了基础[198]。

随后，TCGA 泛癌症图谱收集并分析了来自 33 种不同主要癌症类型的超过 11 000 个样本，在 *Cell Press* 期刊发表了 30 篇论文，其中包括三篇顶级论文，分别聚焦于"起源细胞"[199]"致癌过程"[200]和"信号通路"[201]这三大主题（表 7-1）。在"起源细胞"这一主要主题下，基于器

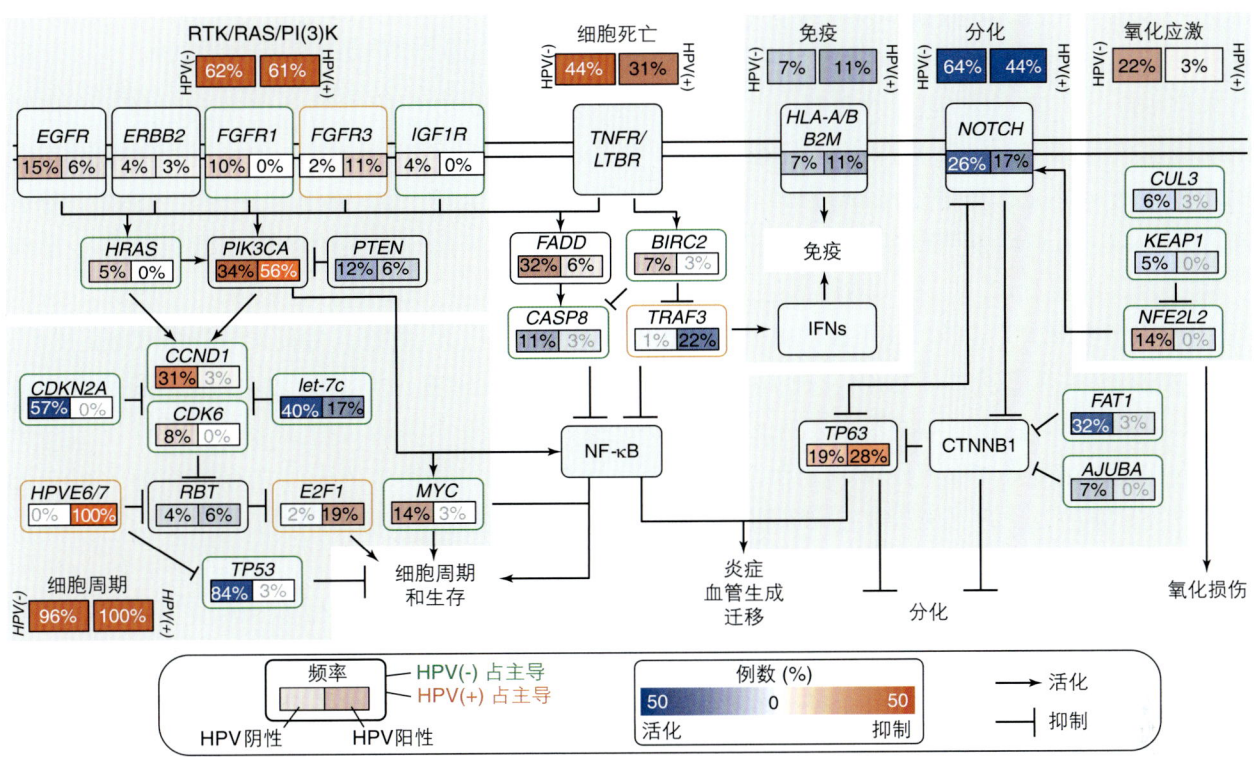

图7-5 信号通路和转录因子的失调。主要受影响的通路、组件及推断功能在正文中已有总结，共涉及279个样本。HPV阴性肿瘤和HPV阳性肿瘤的基因改变频率（%）在子面板中分别展示并突出显示。通路改变包括纯合缺失、局部扩增和体细胞突变。激活和失活的通路/基因以及激活或抑制的符号基于基因组改变和（或）通路功能的预测效应

官系统或分化状态，我们主持并领导了泛鳞状细胞癌项目（PanSCC），研究基于鳞状细胞癌的组织学亚型的肿瘤聚集情况，涵盖了来自头颈部、肺部、食管、宫颈和膀胱的鳞状细胞癌[190]。大多数鳞状细胞癌的发病机制与吸烟和（或）HPV感染相关，我们观察到这些肿瘤共享并携带3q、5p和11q的重复染色体拷贝数变异（CNV）。

另一个主题是"致癌过程"[200]，该主题概述了跨越33种主要癌症类型的致癌分子过程。该项目聚焦于癌症突变状态，并揭示了：① 生殖系基因组如何以通路依赖的方式影响体细胞基因组景观；② 基因组突变如何影响基因表达、信号传导及多组学特征；③ 突变负荷和驱动基因如何影响微环境中的免疫细胞组成。有趣的是，驱动突变对HNSCC肿瘤微环境（TME）中的免疫通信网络影响显著，位列高影响癌种之列[202]。大多数HNSCC样本高表达IFN-γ主导以及创伤愈合相关的基因[203]。第三个主题是"信号通路"[201]，该主题生成了十个信号通路的改变图谱。作者开发了一个可重复使用的、经过策划的通路模板，其中包含了驱动基因的目录，显示57%的肿瘤在这些通路中至少存在一个潜在可操作的药物靶点改变。

使用高通量技术对人类细胞系的景观特征进行表征

癌症细胞系百科全书（cancer cell line encyclopedia, CCLE）项目与TCGA研究同步启动，旨在对大量人类癌症模型进行详细的遗传和药理特征分析[204]。截至目前，该项目已收集了来自超过30种主要癌症类型的1700多个细胞系，并进行了综合的计算分析，将不同的基因组模式与药理药物敏感性联系起来[205]（表7-1）。对于HNSCC，大多数分析的细胞系来自口腔及其他头颈部部位的肿瘤，缺乏完整和详细的临床及病理信息，例如HPV状态。密歇根大学建立

了另一大批HNSCC细胞系,以填补这些空白,这些细胞系被命名为UM-SCC系列。该系列包含来自100多名HNSCC患者的肿瘤,具有详细的临床和病理信息,包括HPV感染状态。我们的实验室通过外显子测序(exome-seq)和RNA测序(RNA-seq)对26条HNSCC细胞系进行了表征,其中包括15条HPV阴性细胞系和11条HPV阳性细胞系,其中18条为UM-SCC细胞系[158]。在这项研究中,我们发现3q、5p和11q染色体的拷贝数增加与癌基因表达的增加有关,包括来自3q的 TP63、PIK3CA 和 ACTL6A 以及来自11q位点的 YAP1、CCND1 和 FADD/BIRC2/3,这与TCGA数据一致。因此,这些细胞系重现了更具侵袭性的HNSCC肿瘤亚型的基因组改变,其中3q26.3的同时扩增和 TP53 突变与较差的生存率相关。此外,Ludwig等人研究了来自口腔的14条UM-SCC细胞系,以确定每条细胞系的突变谱、拷贝数变异(CNV)以及基因和蛋白表达[206]。他们发现 PIK3CA 扩增、CDKN2A 缺失以及 TP53 和 CASP8 突变的高频率是HNSCC主要的遗传改变。此外,该团队还研究了一组来自喉鳞状细胞癌的16条细胞系[207]。发现主要的遗传异常包括 PIK3CA、EGFR、CDKN2A、TP53、NOTCH 和 FAT1 基因。此外,van Harten等人对24条HNSCC细胞系(包括9条UM-SCC细胞系)进行了遗传表征,这些细胞系代表了HPV阳性、HPV阴性以及具有遗传易感性的细胞系,如范可尼贫血(Fanconi anemia, FA)[208]。这些来源于FA的细胞系在拷贝数变异和突变模式上与散发性HPV阴性HNSCC相似。相反,一类CN沉默、HPV阴性、TP53 野生型及 CASP8 突变的HNSCC细胞系与大多数HNSCC肿瘤不同并且类似于TCGA的84例HNSCC病例,这些病例表现为CN沉默且女性比例较高,HRAS 和 CASP8 突变丰富。这些HNSCC细胞系的基因组特征表征为生物标志物的深入机制研究和新治疗策略的识别提供了有用的临床前模型。

基因组范围的扰动与功能分析

为了研究细胞系的功能基因组学,开展了DRIVE项目,即"癌症中RNA干扰对生存影响的深度探究"[209]。该项目评估了7 837个基因在398个癌症细胞系中的敲低效果,每个基因使用约20个shRNA,包括10个HNSCC细胞系(表7-1)。最近,借助CRISPR-Cas9技术,对来自30种癌症类型的324个人类癌症细胞系中的18 009个基因进行了敲低,并开发了一个数据驱动的框架来优先筛选癌症治疗的候选靶点[210]。在这些细胞系中,筛选了34个HNSCC细胞系,并使用已批准的药物(如 EGFR、TUBB4B、TYMS、CDK6 和 HMGCR)确定了优先治疗靶点。该数据集提供了丰富的癌症驱动基因资源以及优先考虑的已知和预测的癌症药物靶点。

该项目还利用213种抗体在899个CCLE细胞系中生成了反向相位蛋白质阵列(RPPA)数据,并研究了蛋白质表达与基因依赖性或药物敏感性的关系[205]。这些数据集汇集在DepMap("探索癌症依赖图谱")平台上(https://depmap.org/portal/)。该数据集开放获取关键的癌症依赖性信息,旨在增加研究社区发现与癌症脆弱性相关的新知识(表7-1)。DepMap门户还整合了被称为PRISM("混合物中相对抑制的谱系分析")的药物筛选数据[211-213]。这种综合分析为识别更好的预测性生物标志物和遗传依赖性提供了强大的工具,进而研究癌症相关的炎症,开发新的治疗策略,为肿瘤精准治疗提供更为有效的治疗方案。

HNSCC TCGA数据集提供了一种独特的方法来研究由肿瘤微环境中异常NF-κB激活调控的炎症基因表达。同时,我们分析了来自TCGA队列的279个HNSCC标本的基因组和转录组改变,并确定了61个参与NF-κB和炎症通路的基因[214]。最常见的30个改变基因分布在96%的HNSCC样本中,其表达与基因组拷贝数变化相关。我们将TCGA数据中的NF-κB及促炎相关基因列表与上述 26 个 HNSCC 细胞系进行了比较，观察到大多数研究的表达特征在 TCGA 数据和 HNSCC 细胞系之间是一致的。通过使用 NF-κB 报告基因系的 RNAi 筛选，我们观察到敲低 TNFR、LTBR 或选定的下游信号组件揭示了经典 NF-κB 通路与替代 NF-κB 通路之间的串扰。在 T 细胞激活、免疫检查点以及由 NF-κB 和促炎基因调控的 IFN-γ 和 STAT 通路基因表达升高的 HNSCC 患者中，观察到了生存率的提高。NF-κB 激活和促炎基因特征的基因签名可以作为潜在的生物标志物，用于在进一步的临床前和临床研究中识别治疗和预后靶点。

总之，基因组学、转录组学和蛋白质组学的高通量技术，结合大规模数据集的计算分析，使我们能够实现对每种癌症类型的全面基因组范围表征，显著加速了癌症研究。TCGA 和泛癌症图谱项目交叉分析了来自 33 种主要癌症的超过 11 000 个肿瘤，使得此前未被识别的分子生物标志物被发现，以及对每种癌症类型中新亚组进行了更准确的分类。此外，CCLE 项目通过整合基因组范围的基因扰动与功能和药理药物敏感性分析，提供了详细的人类癌症模型大规模目录。这些在 HNSCC 人类组织和细胞系大规模研究中识别的 NF-κB 和促炎特征与我们之前的实验室观察结果一致。这些大规模的开源数据集提供了独特的信息代码，能够将肿瘤的遗传或表达缺陷与患者结果具体匹配，从而有望实现量身定制的精准医学，包括诊断和治疗。

总体结论和未来方向

在头颈癌中炎症因子失调，NF-κB 的异常激活是其对肿瘤细胞和肿瘤微环境（TME）产生多种影响的基础。TCGA 发现的基因组改变经常影响涉及 NF-κB 异常激活的通路，这些改变存在于用于机制研究和临床前研究的肿瘤细胞系中，以识别预防或治疗的潜在靶点。肿瘤坏死因子（TNF）是细胞毒性治疗和免疫反应的关键介质，HNSCC 通过 NF-κB 调控的促存活介质对其产生抗性。将 TCGA 的结构基因组学数据、这些细胞系模型以及使用 siRNA、CRISPR 或药物库对抑制 TNF 诱导的 NF-κB 促炎和促存活信号分子的功能筛选整合起来，可以帮助识别具有与 TNF 合成致死活性的关键驱动因子、介质和可药物化的靶点，从而中断它们对恶性表型和免疫的不利影响。我们已经开发了一个 NF-κB 报告基因筛选平台，并完成了全基因组 siRNA 筛选，发现了一些意想不到的候选靶点，目前正在对其进行验证、机制研究和潜在治疗药物的临床前研究。

致谢：作者感谢 Nyall London, Jr. 博士（HNSB, NIDCD/NIH）和 Georgia Z Chen 博士（埃默里大学，亚特兰大，佐治亚州）阅读本综述文章并提供有益的评论和建议。

作者贡献：Jun Jeon 撰写了细胞因子部分，Ramya Viswanathan 撰写了 NF-κB 部分，Ethan Morgan 撰写了泛素化部分，Zhong Chen 撰写了基因组学部分，Carter Van Waes 撰写了引言和总体结论部分。Zhong Chen、Ramya Viswanathan 和 Ethan Morgan 设计并绘制了图表。Zhong Chen 制作了表格。Ramya Viswanathan 管理了文献引用。所有作者均对手稿的最终版本进行了修订和确认。

资金信息：本项目由 NIDCD 内部项目 Z01-DC-00016、73、74 资助。本研究得益于 NIH 医学研究学者计划，这是一个由 NIH 与多萝西·杜克慈善基金会（DDCF 资助号 #2014194）、美国牙科研究协会、高露洁棕榄公司、基因泰克、爱思唯尔及其他私人捐助者共同支持的公私合作伙伴关系。

参 考 文 献

[1] Elenbaas B, Weinberg RA. Heterotypic signaling between epithelial tumor cells and fibroblasts in carcinoma formation. Exp Cell Res. 2001; 264(1): 169–84.
[2] Folkman J. Role of angiogenesis in tumor growth and metastasis. Semin Oncol. 2002; 29(6, Supplement 16): 15–8.
[3] Peltanova B, Raudenska M, Masarik M. Effect of tumor microenvironment on pathogenesis of the head and neck squamous cell carcinoma: a systematic review. Mol Cancer. 2019; 18: 63.
[4] Richmond A. Nf-kappa B, chemokine gene transcription and tumour growth. Nat Rev Immunol. 2002; 2(9): 664–74.
[5] Setrerrahmane S, Xu H. Tumor-related interleukins: old validated targets for new anti-cancer drug development. Mol Cancer. 2017; 16: 153.
[6] Baker KJ, Houston A, Brint E. IL-1 family members in cancer; two sides to every story. Front Immunol. 2019; 10: 1197.
[7] Weber A, Wasiliew P, Kracht M. Interleukin-1 (IL-1) pathway. Sci Signal. 2010; 3(105): cm1.
[8] Zhu W, London NR, Gibson CC, Davis CT, Tong Z, Sorensen LK, et al. Interleukin receptor activates a MYD88-ARNO-ARF6 cascade to disrupt vascular stability. Nature. 2012; 492(7428): 252–5.
[9] Dong G, Chen Z, Kato T, Van Waes C. The host environment promotes the constitutive activation of nuclear factor-kappaB and proinflammatory cytokine expression during metastatic tumor progression of murine squamous cell carcinoma. Cancer Res. 1999; 59(14): 3495–504.
[10] Loukinova E, Chen Z, Van Waes C, Dong G. Expression of proangiogenic chemokine Gro 1 in low and high metastatic variants of Pam murine squamous cell carcinoma is differentially regulated by IL-1alpha, EGF and TGF-beta1 through NF-kappaB dependent and independent mechanisms. Int J Cancer. 2001; 94(5): 637–44.
[11] Smith CW, Chen Z, Dong G, Loukinova E, Pegram MY, Nicholas-Figueroa L, et al. The host environment promotes the development of primary and metastatic squamous cell carcinomas that constitutively express proinflammatory cytokines IL-1alpha, IL-6, GM-CSF, and KC. Clin Exp Metastasis. 1998; 16(7): 655–64.
[12] Thomas GR, Chen Z, Leukinova E, Van Waes C, Wen J. Cytokines IL-1α, IL-6, and GM-CSF constitutively secreted by oral squamous carcinoma induce down-regulation of CD80 costimulatory molecule expression: restoration by interferon γ. Cancer Immunol Immunother. 2004; 53(1): 33–40.
[13] Allen C, Duffy S, Teknos T, Islam M, Chen Z, Albert PS, et al. Nuclear factor-kappaB-related serum factors as longitudinal biomarkers of response and survival in advanced oropharyngeal carcinoma. Clin Cancer Res. 2007; 13(11): 3182–90.
[14] Chen Z, Colon I, Ortiz N, Callister M, Dong G, Pegram MY, et al. Effects of interleukin-1alpha, interleukin-1 receptor antagonist, and neutralizing antibody on proinflammatory cytokine expression by human squamous cell carcinoma lines. Cancer Res. 1998; 58(16): 3668–76.
[15] Chen Z, Malhotra PS, Thomas GR, Ondrey FG, Duffey DC, Smith CW, et al. Expression of proinflammatory and proangiogenic cytokines in patients with head and neck cancer. Clin Cancer Res. 1999; 5(6): 1369–79.
[16] Duffey DC, Chen Z, Dong G, Ondrey FG, Wolf JS, Brown K, et al. Expression of a dominant-negative mutant inhibitor-kappaBalpha of nuclear factor-kappaB in human head and neck squamous cell carcinoma inhibits survival, proinflammatory cytokine expression, and tumor growth in vivo. Cancer Res. 1999; 59(14): 3468–74.
[17] Wolf JS, Chen Z, Dong G, Sunwoo JB, Bancroft CC, Capo DE, et al. IL (interleukin)-1alpha promotes nuclear factor-kappaB and AP-1-induced IL-8 expression, cell survival, and proliferation in head and neck squamous cell carcinomas. Clin Cancer Res. 2001; 7(6): 1812–20.
[18] Derakhshan A, Chen Z, Van Waes C. Therapeutic small molecules target inhibitor of apoptosis proteins in cancers with deregulation of extrinsic and intrinsic cell death pathways. Clin Cancer Res. 2017; 23(6): 1379–87.
[19] Choudhary MM, France TJ, Teknos TN, Kumar P. Interleukin-6 role in head and neck squamous cell carcinoma progression. World J Otorhinolaryngol Head Neck Surg. 2016; 2(2): 90–7.
[20] Hong SH, Ondrey FG, Avis IM, Chen Z, Loukinova E, Cavanaugh PF, et al. Cyclooxygenase regulates human oropharyngeal carcinomas via the proinflammatory cytokine IL-6: a general role for inflammation? FASEB J. 2000; 14(11): 1499–507.
[21] Lee TL, Yeh J, Van Waes C, Chen Z. Epigenetic modification of SOCS-1 differentially regulates STAT3 activation in response to interleukin-6 receptor and epidermal growth factor receptor signaling through JAK and/or MEK in head and neck squamous cell carcinomas. Mol Cancer Ther. 2006; 5(1): 8–19.
[22] da Silva JM, Soave DF, Moreira dos Santos TP, Batista AC, Russo RC, Teixeira MM, et al. Significance of chemokine and chemokine receptors in head and neck squamous cell carcinoma: a critical review. Oral Oncol. 2016; 56: 8–16.
[23] Chan L-P, Wang L-F, Chiang F-Y, Lee K-W, Kuo P-L, Liang C-H. IL-8 promotes HNSCC progression on CXCR1/2-meidated NOD1/RIP2 signaling pathway. Oncotarget. 2016; 7(38): 61820–31.
[24] Loukinova E, Dong G, Enamorado-Ayalya I, Thomas GR, Chen Z, Schreiber H, et al. Growth regulated oncogene-alpha expression by

murine squamous cell carcinoma promotes tumor growth, metastasis, leukocyte infiltration and angiogenesis by a host CXC receptor-2 dependent mechanism. Oncogene. 2000; 19(31): 3477–86.

[25] Bancroft CC, Chen Z, Dong G, Sunwoo JB, Yeh N, Park C, et al. Coexpression of proangiogenic factors IL-8 and VEGF by human head and neck squamous cell carcinoma involves coactivation by MEK-MAPK and IKK-NF-kappaB signal pathways. Clin Cancer Res. 2001; 7(2): 435–42.

[26] Bancroft CC, Chen Z, Yeh J, Sunwoo JB, Yeh NT, Jackson S, et al. Effects of pharmacologic antagonists of epidermal growth factor receptor, PI3K and MEK signal kinases on NF-kappaB and AP-1 activation and IL-8 and VEGF expression in human head and neck squamous cell carcinoma lines. Int J Cancer. 2002; 99(4): 538–48.

[27] Vandercappellen J, Van Damme J, Struyf S. The role of CXC chemokines and their receptors in cancer. Cancer Lett. 2008; 267(2): 226–44.

[28] Dong G, Chen Z, Li ZY, Yeh NT, Bancroft CC, Van Waes C. Hepatocyte growth factor/scatter factor-induced activation of MEK and PI3K signal pathways contributes to expression of proangiogenic cytokines interleukin-8 and vascular endothelial growth factor in head and neck squamous cell carcinoma. Cancer Res. 2001; 61(15): 5911–8.

[29] Dong G, Lee TL, Yeh NT, Geoghegan J, Van Waes C, Chen Z. Metastatic squamous cell carcinoma cells that overexpress c-Met exhibit enhanced angiogenesis factor expression, scattering and metastasis in response to hepatocyte growth factor. Oncogene. 2004; 23(37): 6199–208.

[30] Worden B, Yang XP, Lee TL, Bagain L, Yeh NT, Cohen JG, et al. Hepatocyte growth factor/scatter factor differentially regulates expression of proangiogenic factors through Egr-1 in head and neck squamous cell carcinoma. Cancer Res. 2005; 65(16): 7071–80.

[31] Siemeister G, Martiny-Baron G, Marme D. The pivotal role of VEGF in tumor angiogenesis: molecular facts and therapeutic opportunities. Cancer Metastasis Rev. 1998; 17(2): 241–8.

[32] Kowanetz M, Ferrara N. Vascular endothelial growth factor signaling pathways: therapeutic perspective. Clin Cancer Res. 2006; 12(17): 5018–22.

[33] Lalla RV, Boisoneau DS, Spiro JD, Kreutzer DL. Expression of vascular endothelial growth factor receptors on tumor cells in head and neck squamous cell carcinoma. Arch Otolaryngol Head Neck Surg. 2003; 129(8): 882–8.

[34] Arnold L, Enders J, Thomas SM. Activated HGF-c-Met axis in head and neck cancer. Cancers (Basel). 2017; 9(12): 169.

[35] Aebersold DM, Landt O, Berthou S, Gruber G, Beer KT, Greiner RH, et al. Prevalence and clinical impact of Met Y1253D-activating point mutation in radiotherapy-treated squamous cell cancer of the oropharynx. Oncogene. 2003; 22(52): 8519–23.

[36] Hong IS. Stimulatory versus suppressive effects of GM-CSF on tumor progression in multiple cancer types. Exp Mol Med. 2016; 48(7): e242.

[37] Hansen G, Hercus TR, McClure BJ, Stomski FC, Dottore M, Powell J, et al. The structure of the GM-CSF receptor complex reveals a distinct mode of cytokine receptor activation. Cell. 2008; 134(3): 496–507.

[38] Suh HS, Kim MO, Lee SC. Inhibition of granulocyte-macrophage colony-stimulating factor signaling and microglial proliferation by anti-CD45RO: role of Hck tyrosine kinase and phosphatidylinositol 3-kinase/Akt. J Immunol. 2005; 174(5): 2712–9.

[39] Ninck S, Reisser C, Dyckhoff G, Helmke B, Bauer H, Herold-Mende C. Expression profiles of angiogenic growth factors in squamous cell carcinomas of the head and neck. Int J Cancer. 2003; 106(1): 34–44.

[40] Gutschalk CM, Herold-Mende CC, Fusenig NE, Mueller MM. Granulocyte colony-stimulating factor and granulocyte-macrophage colony-stimulating factor promote malignant growth of cells from head and neck squamous cell carcinomas in vivo. Cancer Res. 2006; 66(16): 8026–36.

[41] Cohen RF, Contrino J, Spiro JD, Mann EA, Chen LL, Kreutzer DL. Interleukin-8 expression by head and neck squamous cell carcinoma. Arch Otolaryngol Head Neck Surg. 1995; 121(2): 202–9.

[42] Mann EA, Spiro JD, Chen LL, Kreutzer DL. Cytokine expression by head and neck squamous cell carcinomas. Am J Surg. 1992; 164(6): 567–73.

[43] Woods KV, El-Naggar A, Clayman GL, Grimm EA. Variable expression of cytokines in human head and neck squamous cell carcinoma cell lines and consistent expression in surgical specimens. Cancer Res. 1998; 58(14): 3132–41.

[44] Yamamura M, Modlin RL, Ohmen JD, Moy RL. Local expression of antiinflammatory cytokines in cancer. J Clin Invest. 1993; 91(3): 1005–10.

[45] Woodford D, Johnson SD, De Costa A-MA, Young MRI. An inflammatory cytokine milieu is prominent in premalignant oral lesions, but subsides when lesions progress to squamous cell carcinoma. J Clin Cell Immunol. 2014; 5(3): 230.

[46] Johnson SD, De Costa A-MA, Young MRI. Effect of the premalignant and tumor microenvironment on immune cell cytokine production in head and neck cancer. Cancers (Basel). 2014; 6(2): 756–70.

[47] Juretić M, Cerović R, Belušić-Gobić M, Brekalo Pršo I, Kqiku L, Špalj S, et al. Salivary levels of TNF-α and IL-6 in patients with oral premalignant and malignant lesions. Folia Biol (Praha). 2013; 59(2): 99–102.

[48] Shkeir O, Athanassiou M, Lapadatescu M, Papagerakis P, Czerwinski MJ, Bradford CR, et al. In vitro cytokines release profile: predictive value for metastatic potential in head and neck squamous cell carcinomas. Head Neck. 2013; 35(11): 1542–50.

[49] Duffey DC, Crowl-Bancroft CV, Chen Z, Ondrey FG, Nejad-Sattari M, Dong G, et al. Inhibition of transcription factor nuclear factor-kappaB by a mutant inhibitor-kappaBalpha attenuates resistance of human head and neck squamous cell carcinoma to TNF-alpha caspase-mediated cell death. Br J Cancer. 2000; 83(10): 1367–74.

[50] Eytan DF, Snow GE, Carlson SG, Schiltz S, Chen Z, Van Waes C. Combination effects of SMAC mimetic birinapant with TNFalpha, TRAIL, and docetaxel in preclinical models of HNSCC. Laryngoscope. 2015; 125(3): E118–24.

[51] Lu H, Yan C, Quan XX, Yang X, Zhang J, Bian Y, et al. CK2 phosphorylates and inhibits TAp73 tumor suppressor function to promote expression of cancer stem cell genes and phenotype in head and neck cancer. Neoplasia. 2014; 16(10): 789–800.

[52] Lu H, Yang X, Duggal P, Allen CT, Yan B, Cohen J, et al. TNF-alpha promotes c-REL/DeltaNp63alpha interaction and TAp73 dissociation from key genes that mediate growth arrest and apoptosis in head and neck cancer. Cancer Res. 2011; 71(21): 6867–77.

[53] Druzgal CH, Chen Z, Yeh NT, Thomas GR, Ondrey FG, Duffey DC, et al. A pilot study of longitudinal serum cytokine and angiogenesis factor levels as markers of therapeutic response and survival in patients with head and neck squamous cell carcinoma. Head Neck. 2005; 27(9): 771–84.

[54] Astradsson T, Sellberg F, Berglund D, Ehrsson YT, Laurell GFE. Systemic inflammatory reaction in patients with head and neck cancer—an explorative study. Front Oncol. 2019; 9: 1177.

[55] Stanam A, Gibson-Corley KN, Love-Homan L, Ihejirika N, Simons AL. Interleukin-1 blockade overcomes erlotinib resistance in head and neck squamous cell carcinoma. Oncotarget. 2016; 7(46): 76087–100.

[56] Braunschweiger PG, Basrur VS, Cameron D, Sharpe L, Santos O, Perras JP, et al. Modulation of cisPlatin cytotoxicity by interleukin-1 alpha and resident tumor macrophages. Biotherapy. 1997; 10(2): 129–37.

[57] Freund-Brown J, Chirino L, Kambayashi T. Strategies to enhance NK cell function for the treatment of tumors and infections. Crit Rev Immunol. 2018; 38(2): 105–30.

[58] Bier H, Hoffmann T, Haas I, van Lierop A. Anti-(epidermal growth factor) receptor monoclonal antibodies for the induction of antibody-dependent cell-mediated cytotoxicity against squamous cell carcinoma lines of the head and neck. Cancer Immunol Immunother. 1998; 46(3): 167–73.

[59] Espinosa-Cotton M, Rodman Iii SN, Ross KA, Jensen IJ, Sangodeyi-Miller K, McLaren AJ, et al. Interleukin-1 alpha increases anti-tumor efficacy of cetuximab in head and neck squamous cell carcinoma. J Immunother Cancer. 2019; 7(1): 79.

[60] Jinno T, Kawano S, Maruse Y, Matsubara R, Goto Y, Sakamoto T, et al. Increased expression of interleukin-6 predicts poor response to chemoradiotherapy and unfavorable prognosis in oral squamous cell carcinoma. Oncol Rep. 2015; 33(5): 2161–8.

[61] Lee TL, Yeh J, Friedman J, Yan B, Yang X, Yeh NT, et al. A signal network involving coactivated NF-kappaB and STAT3 and altered p53 modulates BAX/BCL-XL expression and promotes cell survival of head and neck squamous cell carcinomas. Int J Cancer. 2008; 122(9): 1987–98.

[62] Sriuranpong V, Park JI, Amornphimoltham P, Patel V, Nelkin BD, Gutkind JS. Epidermal growth factor receptor-independent constitutive activation of STAT3 in head and neck squamous cell carcinoma is mediated by the autocrine/paracrine stimulation of the interleukin 6/gp130 cytokine system. Cancer Res. 2003; 63(11): 2948–56.

[63] Bu LL, Yu GT, Wu L, Mao L, Deng WW, Liu JF, et al. STAT3 induces immunosuppression by upregulating PD-1/PD-L1 in HNSCC. J Dent Res. 2017; 96(9): 1027–34.

[64] Liu Q, Yu S, Li A, Xu H, Han X, Wu K. Targeting interlukin-6 to relieve immunosuppression in tumor microenvironment. Tumour Biol. 2017; 39(6): 1010428317712445.

[65] Park SJ, Nakagawa T, Kitamura H, Atsumi T, Kamon H, Sawa S, et al. IL-6 regulates in vivo dendritic cell differentiation through STAT3 activation. J Immunol. 2004; 173(6): 3844–54.

[66] Wang T, Niu G, Kortylewski M, Burdelya L, Shain K, Zhang S, et al. Regulation of the innate and adaptive immune responses by Stat-3 signaling in tumor cells. Nat Med. 2004; 10(1): 48–54.

[67] Johnson DE, O'Keefe RA, Grandis JR. Targeting the IL-6/JAK/STAT3 signalling axis in cancer. Nat Rev Clin Oncol. 2018; 15(4): 234–48.

[68] Leong PL, Andrews GA, Johnson DE, Dyer KF, Xi S, Mai JC, et al. Targeted inhibition of Stat3 with a decoy oligonucleotide abrogates head and neck cancer cell growth. Proc Natl Acad Sci U S A. 2003; 100(7): 4138–43.

[69] Sen M, Thomas SM, Kim S, Yeh JI, Ferris RL, Johnson JT, et al. First-in-human trial of a STAT3 decoy oligonucleotide in head and neck tumors: implications for cancer therapy. Cancer Discov. 2012; 2(8): 694–705.

[70] Liu H, Shen J, Lu K. IL-6 and PD-L1 blockade combination inhibits hepatocellular carcinoma cancer development in mouse model. Biochem Biophys Res Commun. 2017; 486(2): 239–44.

[71] Lu C, Talukder A, Savage NM, Singh N, Liu K. JAK-STAT-mediated chronic inflammation impairs cytotoxic T lymphocyte activation to decrease anti-PD-1 immunotherapy efficacy in pancreatic cancer. Onco Targets Ther. 2017; 6(3): e1291106.

[72] Mace TA, Shakya R, Pitarresi JR, Swanson B, McQuinn CW, Loftus S, et al. IL-6 and PD-L1 antibody blockade combination therapy reduces tumour progression in murine models of pancreatic cancer. Gut. 2018; 67(2): 320–32.

[73] Cohen EEW, Harrington KJ, Hong DS, Mesia R, Brana I, Perez Segura P, et al. A phase Ib/II study (SCORES) of durvalumab (D) plus danvatirsen (DAN; AZD9150) or AZD5069 (CX2i) in advanced solid malignancies and recurrent/metastatic head and neck squamous cell carcinoma (RM-HNSCC): updated results. Ann Oncol. 2018; 29(Supplement 8): viii372–99.

[74] Schalper KA, Carleton M, Zhou M, Chen T, Feng Y, Huang SP, et al. Elevated serum interleukin-8 is associated with enhanced intratumor neutrophils and reduced clinical benefit of immune-checkpoint inhibitors. Nat Med. 2020; 26(5): 688–92.

[75] Yuen KC, Liu LF, Gupta V, Madireddi S, Keerthivasan S, Li C, et al. High systemic and tumor-associated IL-8 correlates with reduced clinical benefit of PD-L1 blockade. Nat Med. 2020; 26(5): 693–8.

[76] Sanmamed MF, Perez-Gracia JL, Schalper KA, Fusco JP, Gonzalez A, Rodriguez-Ruiz ME, et al. Chavnges in serum interleukin-8 (IL-8) levels reflect and predict response to anti-PD-1 treatment in melanoma and non-small-cell lung cancer patients. Ann Oncol. 2017; 28(8): 1988–95.

[77] Greene S, Robbins Y, Mydlarz WK, Huynh AP, Schmitt NC, Friedman J, et al. Inhibition of MDSC trafficking with SX-682, a CXCR1/2 inhibitor, enhances NK-cell immunotherapy in head and neck cancer models. Clin Cancer Res. 2020; 26(6): 1420–31.

[78] Sun SC. The noncanonical NF-kappaB pathway. Immunol Rev. 2012; 246(1): 125–40.

[79] Zhang Q, Lenardo MJ, Baltimore D. 30 years of NF-kappaB: a blossoming of relevance to human pathobiology. Cell. 2017; 168(1–2): 37–57.

[80] House CD, Grajales V, Ozaki M, Jordan E, Wubneh H, Kimble DC, et al. IKappaKappaepsilon cooperates with either MEK or non-canonical NF-κB driving growth of triple-negative breast cancer cells in different contexts. BMC Cancer. 2018; 18(1): 595.

[81] Khongthong P, Roseweir AK, Edwards J. The NF-κB pathway and endocrine therapy resistance in breast cancer. Endocr Relat Cancer. 2019; 26(6): R369–R80.

[82] Sakamoto K, Maeda S. Targeting NF-kappaB for colorectal cancer. Expert Opin Ther Targets. 2010; 14(6): 593–601.

[83] Soleimani A, Rahmani F, Ferns GA, Ryzhikov M, Avan A, Hassanian SM. Role of the NF-kappaB signaling pathway in the pathogenesis of colorectal cancer. Gene. 2020; 726: 144132.

[84] Taniguchi K, Karin M. NF-kappaB, inflammation, immunity and cancer: coming of age. Nat Rev Immunol. 2018; 18(5): 309–24.

[85] Van Waes C. Nuclear factor-kappaB in development, prevention, and therapy of cancer. Clin Cancer Res. 2007; 13(4): 1076–82.

[86] Giuliani C, Bucci I, Napolitano G. The role of the transcription factor nuclear factor-kappa B in thyroid autoimmunity and cancer. Front Endocrinol (Lausanne). 2018; 9: 471.

[87] Liu T, Zhang L, Joo D, Sun SC. NF-kappaB signaling in inflammation. Signal Transduct Target Ther. 2017; 2: 17023.

[88] Cartwright T, Perkins ND, Wilson CL. NFKB1: a suppressor of inflammation, ageing and cancer. FEBS J. 2016; 283(10): 1812–22.

[89] Kaltschmidt B, Greiner JFW, Kadhim HM, Kaltschmidt C. Subunit-specific role of NF-kappaB in cancer. Biomedicines. 2018; 6(2): 44.

[90] Vander Broek R, Snow GE, Chen Z, Van Waes C. Chemoprevention of head and neck squamous cell carcinoma through inhibition of NF-kappaB signaling. Oral Oncol. 2014; 50(10): 930–41.

[91] Ben-Neriah Y. Regulatory functions of ubiquitination in the immune system. Nat Immunol. 2002; 3(1): 20–6.

[92] Christian F, Smith EL, Carmody RJ. The regulation of NF-kappaB subunits by phosphorylation. Cells. 2016; 5(1): 12.

[93] Arun P, Brown MS, Ehsanian R, Chen Z, Van Waes C. Nuclear NF-kappaB p65 phosphorylation at serine 276 by protein kinase A contributes to the malignant phenotype of head and neck cancer. Clin Cancer Res. 2009; 15(19): 5974–84.

[94] Sakurai H, Chiba H, Miyoshi H, Sugita T, Toriumi W. IkappaB kinases phosphorylate NF-kappaB p65 subunit on serine 536 in the transactivation domain. J Biol Chem. 1999; 274(43): 30353–6.

[95] Ondrey FG, Dong G, Sunwoo J, Chen Z, Wolf JS, Crowl-Bancroft CV, et al. Constitutive activation of transcription factors NF-(kappa)B, AP-1, and NF-IL6 in human head and neck squamous cell carcinoma cell lines that express pro-inflammatory and pro-angiogenic cytokines. Mol Carcinog. 1999; 26(2): 119–29.

[96] Dong G, Loukinova E, Chen Z, Gangi L, Chanturita TI, Liu ET, et al. Molecular profiling of transformed and metastatic murine squamous carcinoma cells by differential display and cDNA microarray reveals altered expression of multiple genes related to growth, apoptosis, angiogenesis, and the NF-kappaB signal pathway. Cancer Res. 2001; 61(12): 4797–808.

[97] Loercher A, Lee TL, Ricker JL, Howard A, Geoghegen J, Chen Z, et al. Nuclear factor-kappaB is an important modulator of the altered gene expression profile and malignant phenotype in squamous cell carcinoma. Cancer Res. 2004; 64(18): 6511–23.

[98] Cancer Genome Atlas Network. Comprehensive genomic characterization of head and neck squamous cell carcinomas. Nature. 2015; 517(7536): 576–82.

[99] Zhang J, Chen T, Yang X, Cheng H, Spath SS, Clavijo PE, et al. Attenuated TRAF3 fosters activation of alternative NF-kappaB and reduced expression of antiviral interferon, TP53, and RB to promote HPV-positive head and neck cancers. Cancer Res. 2018; 78(16): 4613–26.

[100] Chen T, Zhang J, Chen Z, Van Waes C. Genetic alterations in TRAF3 and CYLD that regulate nuclear factor kappaB and interferon signaling define head and neck cancer subsets harboring human papillomavirus. Cancer. 2017; 123(10): 1695–8.

[101] Mishra A, Bharti AC, Varghese P, Saluja D, Das BC. Differential expression and activation of NF-kappaB family proteins during oral carcinogenesis: role of high risk human papillomavirus infection. Int J Cancer. 2006; 119(12): 2840–50.

[102] Gupta S, Kumar P, Kaur H, Sharma N, Gupta S, Saluja D, et al. Constitutive activation and overexpression of NF-kappaB/c-Rel in conjunction with p50 contribute to aggressive tongue tumorigenesis. Oncotarget. 2018; 9(68): 33011–29.

[103] Freudlsperger C, Burnett JR, Friedman JA, Kannabiran VR, Chen Z, Van Waes C. EGFR-PI3K-AKT-mTOR signaling in head and neck squamous cell carcinomas: attractive targets for molecular-oriented therapy. Expert Opin Ther Targets. 2011; 15(1): 63–74.

[104] Vivanco I, Sawyers CL. The phosphatidylinositol 3-kinase AKT pathway in human cancer. Nat Rev Cancer. 2002; 2(7): 489–501.

[105] Dan HC, Cooper MJ, Cogswell PC, Duncan JA, Ting JP, Baldwin AS. Akt-dependent regulation of NF-κB is controlled by mTOR and Raptor in association with IKK. Genes Dev. 2008; 22(11): 1490–500.

[106] Dan HC, Ebbs A, Pasparakis M, Van Dyke T, Basseres DS, Baldwin AS. Akt-dependent activation of mTORC1 complex involves phosphorylation of mTOR (mammalian target of rapamycin) by IkappaB kinase alpha (IKKalpha). J Biol Chem. 2014; 289(36): 25227–40.

[107] Tanaka K, Babic I, Nathanson D, Akhavan D, Guo D, Gini B, et al. Oncogenic EGFR signaling activates an mTORC2-NF-kappaB

pathway that promotes chemotherapy resistance. Cancer Discov. 2011; 1(6): 524–38.

[108] Wilson W 3rd, Baldwin AS. Maintenance of constitutive IkappaB kinase activity by glycogen synthase kinase-3alpha/beta in pancreatic cancer. Cancer Res. 2008; 68(19): 8156–63.

[109] Nottingham LK, Yan CH, Yang X, Si H, Coupar J, Bian Y, et al. Aberrant IKKalpha and IKKbeta cooperatively activate NF-kappaB and induce EGFR/AP1 signaling to promote survival and migration of head and neck cancer. Oncogene. 2014; 33(9): 1135–47.

[110] Freudlsperger C, Bian Y, Contag Wise S, Burnett J, Coupar J, Yang X, et al. TGF-beta and NF-kappaB signal pathway cross-talk is mediated through TAK1 and SMAD7 in a subset of head and neck cancers. Oncogene. 2013; 32(12): 1549–59.

[111] Shaulian E, Karin M. AP-1 as a regulator of cell life and death. Nat Cell Biol. 2002; 4(5): E131–6.

[112] Atsaves V, Leventaki V, Rassidakis GZ, Claret FX. AP-1 transcription factors as regulators of immune responses in cancer. Cancers (Basel). 2019; 11(7): 1037.

[113] Hussain S, Bharti AC, Salam I, Bhat MA, Mir MM, Hedau S, et al. Transcription factor AP-1 in esophageal squamous cell carcinoma: alterations in activity and expression during human papillomavirus infection. BMC Cancer. 2009; 9: 329.

[114] Mishra A, Bharti AC, Saluja D, Das BC. Transactivation and expression patterns of Jun and Fos/AP-1 super-family proteins in human oral cancer. Int J Cancer. 2010; 126(4): 819–29.

[115] Gupta S, Kumar P, Kaur H, Sharma N, Saluja D, Bharti AC, et al. Selective participation of c-Jun with Fra-2/c-Fos promotes aggressive tumor phenotypes and poor prognosis in tongue cancer. Sci Rep. 2015; 5: 16811.

[116] Faust RA, Gapany M, Tristani P, Davis A, Adams GL, Ahmed K. Elevated protein kinase CK2 activity in chromatin of head and neck tumors: association with malignant transformation. Cancer Lett. 1996; 101(1): 31–5.

[117] Gapany M, Faust RA, Tawfic S, Davis A, Adams GL, Ahmed K. Association of elevated protein kinase CK2 activity with aggressive behavior of squamous cell carcinoma of the head and neck. Mol Med. 1995; 1(6): 659–66.

[118] Yu M, Yeh J, Van Waes C. Protein kinase casein kinase 2 mediates inhibitor-kappaB kinase and aberrant nuclear factor-kappaB activation by serum factor(s) in head and neck squamous carcinoma cells. Cancer Res. 2006; 66(13): 6722–31.

[119] Brown MS, Diallo OT, Hu M, Ehsanian R, Yang X, Arun P, et al. CK2 modulation of NF-kappaB, TP53, and the malignant phenotype in head and neck cancer by anti-CK2 oligonucleotides in vitro or in vivo via sub-50-nm nanocapsules. Clin Cancer Res. 2010; 16(8): 2295–307.

[120] Bian Y, Han J, Kannabiran V, Mohan S, Cheng H, Friedman J, et al. MEK inhibitor PD-0325901 overcomes resistance to CK2 inhibitor CX-4945 and exhibits anti-tumor activity in head and neck cancer. Int J Biol Sci. 2015; 11(4): 411–22.

[121] Chen Z, Yan B, Van Waes C. The role of the NF-kappaB transcriptome and proteome as biomarkers in human head and neck squamous cell carcinomas. Biomark Med. 2008; 2(4): 409–26.

[122] Allen CT, Conley B, Sunwoo JB, Van Waes C. CCR 20th anniversary commentary: preclinical study of proteasome inhibitor bortezomib in head and neck cancer. Clin Cancer Res. 2015; 21(5): 942–3.

[123] Allen C, Saigal K, Nottingham L, Arun P, Chen Z, Van Waes C. Bortezomib-induced apoptosis with limited clinical response is accompanied by inhibition of canonical but not alternative nuclear factor-κB subunits in head and neck cancer. Clin Cancer Res. 2008; 14(13): 4175–85.

[124] Gaykalova DA, Manola JB, Ozawa H, Zizkova V, Morton K, Bishop JA, et al. NF-kappaB and stat3 transcription factor signatures differentiate HPV-positive and HPV-negative head and neck squamous cell carcinoma. Int J Cancer. 2015; 137(8): 1879–89.

[125] Liu Y, Denlinger CE, Rundall BK, Smith PW, Jones DR. Suberoylanilide hydroxamic acid induces Akt-mediated phosphorylation of p300, which promotes acetylation and transcriptional activation of RelA/p65. J Biol Chem. 2006; 281(42): 31359–68.

[126] Webster GA, Perkins ND. Transcriptional cross talk between NF-kappaB and p53. Mol Cell Biol. 1999; 19(5): 3485–95.

[127] Herzog A, Bian Y, Vander Broek R, Hall B, Coupar J, Cheng H, et al. PI3K/mTOR inhibitor PF-04691502 antitumor activity is enhanced with induction of wild-type TP53 in human xenograft and murine knockout models of head and neck cancer. Clin Cancer Res. 2013; 19(14): 3808–19.

[128] Leiker AJ, DeGraff W, Choudhuri R, Sowers AL, Thetford A, Cook JA, et al. Radiation enhancement of head and neck squamous cell carcinoma by the dual PI3K/mTOR inhibitor PF-05212384. Clin Cancer Res. 2015; 21(12): 2792–801.

[129] Mohan S, Vander Broek R, Shah S, Eytan DF, Pierce ML, Carlson SG, et al. MEK inhibitor PD-0325901 overcomes resistance to PI3K/mTOR inhibitor PF-5212384 and potentiates antitumor effects in human head and neck squamous cell carcinoma. Clin Cancer Res. 2015; 21(17): 3946–56.

[130] Day TA, Shirai K, O'Brien PE, Matheus MG, Godwin K, Sood AJ, et al. Inhibition of mTOR signaling and clinical activity of rapamycin in head and neck cancer in a window of opportunity trial. Clin Cancer Res. 2019; 25(4): 1156–64.

[131] Vermorken JB, Herbst RS, Leon X, Amellal N, Baselga J. Overview of the efficacy of cetuximab in recurrent and/or metastatic squamous cell carcinoma of the head and neck in patients who previously failed platinum-based therapies. Cancer. 2008; 112(12): 2710–9.

[132] Van Waes C, Allen CT, Citrin D, Gius D, Colevas AD, Harold NA, et al. Molecular and clinical responses in a pilot study of gefitinib with paclitaxel and radiation in locally advanced head-and-neck cancer. Int J Radiat Oncol Biol Phys. 2010; 77(2): 447–54.

[133] Pernas FG, Allen CT, Winters ME, Yan B, Friedman J, Dabir B, et al. Proteomic signatures of epidermal growth factor receptor and survival signal pathways correspond to gefitinib sensitivity in head and neck cancer. Clin Cancer Res. 2009; 15(7): 2361–72.

[134] Kuriakose MA, Ramdas K, Dey B, Iyer S, Rajan G, Elango KK, et al. A randomized double-blind placebo-controlled phase IIB trial of

curcumin in oral leukoplakia. Cancer Prev Res (Phila). 2016; 9(8): 683–91.
[135] Hanahan D, Weinberg RA. Hallmarks of cancer: the next generation. Cell. 2011; 144(5): 646–74.
[136] Corn JE, Vucic D. Ubiquitin in inflammation: the right linkage makes all the difference. Nat Struct Mol Biol. 2014; 21(4): 297–300.
[137] Hu H, Sun S-C. Ubiquitin signaling in immune responses. Cell Res. 2016; 26(4): 457–83.
[138] Komander D, Clague MJ, Urbé S. Breaking the chains: structure and function of the deubiquitinases. Nat Rev Mol Cell Biol. 2009; 10(8): 550–63.
[139] Ji Z, He L, Regev A, Struhl K. Inflammatory regulatory network mediated by the joint action of NF-κB, STAT3, and AP-1 factors is involved in many human cancers. Proc Natl Acad Sci U S A. 2019; 116(19): 9453–62.
[140] Wang G, Gao Y, Li L, Jin G, Cai Z, Chao J-I, et al. K63-linked ubiquitination in kinase activation and cancer. Front Oncol. 2012; 2: 5.
[141] Ea C-K, Deng L, Xia Z-P, Pineda G, Chen ZJ. Activation of IKK by TNFalpha requires site-specific ubiquitination of RIP1 and polyubiquitin binding by NEMO. Mol Cell. 2006; 22(2): 245–57.
[142] Wang C, Deng L, Hong M, Akkaraju GR, Inoue J, Chen ZJ. TAK1 is a ubiquitin-dependent kinase of MKK and IKK. Nature. 2001; 412(6844): 346–51.
[143] Winston JT, Strack P, Beer-Romero P, Chu CY, Elledge SJ, Harper JW. The SCFbeta-TRCP-ubiquitin ligase complex associates specifically with phosphorylated destruction motifs in IkappaBalpha and beta-catenin and stimulates IkappaBalpha ubiquitination in vitro. Genes Dev. 1999; 13(3): 270–83.
[144] Li X, Commane M, Jiang Z, Stark GR. IL-1-induced NFkappa B and c-Jun N-terminal kinase (JNK) activation diverge at IL-1 receptor-associated kinase (IRAK). Proc Natl Acad Sci U S A. 2001; 98(8): 4461–5.
[145] Griesinger AM, Josephson RJ, Donson AM, Mulcahy Levy JM, Amani V, Birks DK, et al. Interleukin-6/STAT3 pathway signaling drives an inflammatory phenotype in Group A ependymoma. Cancer Immunol Res. 2015; 3(10): 1165–74.
[146] Haas TL, Emmerich CH, Gerlach B, Schmukle AC, Cordier SM, Rieser E, et al. Recruitment of the linear ubiquitin chain assembly complex stabilizes the TNF-R1 signaling complex and is required for TNF-mediated gene induction. Mol Cell. 2009; 36(5): 831–44.
[147] Tokunaga F, Sakata S-I, Saeki Y, Satomi Y, Kirisako T, Kamei K, et al. Involvement of linear polyubiquitylation of NEMO in NF-kappaB activation. Nat Cell Biol. 2009; 11(2): 123–32.
[148] Harhaj EW, Dixit VM. Deubiquitinases in the regulation of NF-κB signaling. Cell Res. 2011; 21(1): 22–39.
[149] Catrysse L, Vereecke L, Beyaert R, van Loo G. A20 in inflammation and autoimmunity. Trends Immunol. 2014; 35(1): 22–31.
[150] Shembade N, Ma A, Harhaj EW. Inhibition of NF-kappaB signaling by A20 through disruption of ubiquitin enzyme complexes. Science. 2010; 327(5969): 1135–9.
[151] Iliopoulos D, Jaeger SA, Hirsch HA, Bulyk ML, Struhl K. STAT3 activation of miR-21 and miR-181b-1 via PTEN and CYLD are part of the epigenetic switch linking inflammation to cancer. Mol Cell. 2010; 39(4): 493–506.
[152] Hrdinka M, Fiil BK, Zucca M, Leske D, Bagola K, Yabal M, et al. CYLD limits Lys63- and Met1-linked ubiquitin at receptor complexes to regulate innate immune signaling. Cell Rep. 2016; 14(12): 2846–58.
[153] Enesa K, Zakkar M, Chaudhury H, Luong LA, Rawlinson L, Mason JC, et al. NF-kappaB suppression by the deubiquitinating enzyme Cezanne: a novel negative feedback loop in pro-inflammatory signaling. J Biol Chem. 2008; 283(11): 7036–45.
[154] Xu G, Tan X, Wang H, Sun W, Shi Y, Burlingame S, et al. Ubiquitin-specific peptidase 21 inhibits tumor necrosis factor alpha-induced nuclear factor kappaB activation via binding to and deubiquitinating receptor-interacting protein 1. J Biol Chem. 2010; 285(2): 969–78.
[155] Goncharov T, Niessen K, de Almagro MC, Izrael-Tomasevic A, Fedorova AV, Varfolomeev E, et al. OTUB1 modulates c-IAP1 stability to regulate signalling pathways. EMBO J. 2013; 32(8): 1103–14.
[156] Wiener R, Zhang X, Wang T, Wolberger C. The mechanism of OTUB1-mediated inhibition of ubiquitination. Nature. 2012; 483(7391): 618–22.
[157] Sun W, Tan X, Shi Y, Xu G, Mao R, Gu X, et al. USP11 negatively regulates TNFalpha-induced NF-kappaB activation by targeting on IkappaBalpha. Cell Signal. 2010; 22(3): 386–94.
[158] Cheng H, Yang X, Si H, Saleh AD, Xiao W, Coupar J, et al. Genomic and transcriptomic characterization links cell lines with aggressive head and neck cancers. Cell Rep. 2018; 25(5): 1332–45.e5.
[159] Morgan EL, Chen Z, Van Waes C. Regulation of NFκB Signalling by Ubiquitination: A Potential Therapeutic Target in Head and Neck Squamous Cell Carcinoma?. Cancers (Basel). 2020; 12(10): 2877.
[160] Hajek M, Sewell A, Kaech S, Burtness B, Yarbrough WG, Issaeva N. TRAF3/CYLD mutations identify a distinct subset of human papillomavirus-associated head and neck squamous cell carcinoma. Cancer. 2017; 123(10): 1778–90.
[161] Ge Z, Leighton JS, Wang Y, Peng X, Chen Z, Chen H, et al. Integrated genomic analysis of the ubiquitin pathway across cancer types. Cell Rep. 2018; 23(1): 213–26.e3.
[162] Arabi A, Ullah K, Branca RMM, Johansson J, Bandarra D, Haneklaus M, et al. Proteomic screen reveals Fbw7 as a modulator of the NF-κB pathway. Nat Commun. 2012; 3(1): 976–11.
[163] Nateri AS, Riera-Sans L, Da Costa C, Behrens A. The ubiquitin ligase SCFFbw7 antagonizes apoptotic JNK signaling. Science. 2004; 303(5662): 1374–8.
[164] Davis RJ, Welcker M, Clurman BE. Tumor suppression by the Fbw7 ubiquitin ligase: mechanisms and opportunities. Cancer Cell. 2014; 26(4): 455–64.
[165] Lee D-F, Kuo H-P, Liu M, Chou C-K, Xia W, Du Y, et al. KEAP1 E3 ligase-mediated downregulation of NF-kappaB signaling by

targeting IKKbeta. Mol Cell. 2009; 36(1): 131–40.

[166] Drainas AP, Lambuta RA, Ivanova I, Serçin Ö, Sarropoulos I, Smith ML, et al. Genome-wide screens implicate loss of cullin ring ligase 3 in persistent proliferation and genome instability in TP53-deficient cells. Cell Rep. 2020; 31(1): 107465.

[167] Liu J, Shaik S, Dai X, Wu Q, Zhou X, Wang Z, et al. Targeting the ubiquitin pathway for cancer treatment. Biochim Biophys Acta. 2015; 1855(1): 50–60.

[168] Hideshima T, Richardson PG, Anderson KC. Mechanism of action of proteasome inhibitors and deacetylase inhibitors and the biological basis of synergy in multiple myeloma. Mol Cancer Ther. 2011; 10(11): 2034–42.

[169] Oerlemans R, Franke NE, Assaraf YG, Cloos J, van Zantwijk I, Berkers CR, et al. Molecular basis of bortezomib resistance: proteasome subunit beta5 (PSMB5) gene mutation and overexpression of PSMB5 protein. Blood. 2008; 112(6): 2489–99.

[170] Siegel DS, Martin T, Wang M, Vij R, Jakubowiak AJ, Lonial S, et al. A phase 2 study of single-agent carfilzomib (PX-171-003-A1) in patients with relapsed and refractory multiple myeloma. Blood. 2012; 120(14): 2817–25.

[171] Chen Z, Ricker JL, Malhotra PS, Nottingham L, Bagain L, Lee TL, et al. Differential bortezomib sensitivity in head and neck cancer lines corresponds to proteasome, nuclear factor-kappaB and activator protein-1 related mechanisms. Mol Cancer Ther. 2008; 7(7): 1949–60.

[172] Sunwoo JB, Chen Z, Dong G, Yeh N, Crowl Bancroft C, Sausville E, et al. Novel proteasome inhibitor PS-341 inhibits activation of nuclear factor-kappaB, cell survival, tumor growth, and angiogenesis in squamous cell carcinoma. Clin Cancer Res. 2001; 7(5): 1419–28.

[173] Kim J, Guan J, Chang I, Chen X, Han D, Wang C-Y. PS-341 and histone deacetylase inhibitor synergistically induce apoptosis in head and neck squamous cell carcinoma cells. Mol Cancer Ther. 2010; 9(7): 1977–84.

[174] Fulda S, Vucic D. Targeting IAP proteins for therapeutic intervention in cancer. Nat Rev Drug Discov. 2012; 11(2): 109–24.

[175] Varfolomeev E, Blankenship JW, Wayson SM, Fedorova AV, Kayagaki N, Garg P, et al. IAP antagonists induce autoubiquitination of c-IAPs, NF-kappaB activation, and TNFalpha-dependent apoptosis. Cell. 2007; 131(4): 669–81.

[176] Shiozaki EN, Chai J, Rigotti DJ, Riedl SJ, Li P, Srinivasula SM, et al. Mechanism of XIAP-mediated inhibition of caspase-9. Mol Cell. 2003; 11(2): 519–27.

[177] Eytan DF, Snow GE, Carlson S, Derakhshan A, Saleh A, Schiltz S, et al. SMAC mimetic birinapant plus radiation eradicates human head and neck cancers with genomic amplifications of cell death genes FADD and BIRC2. Cancer Res. 2016; 76(18): 5442–54.

[178] Perimenis P, Galaris A, Voulgari A, Prassa M, Pintzas A. IAP antagonists Birinapant and AT-406 efficiently synergise with either TRAIL, BRAF, or BCL-2 inhibitors to sensitise BRAFV600E colorectal tumour cells to apoptosis. BMC Cancer. 2016; 16(1): 624–16.

[179] Fulda S. Promises and challenges of Smac mimetics as cancer therapeutics. Clin Cancer Res. 2015; 21(22): 5030–6.

[180] Tolcher AW, Bendell JC, Papadopoulos KP, Burris HA, Patnaik A, Fairbrother WJ, et al. A phase I dose-escalation study evaluating the safety tolerability and pharmacokinetics of CUDC-427, a potent, oral, monovalent IAP antagonist, in patients with refractory solid tumors. Clin Cancer Res. 2016; 22(18): 4567–73.

[181] Hurwitz HI, Smith DC, Pitot HC, Brill JM, Chugh R, Rouits E, et al. Safety, pharmacokinetics, and pharmacodynamic properties of oral DEBIO1143 (AT-406) in patients with advanced cancer: results of a first-in-man study. Cancer Chemother Pharmacol. 2015; 75(4): 851–9.

[182] Zhao X-Y, Wang X-Y, Wei Q-Y, Xu Y-M, Lau ATY. Potency and selectivity of SMAC/DIABLO mimetics in solid tumor therapy. Cell. 2020; 9(4): 1012.

[183] Matzinger O, Viertl D, Tsoutsou P, Kadi L, Rigotti S, Zanna C, et al. The radiosensitizing activity of the SMAC-mimetic, Debio 1143, is TNFα-mediated in head and neck squamous cell carcinoma. Radiother Oncol. 2015; 116(3): 495–503.

[184] Pierce JW, Schoenleber R, Jesmok G, Best J, Moore SA, Collins T, et al. Novel inhibitors of cytokine-induced IkappaBalpha phosphorylation and endothelial cell adhesion molecule expression show anti-inflammatory effects in vivo. J Biol Chem. 1997; 272(34): 21096–103.

[185] Yang L, Kumar B, Shen C, Zhao S, Blakaj D, Li T, et al. LCL161, a SMAC-mimetic, preferentially radiosensitizes human papillomavirus-negative head and neck squamous cell carcinoma. Mol Cancer Ther. 2019; 18(6): 1025–35.

[186] Xiao R, An Y, Ye W, Derakhshan A, Cheng H, Yang X, et al. Dual antagonist of cIAP/XIAP ASTX660 sensitizes HPV− and HPV+ head and neck cancers to TNFα, TRAIL, and radiation therapy. Clin Cancer Res. 2019; 25(21): 6463–74.

[187] Ye W, Gunti S, Allen CT, Hong Y, Clavijo PE, Van Waes C, et al. ASTX660, an antagonist of cIAP1/2 and XIAP, increases antigen processing machinery and can enhance radiation-induced immunogenic cell death in preclinical models of head and neck cancer. Onco Targets Ther. 2020; 9(1): 1710398.

[188] Stratton MR, Campbell PJ, Futreal PA. The cancer genome. Nature. 2009; 458(7239): 719–24.

[189] Lawrence MS, Stojanov P, Polak P, Kryukov GV, Cibulskis K, Sivachenko A, et al. Mutational heterogeneity in cancer and the search for new cancer-associated genes. Nature. 2013; 499(7457): 214–8.

[190] Campbell JD, Yau C, Bowlby R, Liu Y, Brennan K, Fan H, et al. Genomic, pathway network, and immunologic features distinguishing squamous carcinomas. Cell Rep. 2018; 23(1): 194–212.e6.

[191] Hutter C, Zenklusen JC. The Cancer Genome Atlas: creating lasting value beyond its data. Cell. 2018; 173(2): 283–5.

[192] The TCGA Legacy. Cell. 2018; 173(2): 281–2.

[193] Consortium GT, Laboratory DA, Coordinating Center-Analysis Working G, Statistical Methods groups-Analysis Working G, Enhancing Gg, Fund NIHC, et al. Genetic effects on gene expression across human tissues. Nature. 2017; 550(7675): 204-13.

[194] Tsherniak A, Vazquez F, Montgomery PG, Weir BA, Kryukov G, Cowley GS, et al. Defining a Cancer Dependency Map. Cell. 2017; 170(3): 564–76. e16.

[195] Iorio F, Knijnenburg TA, Vis DJ, Bignell GR, Menden MP, Schubert M, et al. A Landscape of Pharmacogenomic Interactions in Cancer. Cell. 2016; 166(3): 740-54.

[196] Uhlen M, Fagerberg L, Hallstrom BM, Lindskog C, Oksvold P, Mardinoglu A, et al. Proteomics. Tissue-based map of the human proteome. Science. 2015; 347(6220): 1260419.

[197] Parfenov M, Pedamallu CS, Gehlenborg N, Freeman SS, Danilova L, Bristow CA, et al. Characterization of HPV and host genome interactions in primary head and neck cancers. Proc Natl Acad Sci U S A. 2014; 111(43): 15544–9.

[198] Hoadley KA, Yau C, Wolf DM, Cherniack AD, Tamborero D, Ng S, et al. Multiplatform analysis of 12 cancer types reveals molecular classification within and across tissues of origin. Cell. 2014; 158(4): 929–44.

[199] Hoadley KA, Yau C, Hinoue T, Wolf DM, Lazar AJ, Drill E, et al. Cell-of-origin patterns dominate the molecular classification of 10,000 tumors from 33 types of cancer. Cell. 2018; 173(2): 291–304.e6.

[200] Ding L, Bailey MH, Porta-Pardo E, Thorsson V, Colaprico A, Bertrand D, et al. Perspective on oncogenic processes at the end of the beginning of cancer genomics. Cell. 2018; 173(2): 305–20.e10.

[201] Sanchez-Vega F, Mina M, Armenia J, Chatila WK, Luna A, La KC, et al. Oncogenic signaling pathways in the Cancer Genome Atlas. Cell. 2018; 173(2): 321–37.e10.

[202] Bailey MH, Tokheim C, Porta-Pardo E, Sengupta S, Bertrand D, Weerasinghe A, et al. Comprehensive characterization of cancer driver genes and mutations. Cell. 2018; 174(4): 1034–5.

[203] Thorsson V, Gibbs DL, Brown SD, Wolf D, Bortone DS, Ou Yang TH, et al. The immune landscape of cancer. Immunity. 2018; 48(4): 812–30.e14.

[204] Barretina J, Caponigro G, Stransky N, Venkatesan K, Margolin AA, Kim S, et al. The Cancer Cell Line Encyclopedia enables predictive modelling of anticancer drug sensitivity. Nature. 2012; 483(7391): 603–7.

[205] Ghandi M, Huang FW, Jane-Valbuena J, Kryukov GV, Lo CC, McDonald ER 3rd, et al. Next-generation characterization of the Cancer Cell Line Encyclopedia. Nature. 2019; 569(7757): 503–8.

[206] Ludwig ML, Kulkarni A, Birkeland AC, Michmerhuizen NL, Foltin SK, Mann JE, et al. The genomic landscape of UM-SCC oral cavity squamous cell carcinoma cell lines. Oral Oncol. 2018; 87: 144–51.

[207] Mann JE, Kulkarni A, Birkeland AC, Kafelghazal J, Eisenberg J, Jewell BM, et al. The molecular landscape of the University of Michigan laryngeal squamous cell carcinoma cell line panel. Head Neck. 2019; 41(9): 3114–24.

[208] van Harten AM, Poell JB, Buijze M, Brink A, Wells SI, Rene Leemans C, et al. Characterization of a head and neck cancer-derived cell line panel confirms the distinct TP53-proficient copy number-silent subclass. Oral Oncol. 2019; 98: 53–61.

[209] McDonald ER 3rd, de Weck A, Schlabach MR, Billy E, Mavrakis KJ, Hoffman GR, et al. Project DRIVE: a compendium of cancer dependencies and synthetic lethal relationships uncovered by large-scale, deep RNAi screening. Cell. 2017; 170(3): 577–92.e10.

[210] Behan FM, Iorio F, Picco G, Goncalves E, Beaver CM, Migliardi G, et al. Prioritization of cancer therapeutic targets using CRISPR-Cas9 screens. Nature. 2019; 568(7753): 511–6.

[211] Corsello SM, Bittker JA, Liu Z, Gould J, McCarren P, Hirschman JE, et al. The Drug Repurposing Hub: a next-generation drug library and information resource. Nat Med. 2017; 23(4): 405–8.

[212] Corsello SM, Nagari RT, Spangler RD, Rossen J, Kocak M, Bryan JG, et al. Discovering the anticancer potential of non-oncology drugs by systematic viability profiling. Nat Cancer. 2020; 1(2): 235–48.

[213] Yu C, Mannan AM, Yvone GM, Ross KN, Zhang YL, Marton MA, et al. High-throughput identification of genotype-specific cancer vulnerabilities in mixtures of barcoded tumor cell lines. Nat Biotechnol. 2016; 34(4): 419–23.

[214] Yang X, Cheng H, Chen J, Wang R, Saleh A, Si H, et al. Head and neck cancers promote an inflammatory transcriptome through coactivation of classic and alternative NF-kappaB pathways. Cancer Immunol Res. 2019; 7(11): 1760–74.

第 8 章

Justin M. Young and Stephen Thaddeus Connelly

头颈癌相关疼痛
Pain Associated with Head and Neck Cancers

引 言

　　头颈癌是一种起病隐匿的进行性发展的疾病，因其原发病灶位置的不同，可能出现各种各样的症状。病变可能位于各种解剖结构中，如鼻窦、鼻腔、唾液腺、舌、唇、口腔、咽或喉等。当病变侵犯这些解剖结构时，可能会出现或伴随与原发灶解剖位置相关的典型症状，但并不是所有同类型的患者都会出现同样的症状。因此，诊断医生必须意识到，无症状或无疼痛并不意味着没有病变。

　　通常来说，患者本人会在初时发现异常的病变或肿块，或是感到疼痛。在头颈部，包括口腔在内，嘴唇、牙龈、舌头和面颊部是最常见的受累区域。当原发病变位于口腔邻近的解剖结构，如唾液腺、鼻腔或鼻窦时，更易被忽视，且难以通过物理手段明确，往往需要病灶发展至一定的大小或侵犯邻近结构时才会被发现。此外，针对更深处的解剖位置如鼻咽部或喉部，则需要特殊的检查方法来明确病变。但在临床中却较少进行这些特殊检查，除非有明确的相关特殊症状支持检查的必要性。不同的初级保健医生在整理与总结患者病症的相关信息时存在较大的差异，通常根据他们不同的诊断，将患者及时转诊至对应的专科医生处进行治疗。当然，疼痛是最能协助诊断且最直接的症状之一。因此，那些隐匿的或不可见的病灶往往在疾病晚期才会出现症状。

　　在口腔内易于见到结构中（在下文中指嘴唇、牙龈、舌部或面颊上），通常能明显看到一处白色或红色的溃疡。这样的病变通常伴随疼痛，出血或经久不愈等症状，甚至产生炎症反应影响和破坏周围结构组织。典型的症状如下：① 吞咽，呼吸或言语功能障碍；② 进食或吞咽时伴随疼痛（吞咽困难）；③ 慢性咽痛或颈部疼痛（吞咽痛）；④ 频繁的头部疼痛；⑤ 听力困难或耳部异常声响（耳鸣）；⑥ 慢性鼻塞伴或不伴频繁的鼻腔出血（鼻出血）；⑦ 眼周肿胀或视物重影（复视）；⑧ 面部肌肉麻木或乏力；⑨ 异常的声音改变（声音嘶哑）。

　　当然，特殊的症状提示了病变的原发结构可能是哪里。例如，原发于喉部的病变可有声音改变、吞咽困难或疼痛等表现，也可出现咽部肿块及异物感，甚至在早期出现颈部淋巴结肿大。此

J. M. Young
Private Practice, San Francisco, CA, USA

Department of Oral & Maxillofacial Surgery, University of the Pacific, Arthur A. Dugoni School of Dentistry, San Francisco, CA, USA

S. T. Connelly
Department of Oral and Maxillofacial Surgery, University of California San Francisco (UCSF) School of Dentistry, San Francisco, CA, USA

San Francisco VA Health Care System, San Francisco, CA, USA

外，也可能在摄入食物或液体时发生咳嗽或呛咳，从而导致意外吸入少量的反流物质（微量吸入）。因此，一系列的症状表现可能指向原发的病变区域，但这并不绝对。

在口腔中，可能是因刺激物质、有毒物质、酒精或其他致癌物质的长期存在，导致有几个关键部位往往更容易出现病变。根据发生病变的频率排序为舌部及口底，智齿或最后一颗磨牙后的牙龈组织（磨牙后三角），舌侧缘及舌腹。此外，早期也能在牙龈、颊黏膜、嘴唇及腭部发现疼痛刺激或病变。

就目前而言，有关以疼痛作为主诉症状来评估头颈癌，从而进行诊断治疗的研究少之又少。在当前领域中，大多的数据都来自质量较差的报告，如自填式的问卷调查，而不是前瞻性或回顾性的研究[1]。相关研究表明，头颈癌患者普遍存在疼痛反应，其中与某些因素造成疼痛阈值降低或对疼痛更加敏感相关[1-4]。然而，目前对于头颈癌相关疼痛的认知是不足的。从逻辑上来讲，当一个封闭的遍布神经网络的关键解剖结构区域发生变化时，势必会出现疼痛与不适[1]。口腔癌（绝大多数为鳞状细胞癌）的独特之处在于，它们的发生往往伴随着严重的疼痛反应。因此，当病变仅仅为不典型增生或原位发生时，往往不会出现疼痛[2-4]。一旦病变的性质发生转变，其特征表现就是疼痛。通常，疼痛的发生多与局部的功能相关，这是因为口腔周围的肌肉组群和骨骼在我们咀嚼、说话和吞咽时不断运动[3]。但是，发生在口腔外的病变则往往不会出现疼痛，如舌根、鼻窦、喉部和前文提到的其他部位。

综上所述，我们将回顾性分析当代对头颈癌相关疼痛的理论知识，并在此基础上进一步探索与阐述头颈癌相关疼痛的发生机制与模式，同时也将探索与制定头颈癌相关疼痛的治疗方法。

头颈癌相关疼痛的机制

众所周知，大多数头颈癌和口腔鳞状细胞癌（OSCC）患者的首发症状为病变部位出现特异性疼痛[5]。目前，头颈癌相关疼痛广泛发生的主流观点认为，癌细胞能够产生大量的可溶性因子导致病变周围的微环境发生改变，从而在某种程度上触发、强化、敏感化和维持疼痛感受通路的开放[2,4]。此外，对于疼痛的感受是主观的，且可因个体或病变位置的不同而产生较大的差异。与口腔癌疼痛的相关因素可能包括以下几种：① 与原发病变相关，包括组织学类型（如分化）；② 是否存在远处转移；③ 病变是否位于肌肉或骨骼功能部位附近，大多数口腔鳞癌病变便是如此。已有的研究证明，口腔咀嚼功能如咀嚼、饮水、交谈、吞咽等行为将加剧口腔鳞癌患者的疼痛[3]。这种因行为增加疼痛的表现是较为罕见的，与其他类型的头颈鳞状细胞癌（HNSCC）如鼻咽癌和喉癌无关[4]。随着原发病变的进展，其周围的微环境同样发生了相关的变化，这可能会导致口腔癌疼痛的持续或加剧（图8-1）。这些变化发生在病变的邻近细胞中，使周围的微环境倾向于表现为促进组织修复的表型，而不是促炎的表型。由此可以推测，由于肿瘤具有共同的发生发展途径，那么其他类型的HNSCC同样会有相同或相似的表现。因此，与乳腺癌等其他癌症一样，侵袭能力更强的病变往往与细胞组织修复的表型相关。通常，与此相关的细胞如成纤维细胞，巨噬细胞和其他免疫细胞会在微环境改变时参与组织修复，而这些行为可以通过检测这些细胞释放和响应的细胞因子来证实。然而，目前还没充足的证据能够证明它们是如何导致口腔癌相关疼痛的[2,4-9]。

在微环境中的某些其他介质，可能也参与了疼痛的发生过程，包括癌症或微环境中产生的可溶性因子，如内皮素-1、趋化因子、整合素和蛋白酶或其激活受体（PAR-2），以及神经生长因子（NGF）和神经秩蛋白（NRTN）等[2,4,6-10]。

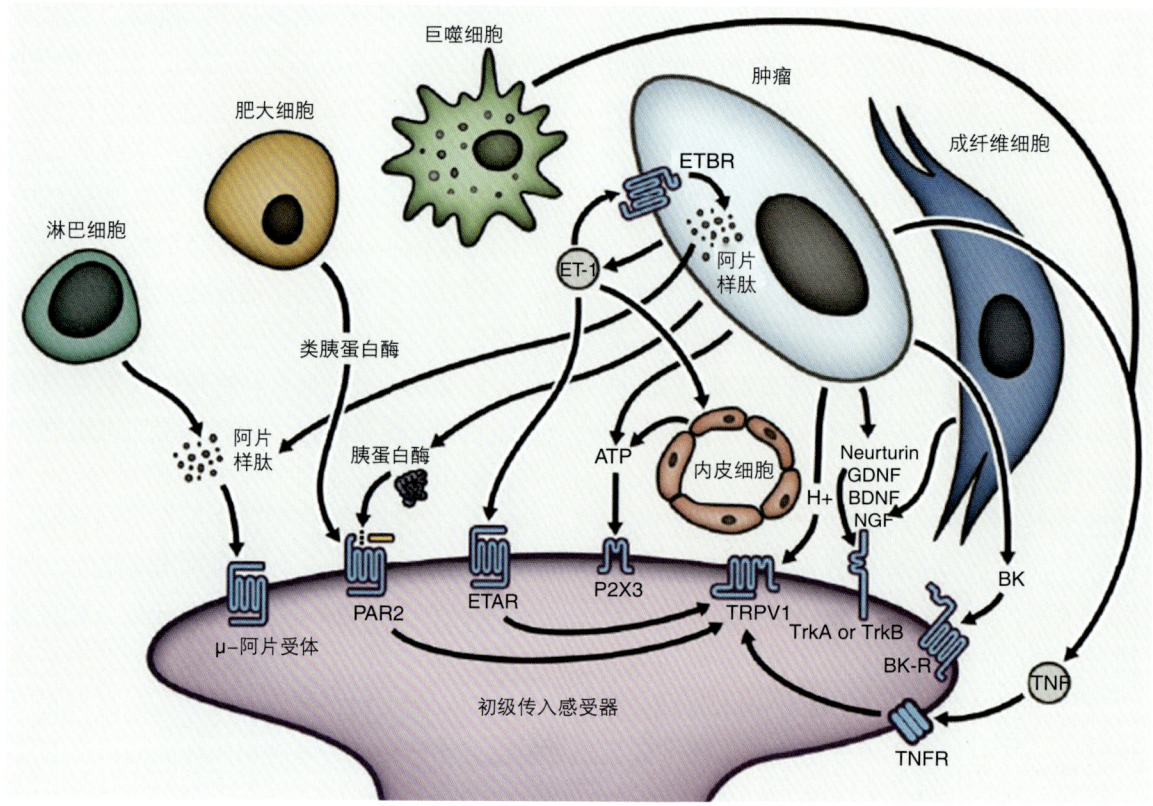

图 8-1 不同中介的再现可能导致了癌症性疼痛。注释：BDNF，脑源性神经营养因子；BK，缓激肽；BK-R，缓激肽受体；ET-1，内皮素-1；ETAR，内皮素 A 受体；ETBR，内皮素 B 受体；GDNF，神经胶质源性神经营养因子；NGF，神经生长因子；PAR2，蛋白酶激活受体；TrkA，酪氨酸激酶受体 A；TrkB，酪氨酸激酶受体 B；TRPV1，瞬时受体电位类香草素 1（经允许引自参考文献[4]）

这些介质间的复杂关系需要在它们相互作用时才能被更好地解读。据目前已知的研究，主要的信号通路如下文所示。

神经生长因子（NGF）

NGF 通常是为促进传入感觉神经元的局部生长而分泌的，通过激活其敏感的高亲和性酪氨酸激酶受体，癌症微环境中较高浓度的 NGF 可使许多类型的癌症增殖、活化和侵袭。此外，还可能出现热痛、机械痛和疼痛过敏。NGF 还可能在免疫调节中发挥作用，影响淋巴细胞，导致肥大细胞脱颗粒，并使脊髓中的 P 物质和降钙素基因相关肽（CGRP）全面增加。这两种物质都参与疼痛信号的传导，并最终导致敏感化。这或许可以解释 NGF 在痛觉过敏中的作用。据报道，NGF 与多种癌症"神经周围"扩散有关，即使在手术切除癌肿后也会导致持续疼痛[10,11]。血管生成和神经发生被认为具有相互关联的激活途径。NGF 本身可能是肿瘤微环境中血管生成的关键因子，而且有大量文件证明它是疼痛的先兆（图 8-2）[2,4,10-12]。

内皮素-1

内皮素-1 mRNA 和蛋白在 HNSCC 癌症微环境中的表达量升高，似乎是一种能产生痛觉的强效血管活性肽，是癌痛的主要调节因子[4,6]。它的下游靶点是两种 G 蛋白偶联受体（A 类和 B 类）。A 类受体主要位于外周感觉神经元上，而 B 类靶点则主要位于坐骨神经的非髓鞘施万细胞和背根神经节卫星细胞。后者与炎性疼痛和血管扩张有关[4-7]。这两种受体之间似乎存在着复杂的、鲜为人知的相互作用，它们可能控制着一个复杂的级联，控制癌症微环境中的痛觉。在动物模型中测试这些受体的激动剂和拮抗剂已经

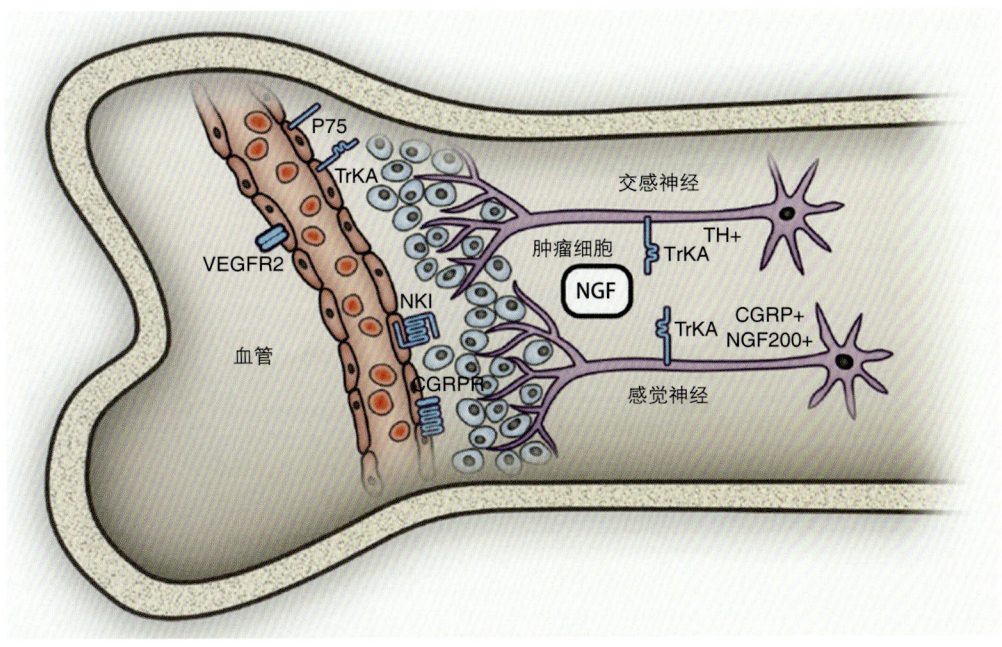

图8-2 NGF可刺激血管生成和神经发生。NGF通过TrkA作用，生成支配癌症微环境的感觉和交感神经纤维。而这两种纤维类型都会导致癌痛。注释：CGRP，降钙素基因相关蛋白；CGRPR，降钙素基因相关蛋白受体；NGF，神经生长因子；NK1，神经激肽-1受体；SP，P物质；TH，酪氨酸羟化酶；TrkA，酪氨酸激酶受体A；VEGF，血管内皮生长因子；VEGFR，血管内皮生长因子受体（经允许引自参考文献[4]）

取得了令人惊喜的结果，但到目前为止，还没有出现与临床相关的治疗机制[8,9]。通常情况下，激动剂会减轻疼痛，而拮抗剂则会引起疼痛。因此，这种效应似乎是多因素和反直觉的，或许表明了刺激这两个靶点之间的平衡状态。

蛋白酶与蛋白酶激活受体

头颈癌的蛋白水解活性是癌症发生、组织侵袭、转移以及癌症疼痛传播的关键机制之一[3]。在多种癌症如肾细胞癌、前列腺癌和结直肠癌中，均已鉴定出蛋白酶和蛋白水解肽（胰蛋白酶、胰酶和丝氨酸蛋白酶）[11]。研究表明，这些肽中的多数能够通过激活与蛋白酶相关的受体（PAR），直接增加痛觉信号传导，最终导致P物质和CGRP从C纤维中释放。PAR-2是其中一种特定的受体，已被详细研究。它位于感觉受体上，当在实验中将其注射至无癌小鼠体内时，其能够介导机械性痛觉过敏[3,13]。这引发了人们的猜测，即PAR类型机制的激活是否会导致口腔鳞状细胞癌（OSCC）中所出现的功能性疼痛或机械性疼痛[3,13]。在头颈癌环境中存在多种蛋白水解过程。其他关键因素包括基质金属蛋白酶（MMP）8和9、神经胰蛋白酶、补体因子B，以及纤溶酶原。特别是对于MMP 8和9，两者在正常组织与癌变组织之间的平衡可提示癌症的侵袭性、生物行为和转移扩散[3]。这是任何涉及补体及其激活或正常炎症级联反应过程的一个已广为人知的方面。而体内靶向蛋白水解过程可能成为未来的治疗靶点[14]。

治疗方式如何导致疼痛

众所周知，头颈癌相关疼痛在成功切除肿瘤后通常会得到缓解。然而，各种治疗方案所带来的后遗症通常会包括显著的疼痛。手术和放疗是目前头颈癌主要的治疗方式，但往往会使大多数患者正常的生物力学、口腔咀嚼功能和生活质量出现紊乱或下降[13,15]。这些情况部分是由黏膜炎、上皮萎缩、神经病变、颞下颌关节紊乱（TMD）或肌筋膜疼痛引起的[3,15]。而单是黏膜炎就对口腔及咀嚼功能、牙齿健康、吞咽功能和唾液分泌产生严重影响。而因为正常的黏膜免疫受到损害，这一过程也使接受放射治疗的患者更容易感染真菌。这些旨在去除原发病灶的必要手段往往会改变个体的生活，并需要较长的恢复时间。根治性切除本身可能会破坏正常结构，导致敏化、中枢疼痛现象和神经性疼痛的发展[15]。在手术治疗后即刻，对于其他方面，如言语不清以及头、颈、肩部区域的活动障碍，会变得更加明显[15]。

慢性疼痛的病理生理学

在这里，我们简要回顾疼痛发生和持续的病理生理学，以便理解何时、何地、为何以及如何进行干预可能对患者有益。在正常功能中，痛觉通过上行和下行信号的精细平衡来调节，这些信号最终由中枢神经系统（CNS）调控。传入信号从外周组织的痛觉感受器通过背根神经节和脊髓背角的初级传入神经传递到大脑。继发信号则被传递到大脑进行处理和响应。这些响应可能表现为调节、恐惧、焦虑、增强或退缩。任何对上行信号和下行调节响应之间平衡的扰动都会使得结果倾向于几种持续疼痛感知的过程。无论是手术还是放射治疗引起的组织损伤通常都会导致急性疼痛，这种疼痛在正常组织愈合期间或之前会得到缓解。目前大多数疼痛控制方式都用于这一阶段。相比之下，当正常体感功能延长且更高的中枢机制参与到疼痛的持续中时，慢性疼痛就会发生（图8-3）[16-19]。

调节

病理性疼痛处理通路的进行是在第二级神经元通过突触释放兴奋性氨基酸和神经肽（如P物质和谷氨酸）进行更长时间和持续刺激的情况下建立的，这些物质结合并激活脊髓背角第二级神经元的突触后受体[20-22]。过度的N-甲基-D-天冬氨酸（NMDA）和α-氨基-3-羟基-5-甲基-4-异噁唑丙酸（AMPA）介导的信号传导呈现出一种过度兴奋状态，这种状态放大了感觉反应，并可能导致更高阶脑区的激活，从而引发"中枢致敏"[17,20-22]。在这种状态下，脑干对下行疼痛调节通路的控制受损，下行抑制和兴奋之间的平衡被改变，兴奋占主导地位。疼痛感知通过上行疼痛通路的敏化得以持续和增强，而下行抑制的受损则导致疼痛抑制的解除。大脑此时接收到的是改变后的、异常的感觉信息。

伤害感受器的激活本身并不一定会产生疼痛。有些人即便有明显的脊柱病变也无症状，而另一些人则在没有明显器质性损伤的情况下经历严重的、慢性的、致残的疼痛[15,20]。患者对镇痛治疗的反应也有很大差异。因此，许多疼痛控制的治疗必须针对个体进行调整。许多典型的治疗方法，如单独使用非甾体抗炎药（NSAID）和阿片类药物可能无效。疼痛反应差异的一个关键因素是疼痛信息在中枢神经系统中的调节方式[15,20]。肿瘤生长已被证明可以直接影响周围神经纤维的形态。因为表皮细胞中的许多纤维都是痛觉感受器，所以这一观点已在表皮细胞中进行了研究论证[23]。存在于大多数头颈部黏膜表面的鳞状上皮细胞也会有这些相同的损害。在肿瘤发展过程中，痛觉感受器的致敏是由神经损伤、炎性介质的释放以及致痛物质的释放共同导致的[2]。

疼痛信号在从其背角进入点到达中枢神经系统并在大脑皮层中被处理和感知的过程中可以被增强或减弱。外周组织损伤或病变和疼痛强度在各种通路中受到调节和干扰[17,21,22,24]。如果不对重复刺激导致的持续性的调解敏化进行治疗和预

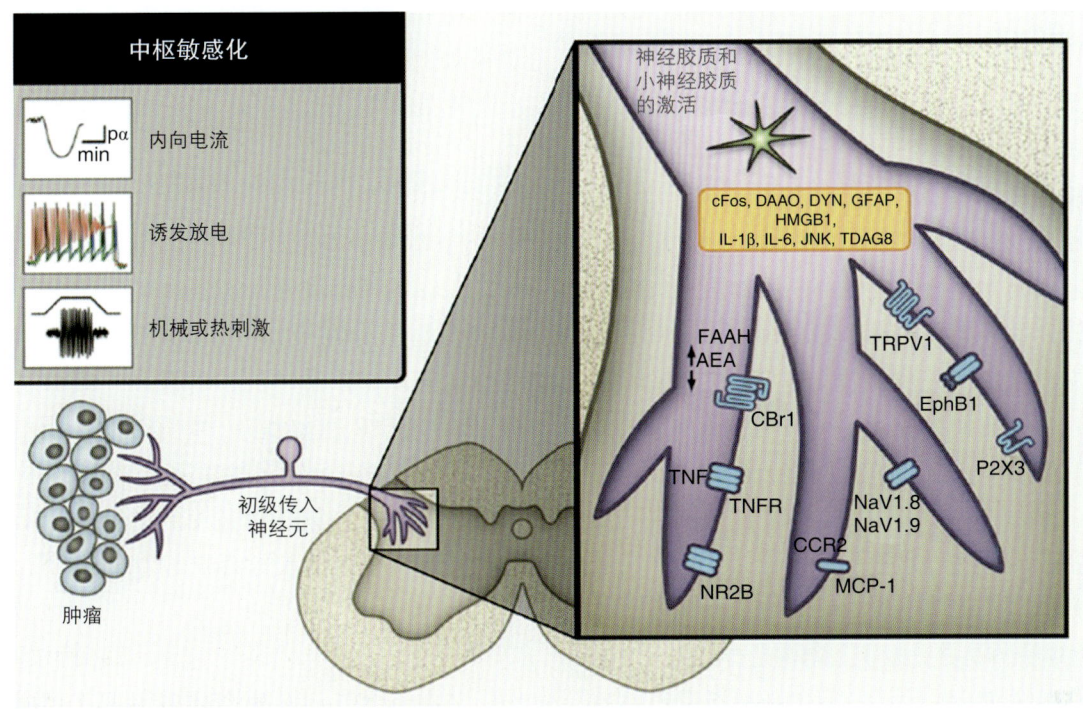

图 8-3 癌症相关疼痛信号上调的总结：有多种途径参与其中。注释：AEA，花生四烯乙醇胺；CBr1，大麻素受体 1；CCR2，趋化因子 C-C 基序受体 2；DAAO，D-氨基酸氧化酶；DYN，强啡肽；EphB1，ephrin B 配体受体；FAAH，脂肪酸酰胺水解酶；GFAP，胶质纤维酸性蛋白；HMGB1，高迁移率族蛋白 1；JNK，c-jun 氨基末端激酶；MCP-1，单核细胞趋化蛋白-1；NR2B，NMDA（N-甲基-D-天冬氨酸）受体亚基；TDAG8，T 细胞死亡相关基因 8；TNF，肿瘤坏死因子；TNFR，肿瘤坏死因子受体；TRPV1，瞬时受体电位香草素 1（经允许引自参考文献 [4]）

防，中枢神经系统的疼痛调节异常将持续存在，并可能对干预产生抵抗[24, 25]。

在头颈癌中，当体感系统的任何部分的神经纤维功能失调或错误传递信号时，即使没有病变或疾病（如区域淋巴结扩散或转移），也可能发展出神经性疼痛[26, 27]。这可能发生在癌症微环境形成之前。当慢性疼痛既不是伤害感受性（如组织损伤），也不是神经性（如神经病理）时，有研究提出了"改变的痛觉感受"的概念来解释这种疼痛机制[21, 26, 28]。自 21 世纪 00 年代初以来，慢性疼痛中的非适应性中枢神经系统神经可塑性已被视为一种独立的疾病过程，并且将其转化为肿瘤学和头颈部癌症手术的临床实践早已势在必行[29]。

新 进 展

我们将探讨当前的治疗方式、未来的研究领域以及新的治疗方法。其中一些治疗方式在其他学科中取得疗效，这些治疗方式的使用有望成为头颈癌疼痛的管理方案。如前所述，迄今为止，头颈癌疼痛管理的主要方法是非甾体药物和阿片类镇痛药。这些治疗方案大多过时、疗效欠佳，疼痛的临床管理仍然难以把握。此外，如前所述，在癌症微环境中引起疼痛和术后疼痛的众多因素需要不断的研究，探索新的治疗模式，为术后和辅助治疗后的头颈癌患者提供最佳生活质量。为此，我们讨论非手术干预的治疗方案。

复合镇痛制剂

局部使用复合镇痛药物在慢性疼痛管理中越来越受欢迎。它们可能更适用于 HNSCC 患者，特别是在潜在放射治疗后的黏膜炎区域，以及相关疼痛部位的治疗。复合镇痛制剂通常结合三种或更多种的止痛药物，使用尽可能低剂量的复合药物成分而不是单种高剂量的药物成分，以实现多种互补作用。一系列病例报道表明局部使用氯胺酮的人工唾液悬浮液可以显著缓解难治性的口腔黏膜炎[30]。其他常用的组合包括氟比洛芬、曲马多、可乐定、环苯扎林、布比卡因、巴氯芬、苯妥英钠、加巴喷丁和利多卡因[31]。

许多小型非对照试验显示复合镇痛制剂的有效性，但这种方法必须权衡局部渗透导致的全身暴露及潜在毒性的问题[32,33]。复方制剂不受 FDA 监管；载体制剂和活性药物浓度应标准化，以提高复合镇痛制剂的安全性和有效性[32,33]。因此，这些复合制剂需要进一步的研究，以确定它们是否可以在 HNSCC 和 OSCC 的动态骨骼肌环境中使用。

他喷他多

他喷他多是一种 μ-阿片类受体激动剂和去甲肾上腺素再摄取抑制剂结合成单个分子的复合制剂[34]。缓释制剂对多种慢性疼痛，伴或不伴有神经性疼痛的患者有疗效[35,36]。研究人员发现，在长期镇痛治疗期间，患者的功能、健康状况和生活质量均有所改善[36]。该药具有良好的安全性，胃肠道耐受性优于其他阿片类药物，且停药后戒断反应风险低[35,36]。在研究中，他喷他多在损伤性和神经性慢性腰痛模型中与羟考酮一样有效，具有更好的胃肠道耐受性和治疗依从性[37]。重要的是，他喷他多的 μ-阿片受体结合亲和力比吗啡低 18 倍，表明其滥用风险低于标准阿片类药物[37]。

西博帕多和 NKTR-181

这两种新型阿片类镇痛药正在开发和测试中，旨在提高标准阿片类药物的药物安全性。西博帕多是一种 μ-阿片受体激动剂和痛觉啡肽/孤啡肽阿片受体激动剂，可提高呼吸抑制的安全性[38]。NKTR-181 是一种长效的 μ-阿片受体激动剂，其结构特性可以降低其渗透血脑屏障的能力，并可能限制药物滥用的可能性，早期研究表明它具有良好的长期疼痛控制作用[39]。

神经化学

考虑到在任何肿瘤微环境中都存在神经化学调节剂，尤其是 OSCC 中，可以肯定地说，尚有许多新的治疗靶点未被发现。肿瘤微环境中的许多可溶性介质因子是通过它们的拮抗剂被发现的[2,4]，并不是所有的拮抗剂都被探索过。似乎在 OSCC 肿瘤微环境中的一些介质之间存在着微妙的平衡。例如，内皮素 A 和 B 受体之间的相互作用，当这些受体分别被激动和拮抗时，会产生不可预测的结果[2,4,9,10]。缓激肽对内皮素-1 的表达有直接影响，但其受体的激动和拮抗作用及其伴随的二阶效应仍不可预测[4]。

肿瘤微环境中介质的调节不属于某一炎症性、神经性或功能失调（肌肉骨骼）的独立范畴，而是具有复杂的、未被探索的相互作用。当受体被激活或失活时，受体翻译后的修饰和细胞内信号通路的持续切换，配体效应和兴奋性的变化使这些治疗靶点不适合长效的治疗[37,38,40]。

未 来 展 望

目前尚有其他几个潜在的治疗方案，例如，microRNA（miRNA）是信使 RNA 的抑制片段，能够阻断引发和保持疼痛信号的蛋白质的翻译过程[37,40]。虽然一些 miRNA 在维持疼痛中起作用，但其他 miRNA 的过表达可能通过调节趋化因子来促进疼痛的缓解。基因治疗疼痛的一个明显的缺陷是我们还不了解长期抑制这些途径的后果，并且基因疗法进入市场的途径是复杂的[37,40]。而抗体或免疫疗法在这个领域更有前景。目前正在进行针对NGF的试验，这是一种可溶性因子，不仅在疼痛中起重要作用，而且也能促进癌症的增殖。当抗体中和它的作用时，NGF的活性会降低。而这种方法的不足是，可能具有在中枢神经系统水平上阻断疼痛感知的主动机制。

表观遗传疗法也正兴起，其作用靶点是异常的遗传因素，这些异常因素会延长导致慢性疼痛的蛋白质异常转录。例如，组蛋白乙酰化的调节已被证明在疼痛的病理生理学中发挥作用[37,38,40]。此外，修饰特定位点的表观遗传状态可能允许转录水平的基因沉默[40]。

总之，随着研究和试验的开展，有希望进一步缓解头颈癌患者群体的疼痛。有了这些，我们将有希望进一步应对外科手术和生物力学治疗带来的不良反应，例如疼痛。这将对那些必须忍受治疗、生活方式改变和功能损害的患者而言更为友好。

参 考 文 献

[1] Macfarlane TV, Wirth T, Ranasinghe S, et al. Head and neck cancer pain: systematic review of prevalence and associated factors. J Oral Maxillofac Res. 2012; 3(1): e1.
[2] Schmidt BL. The neurobiology of cancer pain. J Oral Maxillofac Surg. 2015; 73(12 Suppl): S132-5.
[3] Connelly ST, Schmidt BL. Evaluation of pain in patients with oral squamous cell carcinoma. J Pain. 2004; 5(9): 505-10.
[4] Schmidt BL. The neurobiology of cancer pain. Neuroscientist. 2014; 20(5): 546-62.
[5] Marshall JA, Mahanna GK. Cancer in the differential diagnosis of orofacial pain. Dent Clin North Am. 1997; 41(2): 355-65.
[6] Lam DK, Dang D, Zhang J, Dolan JC, Schmidt BL. Novel animal models of acute and chronic cancer pain: a pivotal role for PAR2. J Neurosci. 2012; 32: 14178.
[7] Nelson J, Bagnato A, Battistini B, Nisen P. The endothelin axis: emerging role in cancer. Nat Rev Cancer. 2003; 3: 110-6.
[8] Pickering V, Jay Gupta R, Quang P, et al. Effect of peripheral endothelin-1 concentration on carcinoma-induced pain in mice. Eur J Pain. 2008; 12: 293.
[9] Quang PN, Schmidt BL. Endothelin-A receptor antagonism attenuates carcinoma-induced pain through opioids in mice. J Pain. 2010; 11(7): 663-71.
[10] Levi-Montalcini R, Skaper SD, Dal Toso R, Petrelli L, Leon A. Nerve growth factor: from neurotrophin to neurokine. Trends Neurosci. 1996; 19(11): 514-20.
[11] Schmidt BL, Hamamoto DT, Simone DA, Wilcox GL. Mechanism of cancer pain. Mol Interv. 2010; 10(3): 164-78.
[12] Nico B, Mangieri D, Benagiano V, Crivellato E, Ribatti D. Nerve growth factor as an angiogenic factor. Microvasc Res. 2008; 75: 135-41.
[13] Yang Y, Zhang P, Li W. Comparison of orofacial pain of patients with different stages of precancer and oral cancer. Sci Rep. 2017; 7(1): 203.
[14] Hardt M, Lam DK, Dolan JC, Schmidt BL. Surveying proteolytic processes in human cancer microenvironments by microdialysis and activity-based mass spectrometry. Proteomics Clin Appl. 2011; 5(11-12): 636-43.
[15] Gellrich NC, Schimming R, Schramm A, Schmalohr D, Bremerich A, Kugler J. Pain, function, and psychologic outcome before, during, and after intraoral tumor resection. J Oral Maxillofac Surg. 2002; 60(7): 772-7.
[16] Fornasari D. Pharmacotherapy for neuropathic pain: a review. Pain Ther. 2017; 6(1): 25-33.
[17] Colloca L, Ludman T, Bouhassira D, et al. Neuropathic pain. Nat Rev Dis Primers. 2017; 3: 17002.
[18] Finnerup NB, Attal N, Haroutounian S, et al. Pharmacotherapy for neuropathic pain in adults: systematic review, meta-analysis and updated NeuPSIG recommendations. Lancet Neurol. 2015; 14(2): 162-73.
[19] Binder A, Baron R. The pharmacological therapy of chronic neuropathic pain. Dtsch Arztebl Int. 2016; 113(37): 616-25.
[20] Rose M. Neck pain in adults. NetCE course reference material #94130.
[21] Baron R, Hans G, Dickenson AH. Peripheral input and its importance for central sensitization. Ann Neurol. 2013; 74(5): 630-6.
[22] Bannister K, Dickenson AH. What the brain tells the spinal cord. Pain. 2016; 157(10): 2148-51.
[23] Simone DA, Nolano M, Johnson T, Wendelschafer-Crabb G, Kennedy WR. Intradermal injection of capsaicin in humans produces degeneration and subsequent reinnervation of epidermal nerve fibers: correlation with sensory function. J Neurosci. 1998; 18(21): 8947-59.
[24] Yarnitsky D. Role of endogenous pain modulation in chronic pain mechanisms and treatment. Pain. 2015; 156(Suppl 1): S24-31.

Fornasari D. Pain mechanisms in patients with chronic pain. Clin Drug Investig. 2012; 32(1): 45–52.

[25] Worley SL. New directions in the treatment of chronic pain. PT. 2016; 41(2): 107–14.

[26] Spahr N, Hodkinson D, Jolly K, Williams S, Howard M, Thacker M. Distinguishing between nociceptive and neuropathic components in chronic low back pain using behavioral evaluation and sensory examination. Musculoskelet Sci Pract. 2017; 27: 40–8.

[27] Fornasari D. Pain mechanisms in patients with chronic pain. Clin Drug Investig. 2012; 32(1): 45–52.

[28] Förster M, Mahn F, Gockel U, et al. Axial low back pain: one painful area — many perceptions and mechanisms. PLoS One. 2013; 8(7): e68273.

[29] Woolf CJ, American College of Physicians, American Physiological Society. Pain: moving from symptom control toward mechanism-specific pharmacologic management. Ann Intern Med. 2004; 140(6): 441–51.

[30] Slatkin NE, Rhiner M. Topical ketamine in the treatment of mucositis pain. Pain Med. 2003; 4(3): 298–303.

[31] Knezevic NN, Tverdohleb T, Nikibin F, Knezevic I, Candido KD. Management of chronic neuropathic pain with single and compounded topical analgesics. Pain Manag. 2017; 7(6): 537–58.

[32] Derry S, Conaghan P, Da Silva JA, et al. Topical NSAIDs for chronic musculoskeletal pain in adults. Cochrane Database Syst Rev. 2016; 4: CD007400.

[33] Hesselink JMK. Topical analgesics: critical issues related to formulation and concentration. J Pain Relief. 2016; 5: 274.

[34] Manion J, Waller MA, Clark T, Massingham JN, Gregory Neely G. Developing modern pain therapies. Front Neurosci. 2019; 13: 1370.

[35] Baron R, Eberhart L, Kern KU, et al. Tapentadol prolonged release for chronic pain: a review of clinical trials and 5 years of routine clinical practice data. Pain Pract. 2017; 17(5): 678–700.

[36] Sánchez Del Águila MJ, Schenk M, Kern KU, Drost T, Steigerwald I. Practical considerations for the use of tapentadol prolonged release for the management of severe chronic pain. Clin Ther. 2015; 37(1): 94–113.

[37] Tramullas M, Francés R, de la Fuente R, Velategui S, Carcelén M, García R, Llorca J, Hurlé MA. MicroRNA-30c-5p modulates neuropathic pain in rodents. Sci Transl Med. 2018; 10(453): eaao6299.

[38] Christoph A, Eerdekens MH, Kok M, Volkers G, Freynhagen R. Cebranopadol, a novel first-in-class analgesic drug candidate: first experience in patients with chronic low back pain in a randomized clinical trial. Pain. 2017; 158(9): 1813–24.

[39] Miyazaki T, Choi IY, Rubas W, et al. NKTR-181: a novel mu-opioid analgesic with inherently low abuse potential. J Pharmacol Exp Ther. 2017; 363(1): 104–13.

[40] Stover JD, Farhang N, Berrett KC, Gertz J, Lawrence B, Bowles RD. CRISPR epigenome editing of AKAP150 in DRG neurons abolishes degenerative IVD-induced neuronal activation. Mol Ther. 2017; 25: 2014–27.

第 9 章

Solange Massa, Ayman Fouad, Mehdi Ebrahimi, and Peter Luke Santa Maria

口腔黏膜黏附给药治疗头颈癌的发展趋势

Emerging Trends in Oral Mucoadhesive Drug Delivery for Head and Neck Cancer

引 言

口腔黏膜黏附给药系统是指设计一类通过与口腔黏膜相互作用，以提高药物活性成分在吸收位点的吸收效率和停留时间的药物制剂递送系统。口腔黏膜为局部或全身药物给药提供了理想的场所。就局部给药而言，黏附系统可以实现药物的定点释放，减少全身副作用，并延长药物在口腔内的停留时间。就全身给药而言，黏附系统可以避免首过代谢，提供直接且无痛的给药方式。唾液通过促进活性成分的水溶性溶解，并与黏膜的黏蛋白相互作用，为药物递送系统提供了表面锚点。然而，开发用于局部或全身给药的黏附系统面临着诸多挑战。口腔黏膜黏附给药面临的局限和挑战包括局部酶的降解、口腔内 pH 的变化、药物的不良味道或气味、给药剂量的限制以及仅适用于被动扩散的药物。此外，还要考虑药物可能被吞咽后经常规口服途径被吸收的情况。相比胃肠道的其他部分，譬如小肠，口腔黏膜的通透性也较低。

当黏附性化合物与黏膜接触后，会依次经历黏附的两个阶段：接触阶段和巩固阶段。黏膜黏附可用多种理论来解释，包括扩散理论、吸附理论、电子理论、断裂理论和润湿理论。通过使用从液体到固体的各种剂型，并结合适当的成分，口腔黏膜黏附给药系统可以在局部和全身给药中实现预期的效果。黏附材料可通过特定的配方设计，进一步提高药物的生物利用度、吸收和转运，同时将全身副作用降到最低。本章首先概述口腔黏膜的组织结构，以便更好地理解口腔黏膜黏附剂的作用机制，随后讨论了现有和新兴的口腔黏膜黏附给药制剂在头颈癌及相关疾病治疗中的应用。

S. Massa · P. L. S. Maria (✉)
Department of Otolaryngology, Head & Neck Surgery, Stanford University, Stanford, CA, USA
e-mail: psm01@stanford.edu

A. Fouad
Department of Otolaryngology, Head & Neck Surgery, Stanford University, Stanford, CA, USA

Department of Otolaryngology, Head & Neck Surgery, Tanta University, Tanta, Egypt

M. Ebrahimi
Department of Oral Rehabilitation, Prince Philip Dental Hospital, The University of Hong Kong, Pok Fu Lam, Hong Kong, China

口腔黏膜的组织结构及唾液成分

口腔黏膜由一系列相互作用的复杂层次构成，这些层次通过细胞黏附相互连接[1]。对口腔黏膜进行组织学检查可发现，其具有三个功能各异的层次：上皮层、基底膜和结缔组织层[2,3]。口腔内不同部位的上皮厚度各不相同。人体中，口底的上皮厚度约为 100 μm，舌侧缘约为 220 μm，硬腭约为 250 μm，颊部约为 300 μm[4]，这些区域也是溃疡和恶性肿瘤等许多口腔病变的主要发生部位。下方的结缔组织层支撑着基底膜，而基底膜则支撑着上皮层[5]（图 9-1）。

■ 上皮层

上皮层的主要功能是作为屏障来保护其下方的结构[6]。一般来说，口腔黏膜的通透性取决于所递送物质的物理和化学性质[3]。基底层是前体细胞的来源，这些细胞会分裂产生新细胞，再经过分裂、分化后向表层迁移。由于这一过程，角质形成细胞从基底层到表层的形状、大小和成熟度各不相同[7]。口腔内的上皮可分为两个明显不同的功能区：① 非角化上皮区；② 角化上皮区。非角化上皮区是黏液分泌区，含有包含硫酸胆固醇和葡萄糖神经酰胺的膜被颗粒[8]，包括口底、舌腹、软腭、颊和唇黏膜。角化上皮区是咀嚼和屏障区，含有由神经酰胺和酰基神经酰胺组成的中性脂质[9]，包括舌背、硬腭和牙龈黏膜。

■ 基底膜

基底膜的主要功能是为上皮层提供支撑，并将其固定在下方的结缔组织上[10]。基底膜由两个不同的层组成：基板和网状结缔组织[11]。基板可以进一步分为透明板和致密板。透明板是紧邻上皮层的一层薄而透明的结构，而致密板则是靠近网状结缔组织的一层厚而致密的结构。透明板主要由肌营养不良蛋白聚糖、巢蛋白、层粘连蛋白和整合素组成，然而关于透明板是否真的存在仍存在争论，有人认为它仅仅是组织切片制备过程中的人工产物[12]。致密板含有富硫酸乙酰肝素串珠蛋白聚糖包被的Ⅳ型胶原蛋白[13]。基底膜通过Ⅶ型胶原与下方的结缔组织层相连接[13,14]。

■ 结缔组织

结缔组织的主要功能是为整个黏膜提供支撑结构，并为位于基底膜下方的固有层（一种基于结缔组织的结构）提供主要营养来源[14]。结缔组织主要有三个组成部分：由胶原蛋白和弹性蛋

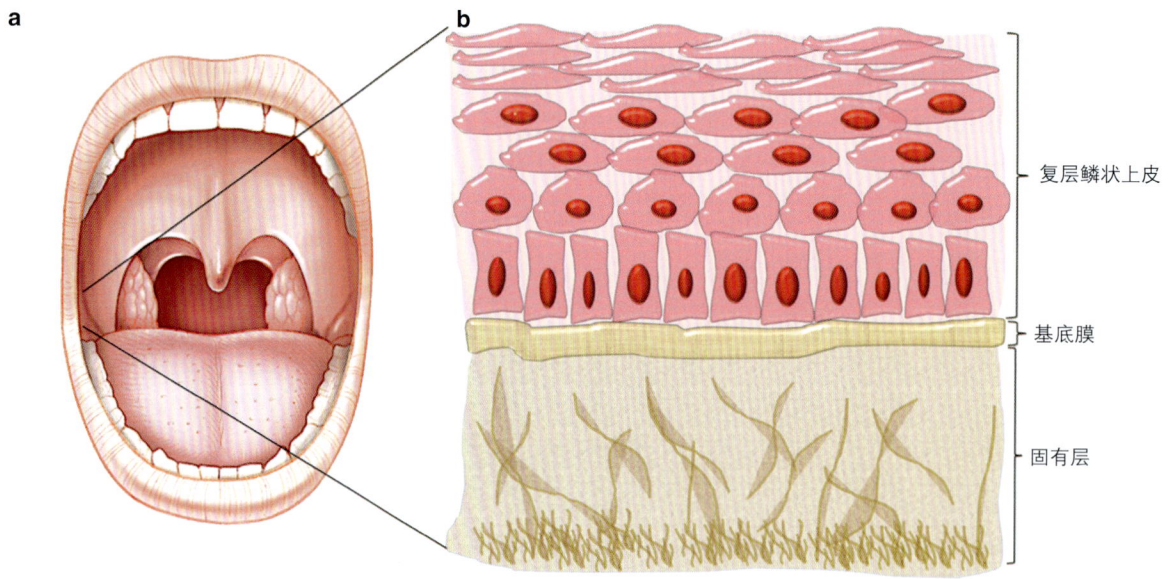

图 9-1　a. 口腔解剖结构图。b. 口腔组织学示意图（经 Chris Gralapp, MA, CMI 的版权许可重制）

白构成的纤维[15]；包括成纤维细胞、脂肪细胞、巨噬细胞、肥大细胞和白细胞等的细胞；以及用于在细胞间隙中保持水分和胶原纤维的糖胺聚糖和蛋白聚糖系统[16,17]。

唾液、黏液和黏蛋白

唾液是口腔的主要润滑剂，其日分泌量为0.5～2 L，pH范围为5.5～7[18]。唾液中超过95%是水，其富含水分的环境正是使用亲水性高分子材料进行经黏膜给药的基础。这种薄而透明且黏稠的分泌物附着在上皮组织上，平均厚度为50～450 μm。唾液由杯状细胞分泌，但也可以由外分泌腺中的特化黏液细胞产生。唾液的成分包括脂类（1%～2%）、矿物盐（1%）、免疫球蛋白、黏蛋白以及其他游离蛋白（0.5%～1%）。唾液的黏稠性源自黏液与黏蛋白纤维的结合，后者具有很强的结合水分的能力，能够影响药物递送[19]。黏蛋白是一类由25%氨基酸和75%碳水化合物组成的糖蛋白[20]，既可以以膜结合型（如MUC1、MUC3和MUC4）存在于口腔上皮中[21]，也可以以游离型存在于唾液中（如MUC2和MUC5AC）。MUC7和MUC5B形成黏液网络，通过与MUC1连接附着于上皮[22]（图9-2）。尽管黏液因唾液酸和硫酸残基而带有负电荷，但给药系统可以据此特性进行设计，不过这也为药物的附着和输递送提出了挑战[23,24]。

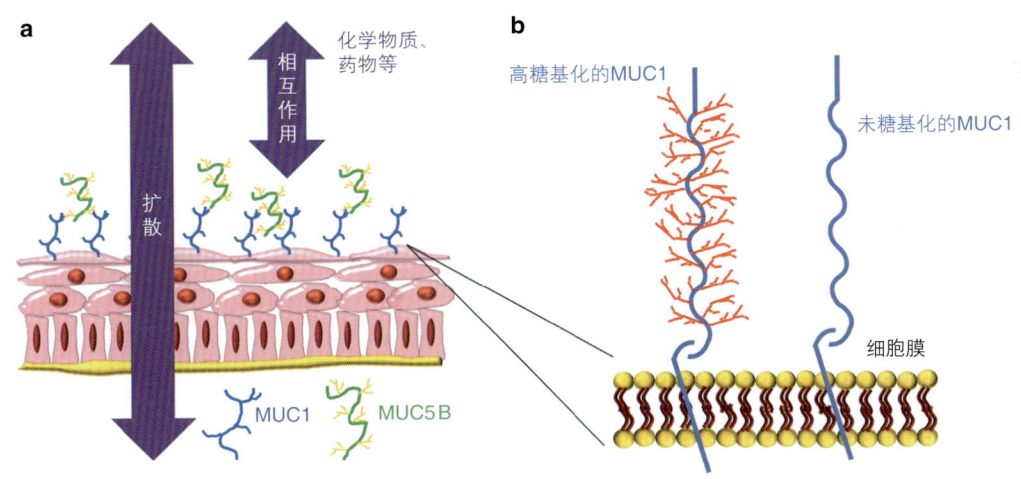

图9-2 a. 口腔黏膜表达的MUC1与唾液黏蛋白MUC5B连接。b. MUC1作为跨膜蛋白表达于黏膜表面

黏膜黏附理论

给药系统与黏膜表面耦合的具体机制尚未完全明确，但通常认为这一过程可分为两个阶段：① 接触阶段；② 巩固阶段。在接触阶段，材料通过膨胀和扩散机制接触黏膜。巩固阶段则由水分触发，此时黏附性化合物通过范德华力和氢键与黏膜表面连接[25]。从物理和化学的角度来看，已有几种结合理论用于解释材料如何表现出黏膜黏附性（图9-3）。

扩散理论

扩散理论的核心是通过黏液糖蛋白和黏膜黏附性聚合物链之间的缠绕，形成半永久性的黏附键[26]。许多因素会影响大分子之间的相互扩散，例如聚合物链适当的柔韧性、两个成分间的溶解性、聚合物的暴露程度、两者化学结构的匹配度，以及生物黏附聚合物的扩散系数。溶解参数

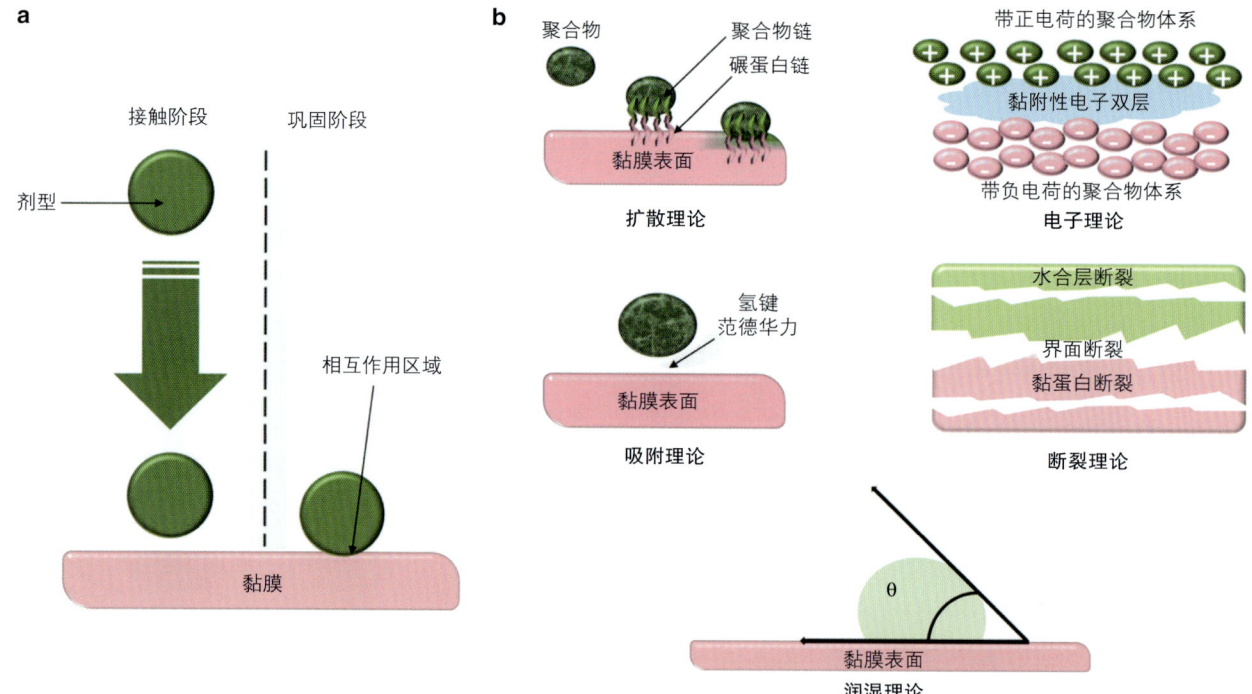

图 9-3 黏膜黏附理论。a. 黏附性化合物与黏膜表面的相互作用可分为两个阶段：接触阶段和巩固阶段。b. 解释黏附表面与递送系统关系的五种黏附理论：扩散理论、电子理论、吸附理论、断裂理论和润湿理论

最接近黏液糖蛋白的材料能够与之形成最强的生物黏附键[27, 28]。

电子理论

电子理论的核心在于当两个电性不同的结构接触时所发生的电子转移。若生物黏附材料和目标生物表面具有不同的电子结构，当这两个表面相互接触时，便会发生电子转移，形成带电的双电层。当这种双电层在黏液和聚合物之间形成时，产生的吸引力会将这两者结合在一起[29, 30]。

吸附理论

吸附理论描述了初次接触后产生的原子表面作用力。在该理论中，发生两种化学键：① 初级共价键，它通常不利，因为它可能会产生永久性的结合；② 次级键，如范德华力、氢键、静电力和疏水作用力[31]。对于聚合物来说，这些系统通常含有羧基，因此氢键是主要的界面作用力。

断裂理论

断裂理论的主要概念是，将两个表面分离所需的断裂力（S_m）等同于黏附力。断裂力（S_m）的计算公式为 $S_m = F_m/A_\theta$。其中，F_m 是将两个表面分离时所施加最大力的比值，A_θ 是表面积[32]。

润湿理论

润湿理论描述了液体与黏膜黏附表面之间的关系，主要通过物质与表面之间的接触角来定义。界面张力可以预测生物黏附性聚合物在生物表面上的铺展行为。铺展系数（S）可以通过杨氏方程来计算：

$$\gamma_{SG} = \gamma_{SL} + \gamma_{LG}\cos\theta$$

其中，γ 表示两种成分之间的界面张力，γ_{SG} 为固体表面张力，γ_{SL} 为固-液界面张力，γ_{LG} 为液体表面张力，θ 为接触角且可以容易地测量[33, 34]。理想情况下，接触角应尽可能接近零，表示良好的铺展性。

用于头颈癌的口腔黏膜黏附给药制剂

市面上已有许多口腔黏膜黏附系统，但专门针对头颈部疾病的却寥寥无几。特别是对于头颈肿瘤，其应用仅局限于疼痛控制以及放射治疗引起的口腔黏膜炎和口干症的管理。表 9-1 总结了现有的用于头颈癌及其他头颈部疾患的口腔黏膜黏附剂。尽管有许多关于口腔黏膜黏附系统的临床试验，但其中很少能顺利通过临床试验并进入市场[35,36]（表 9-2）。

表 9-1 用于头颈部疾病的商业口腔黏膜黏附制剂

编号	应用	药物	制剂形式	商品名
1	头颈癌放射治疗后及干燥综合征等引发的口干症	盐酸毛果芸香碱	片剂，水凝胶颊黏附片	Piolobuc, Salegen
2	阿片类药物依赖患者的麻醉剂	盐酸丁丙诺啡和盐酸纳洛酮	片剂	Subutex
3	疼痛	舒芬太尼	片剂	Dsuvia, Zalviso
4	疼痛	枸橼酸芬太尼	片剂，喷雾剂，薄膜，含片	Abstral, Actiq, Subsys, Fentora, Onsolis
5	疼痛	布托啡诺	片剂，薄膜	Temgesic, Belbuca
6	阿片类药物依赖患者的麻醉剂	丁丙诺啡 + 纳洛酮	薄膜	Suboxone
7	镇静	劳拉西泮	片剂	Ativan, Temesta Expidet Buccal
8	镇静	奥沙西泮	片剂	Seresta Expidet Buccal
9	过敏性鼻炎	变应原提取物	片剂	Grastek, Oralair, Odactra, Ragwitek
10	口腔念珠菌病	制霉菌素	漱口水	Nilstat, Mycostatin
11	口腔念珠菌病	咪康唑	凝胶	Daktarin, Decozol
12	口-咽念珠菌病	咪康唑	片剂	Loramyc, Lauriad
13	口腔溃疡	曲安奈德	糊剂	Kenalog in Orabase, Aftach
14	抗菌漱口水	葡萄糖酸氯己定	口腔黏膜凝胶	Corsodyl gel
15	类固醇	氢化可的松琥珀酸钠	口腔黏膜丸剂	Corlan pellets
16	恶心/呕吐	盐酸丙氯拉嗪	片剂	Buccastem
17	恶心/呕吐	盐酸丙氯拉嗪	片剂	Tementil
18	偏头痛	利扎曲普坦	片剂	Maxalt Wafers
19	癫痫	咪达唑仑	漱口水	Buccolam, Epistatus

表 9-2　头颈肿瘤学相关口腔黏膜黏附制剂的近期和当前临床试验

编号	标题/年份	疾病状况	干预措施	招募人数	试验阶段/参考文献
1	地塞米松治疗口腔扁平苔藓（2005—2008）	口腔扁平苔藓	药物：地塞米松溶液	70	2期[48]
2	BEMA™ 芬太尼用于癌症患者爆发性疼痛的安全性研究（2006—2008）	癌痛	药物：BEMA 芬太尼片	244	3期[49]
3	可乐定 Lauriad® 治疗口腔黏膜炎的有效性和安全性研究（2010—2014）	头颈癌患者放化疗诱发的严重口腔黏膜炎	药物：可乐定 Lauriad® 颊黏附片 药物：安慰剂 Lauriad®	183	2期[50, 51]
4	MuGard 对头颈癌患者口腔黏膜炎缓解效果的研究（MuGard）（2011—2013）	口腔黏膜炎	器械：MuGard 口腔创面冲洗液 器械：水性对照冲洗液	120	4期[52, 53]
5	苯妥英黏附性糊剂在口腔活检后伤口愈合中的临床效果（2012—2013）	疼痛 伤口愈合	药物：苯妥英糊剂 药物：安慰剂	40	1期[54]
6	曲安奈德黏附膜与甘草黏附膜的效果比较（2013—2014）	黏膜炎	药物：曲安奈德膜与甘草膜（Aftogel 贴片）	60	1期和2期[55, 56]
7	曲安奈德黏附膜和甘草黏附膜对扁平苔藓的效果比较（2014—2015）	口腔扁平苔藓	药物：甘草膜（Aftogel 贴片）与曲安奈德膜	60	2期[57]
8	Forrad® 在接受 IMRT 的鼻咽癌患者放射诱发黏膜炎中的疗效和安全性研究（2016—2017）	鼻咽肿瘤 口炎	药物：口腔溃疡漱口液（Forrad®） 水凝胶与四联混合物（地塞米松、庆大霉素、维生素 B_{12} 和普鲁卡因）	90	2期[58]
9	姜黄素治疗口腔黏膜下纤维化的有效性研究（ECOSMF）（2014—2018）	口腔黏膜下纤维化	药物：姜黄素黏附凝胶、姜黄素胶囊、姜黄素黏附凝胶+姜黄素胶囊 药物：安慰剂胶囊	200	2期[59, 60]
10	Aqualief® 作为口干症患者的膳食补充剂的疗效研究（2016—2017）	因唾液腺分泌不足导致的口干症	膳食补充剂：Aqualief 片剂 补充剂：安慰剂	60	不适用[61]
11	地塞米松溶液治疗口腔扁平苔藓（2017—2019）	口腔扁平苔藓	药物：MucoLox™ 地塞米松溶液（Decadron Elixir）	24	2期[62]
12	Rivelin®-CLO 贴片治疗口腔扁平苔藓（2018—2019）	口腔扁平苔藓	药物：丙酸氯倍他索（Rivelin®-CLO 贴片）	140	2期[63]
13	Aqualief® 对因头颈癌放疗导致的口干症患者的疗效（2017—2020）	口干症 无唾液症 唾液减少 口干	膳食补充剂：Aqualief® 片剂（一种基于肌肽和木樨的食品补充剂） 其他：安慰剂	100	不适用[64]
14	局部使用洋甘菊预防化疗诱发的口腔黏膜炎（2019—2020）	化疗诱发的口腔黏膜炎	药物：洋甘菊局部口腔凝胶（Carbopol® 970），咪康唑局部凝胶，BBC 口腔喷雾剂（麻醉剂和抗炎剂），Oracure 凝胶（止痛凝胶）	45	2期[65, 66]

续　表

编号	标题/年份	疾病状况	干预措施	招募人数	试验阶段/参考文献
15	肌肽补充剂对口腔唾液量/质量的影响（PHoral）（2020—2020）	口腔疾病	膳食补充剂：Aqualief 片剂 膳食补充剂：安慰剂片剂	60	不适用[67,68]
16	MucoLox® 制剂缓解头颈癌黏膜炎症状的研究（2018—2021）	头颈癌患者的口腔黏膜炎	药物：MucoLox® 聚合物水凝胶和碳酸氢钠	27	2 期[69]
17	辅酶 Q10 与局部皮质类固醇治疗口腔扁平苔藓的临床和生化评估：随机对照临床试验（2019—2021）	口腔扁平苔藓	药物：辅酶 Q10 黏膜黏附片剂（泛醇）	34	1 期[70,71]

注：BEMA，生物可降解黏膜黏附系统；IMRT，调强放射治疗。

总体而言，现有的口腔黏膜黏附给药制剂包括固体、半固体和液体制剂。第一代黏附剂是天然或合成的亲水性聚合物，包括阳离子、阴离子或非离子型。第二代黏附剂则使用了多功能生物材料，能够同时结合亲水性和亲脂性药物，并具备更智能的黏膜黏附机制。近年来，纳米颗粒给药系统的出现显著提升了黏膜黏附给药的药物渗透性和释放动力学，以及更强的抗酶降解能力和减少全身不良反应的优势[36-38]。

固体制剂

使用固体口服制剂的效果取决于其制造工艺、设计和固相类型[39]。这类制剂适合局部、稳定和持续时间较长的药物递送。

■ 片剂

片剂是黏附性药物系统的固体形式，可通过粉末混合压缩制备。这些片剂可用于局部治疗和全身治疗。对于局部治疗，片剂可以直接应用于目标部位。对于全身治疗，片剂可以保护药物免受酶降解，并通过与黏膜吸收表面紧密接触来避免首过代谢。为了使含片在口腔环境中有效，其理想情况是比口服的片剂溶解速度更快。它的主要缺点包括味道不佳和刺激性，这影响患者的接受度，且药物可能随着唾液扩散，降低局部治疗的效果。片剂可以通过单独使用生物黏附性聚合物或将其与其他物质结合来制备，再加入活性成分形成基质[40,41]。

■ 薄片剂

薄片剂是实现多方面功效的优良给药系统。双层薄片剂可以一侧用于黏附，另一侧则负载药物，实现药物的长效稳定释放。如果薄片剂具备理想的机械和化学特性，它们可能成为治疗口腔感染的理想系统[42]。

■ 生物黏附微球

生物黏附微球可以通过水悬液、气雾剂、糊剂、凝胶或软膏的形式递送。该系统的主要优点是具有较高的膨胀比以及比其他制剂更长的半衰期[43]。由于其体积小且给药方便，通常更容易被患者接受。如有需要，这些系统可设计为在口腔黏膜内滞留，从而减少全身不良反应。

半固体制剂

半固体制剂的结构与片剂类似，区别在于赋形剂，通常以细粉形式溶解或悬浮在水性或非水性基质中。与片剂相比，半固体制剂的优点在于口感更好，并且可以通过注射器或手指直接应用于目标区域。然而，其给药剂量可能不稳定且定位不够精准[44]。

■ 薄膜和贴片

贴片通常通过将聚合物、药物和赋形剂混合后制成铸型，干燥后制备成半固体状。贴片的大小不一，常见尺寸为 1～3 cm，呈椭圆形，以便在颊黏膜上使用。贴片与片剂有类似的优缺点。由于比片剂更薄、更柔软，贴片似乎更易被患者接受。然而，其相对较薄的尺寸使其容易过度水化并丧失生物黏附特性[45]。

- 咀嚼胶

咀嚼胶制剂通常由咀嚼胶基质与增塑剂、填料、色素和活性成分混合而成。虽然这种系统具有良好的储药能力，但由于药物只在咀嚼时释放，其药物吸收率和生物利用度较低[46]。已有多项实验工作来评估这种疗法以绕过肝脏首过效应。

- 软膏或凝胶

与其他制剂相比，凝胶或软膏在减少过敏或刺激的风险上具有一定的优势。它们的制造过程相对简单，活性成分易于添加到给药系统中。此外，凝胶的释放速度比固体系统更快[47]。

液体或悬液制剂

液体制剂的主要优点是其能够分布整个口腔。然而，其主要缺点是无法针对特定区域给药，且给药量无法控制。此外，如果添加的活性成分易受唾液中酶的破坏，这种系统对药物的降解几乎没有保护效果，或保护效果非常有限。

口腔黏膜黏附给药系统的组成成分

在设计口腔黏膜黏附给药系统时，主要目标是通过口腔黏膜递送所需的活性成分，以达到局部或全身的治疗效果。为实现这一目标，制剂需满足以下几项特性，包括：① 选择合适的药物成分；② 设计良好的生物黏附聚合物系统；③ 考虑添加背衬膜、增塑剂和（或）渗透增强剂。

药物成分

黏膜黏附给药系统的设计应基于每种药物的药代动力学特性。理想的药物标准应包括：① 小剂量的常规单次给药；② 理想分子量在 75～100 道尔顿之间；③ 生物半衰期为 2～8 小时；④ 存在首过效应或全身前药物清除；⑤ 尽可能通过被动吸收[72,73]；⑥ 在口腔 pH 环境中具有稳定性。

生物黏附聚合物

在口腔给药系统的设计中，生物黏附聚合物的选择和表征至关重要。理想的黏膜黏附聚合物应具备以下条件：① 高分子量，以促进黏液与聚合物的相互作用；② 良好的膨胀性能，通过高交联度避免解体并保护活性成分；③ 通过灵活的聚合物链促进活性成分黏附于黏膜；④ 适宜的 pH；⑤ 对环境惰性；⑥ 与生物膜相容；⑦ 保质期长，能够长期储存而不分解；⑧ 经济实惠；⑨ 易于添加到药物配方中[74]。另一个理想特性是能够通过将药物嵌入聚合物基质中，控制药物在口腔中的释放[75]。

聚合物可以按来源（天然/合成）、溶解度或所带电荷等进行分类。如果按所带电荷分类，聚合物可分为阴离子聚合物、阳离子聚合物和非离子聚合物。最常用的阴离子聚合物包括黄原胶、海藻酸钠、果胶、壳聚糖-乙二胺四乙酸和聚丙烯酸。阳离子聚合物包括壳聚糖、葡聚糖、氨基葡聚糖和二乙胺乙基葡聚糖等。非离子聚合物包括 Eudragit® 类似物和聚丙烯酰胺。

背衬膜

背衬膜的主要功能是将生物黏附材料贴合在黏膜上。这层膜能防止药物在黏膜外流失，并提高患者的依从性。因此，背衬膜必须是惰性的，对药物不渗透，并能增强药物的渗透性。常用于制备背衬膜的材料包括卡波普、硬脂酸镁、羟丙基甲基纤维素（HPMC）、羟丙基纤维素（HPC）、羧甲基纤维素（CMC）以及聚卡波非[76]。

增塑剂

增塑剂是一种用于增强塑性和柔韧性的物质，

它可以使黏膜黏附性给药系统更柔软，并且可以大量添加到配方中。尤其是对于聚合物来说，它可以通过自身改性（或其单体）实现内部增塑，或者在配方完成后通过外部增塑来增加柔韧性。最常用的增塑剂包括山梨醇、丙二醇和甘油[77]。

渗透增强剂

渗透增强剂是用来增加目标药物黏膜渗透率的化合物。在选择渗透增强剂时，需考虑多种因素，包括药物的理化性质、给药部位，以及载体和其他赋形剂的特性。所有这些增强剂必须安全、可逆、无刺激且化学性质稳定。

渗透增强剂通过以下几种机制发挥作用：① 通过降低黏液和唾液的黏度来改变黏液的流变学特性；② 通过作用于脂质或蛋白质成分，干扰细胞内脂质排列，从而增加脂质双分子层的流动性；③ 改变紧密连接以促进吸收；④ 改变药物的分配系数以增加其溶解度[78]。

常见的渗透增强剂包括：① 甾体类去垢剂，如胆汁盐、皂苷、甘氨胆酸钠、牛磺胆酸钠、糖基二氢夫西地酸钠；② 表面活性剂，包括阳离子型（如十六烷基三甲基溴化铵）、阴离子型（如十二烷基硫酸钠）和非离子型（如蔗糖脂肪酸酯）；③ 脂肪酸，如月桂酸、己酸、油酸；④ 其他物质，如螯合剂（如水杨酸类和亚砜类）[79]。

小 结

黏膜黏附给药系统是传统给药方式的一种很有前景的替代方案。在头颈癌领域，这些系统已经用于口腔黏膜炎、口干症和疼痛控制的管理。其优势包括绕过首过代谢和胃肠道酶降解，从而提高药物的生物利用度；多种剂型选择，如贴片、薄膜、喷雾等；可适用于对常规给药方式无反应或有创伤的患者。活性药物还可以通过控释或缓释的方式释放，从而调整药物的吸收模式。

目前，新的给药系统正在研发，以用于管理口腔潜在的癌前病变。预计包括纳米颗粒形式在内的更多创新制剂将在全面的临床前研究和优化后最终进入临床试验，从而实现更高效的局部和全身给药。

致谢：感谢认证医学插画师 Chris Gralapp 提供了图 9-1a 和图 9-4 中的人类口腔图像。

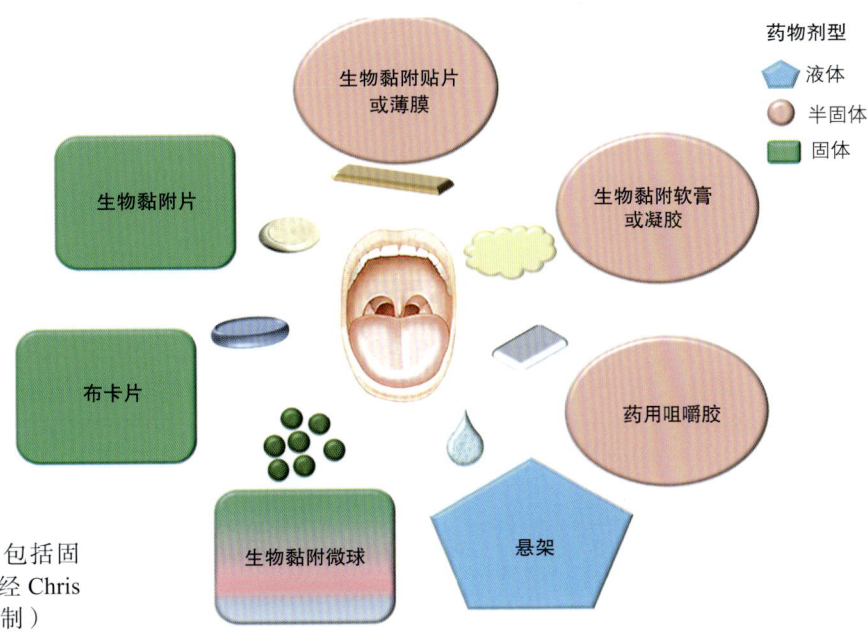

图 9-4 口腔黏膜黏附制剂，包括固体、半固体和液体给药系统（经 Chris Gralapp, MA, CMI 的版权许可重制）

参 考 文 献

[1] Chen J, Ahmad R, Li W, Swain M, Li Q. Biomechanics of oral mucosa. J R Soc Interface. 2015; 12: 20150325. https: //doi.org/10.1098/rsif.2015.0325.
[2] Harris D, Robinson JR. Drug delivery via the mucous membranes of the oral cavity. J Pharm Sci. 1992; 81: 1–10. https: //doi.org/10.1002/jps.2600810102.
[3] Squier CA. The permeability of oral mucosa. Crit Rev Oral Biol Med. 1991; 2: 13–32. https: //doi.org/10.1177/10454411910020010301.
[4] Prestin S, Rothschild SI, Betz CS, Kraft M. Measurement of epithelial thickness within the oral cavity using optical coherence tomography. Head Neck. 2012; 34: 1777–81. https: //doi. org/10.1002/hed.22007.
[5] Redler P, Lustig ES. Control of epithelial development in normal and pathological connective tissue from oral mucosa. Dev Biol. 1970; 22: 84–95. https: //doi. org/10.1016/0012-1606(70)90007-2.
[6] Luke DA. Cell proliferation in epithelium of murine oral mucosa in vivo and in vitro. An autoradiographic study using tritiated thymidine. Virchows Arch B Cell Pathol. 1979; 29: 343–9. https: //doi.org/10.1007/BF02899365.
[7] Jonek T, Gruszeczka B. Histological study of changes in the epithelium of the oral mucosa caused by estrogens in castrated mice. Czas Stomatol. 1976; 29: 767–72. http: //www.ncbi.nlm. nih.gov/pubmed/1067954.
[8] Adams D. The mucus barrier and absorption through the oral mucosa. J Dent Res. 1975; 54 Spec No: B19–26. https: //doi.org/10.1177/00220345750540021601.
[9] Dale BA, Stern IB, Clagett JA. Initial characterization of the proteins of keratinized epithelium of rat oral mucosa. Arch Oral Biol. 1977; 22: 75–82. https: //doi. org/10.1016/0003-9969(77)90081-4.
[10] Watanabe I. Ultrastructure of the basal membrane of the mucosa of the hard palate of rats. Quintessencia. 1981; 8: 57–65. http: //www.ncbi.nlm.nih.gov/pubmed/6954560.
[11] Ricci V, Gasparini G. The structure of the basal membrane of the nasal mucosa in man, under the electron microscope. Boll Soc Ital Biol Sper. 1960; 36: 932–4. http: //www.ncbi.nlm.nih. gov/pubmed/13741218.
[12] Chan FL, Inoue S. Lamina lucida of basement membrane: an artefact. Microsc Res Tech. 1994; 28: 48–59. https: //doi.org/10.1002/jemt.1070280106.
[13] Adachi E, Hopkinson I, Hayashi T. Basement-membrane stromal relationships: interactions between collagen fibrils and the lamina densa. Int Rev Cytol. 1997; 173: 73–156. https: //doi. org/10.1016/s0074-7696(08)62476-6.
[14] Weijs TJ, Goense L, van Rossum PSN, Meijer GJ, van Lier ALHMW, Wessels FJ, Braat MNG, Lips IM, Ruurda JP, Cuesta MA, van Hillegersberg R, Bleys RLAW. The peri-esophageal connective tissue layers and related compartments: visualization by histology and magnetic resonance imaging. J Anat. 2017; 230: 262–71. https: //doi.org/10.1111/joa.12552.
[15] Sauer F, Oswald L, Ariza de Schellenberger A, Tzschätzsch H, Schrank F, Fischer T, Braun J, Mierke CT, Valiullin R, Sack I, Käs JA. Collagen networks determine viscoelastic properties of connective tissues yet do not hinder diffusion of the aqueous solvent. Soft Matter. 2019; 15: 3055–64. https: //doi.org/10.1039/c8sm02264j.
[16] Mourão PA. Proteoglycans, glycosaminoglycans and sulfated polysaccharides from connective tissues. Mem Inst Oswaldo Cruz. 1991; 86(Suppl 3): 13–22. https: //doi. org/10.1590/s0074-02761991000700003.
[17] Muir H. Chemistry and metabolism of connective tissue glycosaminoglycans (mucopolysaccharides). Int Rev Connect Tissue Res. 1964; 2: 101–54. https: //doi.org/10.1016/B978-1-4831-6751-0.50009-4.
[18] Roblegg E, Coughran A, Sirjani D. Saliva: an all-rounder of our body. Eur J Pharm Biopharm. 2019; 142: 133–41. https: //doi.org/10.1016/j.ejpb.2019.06.016.
[19] Teubl BJ, Stojkovic B, Docter D, Pritz E, Leitinger G, Poberaj I, Prassl R, Stauber RH, Fröhlich E, Khinast JG, Roblegg E. The effect of saliva on the fate of nanoparticles. Clin Oral Investig. 2018; 22: 929–40. https: //doi.org/10.1007/s00784-017-2172-5.
[20] Bansil R, Stanley E, LaMont JT. Mucin biophysics. Annu Rev Physiol. 1995; 57: 635–57. https: //doi.org/10.1146/annurev.ph.57.030195.003223.
[21] Kho H-S. Oral epithelial MUC1 and oral health. Oral Dis. 2018; 24: 19–21. https: //doi. org/10.1111/odi.12713.
[22] Frenkel ES, Ribbeck K. Salivary mucins in host defense and disease prevention. J Oral Microbiol. 2015; 7: 29759. https: //doi.org/10.3402/jom.v7.29759.
[23] Agarwal S, Aggarwal S. Mucoadhesive polymeric platform for drug delivery: a comprehensive review. Curr Drug Deliv. 2015; 12: 139–56. https: //doi.org/10.2174/1567201811666140924124722.
[24] Fröhlich E, Roblegg E. Mucus as barrier for drug delivery by nanoparticles. J Nanosci Nanotechnol. 2014; 14: 126–36. https: //doi.org/10.1166/jnn.2014.9015.
[25] Smart JD. The basics and underlying mechanisms of mucoadhesion. Adv Drug Deliv Rev. 2005; 57: 1556–68. https: //doi.org/10.1016/j.addr.2005.07.001.
[26] Andrews GP, Laverty TP, Jones DS. Mucoadhesive polymeric platforms for controlled drug delivery. Eur J Pharm Biopharm. 2009; 71: 505–18. https: //doi.org/10.1016/j.ejpb.2008.09.028.
[27] Fu Y, Kao WJ. Drug release kinetics and transport mechanisms of non-degradable and degradable polymeric delivery systems. Expert

Opin Drug Deliv. 2010; 7: 429–44. https: //doi. org/10.1517/17425241003602259.

[28] Lee JW, Park JH, Robinson JR. Bioadhesive-based dosage forms: the next generation. J Pharm Sci. 2000; 89: 850–66. https: //doi. org/10.1002/1520-6017(200007)89: 7 < 850: : AID-JPS2 > 3.0.CO; 2-G.

[29] Guardado-Alvarez TM, Devi LS, Vabre J-M, Pecorelli TA, Schwartz BJ, Durand J-O, Mongin O, Blanchard-Desce M, Zink JI. Photoredox activated drug delivery systems operating under two photon excitation in the near-IR. Nanoscale. 2014; 6: 4652–8. https: //doi. org/10.1039/c3nr06155h.

[30] Dodou D, Breedveld P, Wieringa PA. Mucoadhesives in the gastrointestinal tract: revisiting the literature for novel applications. Eur J Pharm Biopharm. 2005; 60: 1–16. https: //doi. org/10.1016/j.ejpb.2005.01.007.

[31] McGinty S, Pontrelli G. A general model of coupled drug release and tissue absorption for drug delivery devices. J Control Release. 2015; 217: 327–36. https: //doi.org/10.1016/j. jconrel.2015.09.025.

[32] Smart JD. Theories of mucoadhesion. In: Mucoadhesive mater drug delivery systems. Chichester: Wiley; 2014. p. 159–74. https: //doi. org/10.1002/9781118794203.ch07.

[33] Ugwoke MI, Agu RU, Verbeke N, Kinget R. Nasal mucoadhesive drug delivery: background, applications, trends and future perspectives. Adv Drug Deliv Rev. 2005; 57: 1640–65. https: //doi.org/10.1016/j.addr.2005.07.009.

[34] Cheng Y, Jiao X, Zhao L, Liu Y, Wang F, Wen Y, Zhang X. Wetting transition in nanochannels for biomimetic free-blocking on-demand drug transport. J Mater Chem B. 2018; 6: 6269–77. https: //doi.org/10.1039/C8TB01838C.

[35] Ebrahimi M. Standardization and regulation of biomaterials. In: Handbook biomater. biocompat.: Elsevier; United Kingdom 2020. p. 251–65. https: //dokumen.pub/handbook-of-biomaterials-biocompatibility-woodhead-publishing-series-in-biomaterials-1nbsp ed-0081029675-9780081029671.html.

[36] Hua S. Advances in nanoparticulate drug delivery approaches for sublingual and buccal administration. Front Pharmacol. 2019; 10: 1328. https: //doi.org/10.3389/fphar.2019.01328.

[37] Morales JO, Brayden DJ. Buccal delivery of small molecules and biologics: of mucoadhesive polymers, films, and nanoparticles. Curr Opin Pharmacol. 2017; 36: 22–8. https: //doi. org/10.1016/j.coph.2017.07.011.

[38] Hua S, de Matos MBC, Metselaar JM, Storm G. Current trends and challenges in the clinical translation of nanoparticulate nanomedicines: pathways for translational development and commercialization. Front Pharmacol. 2018; 9: 790. https: //doi.org/10.3389/fphar.2018.00790.

[39] Zhang GGZ, Law D, Schmitt EA, Qiu Y. Phase transformation considerations during process development and manufacture of solid oral dosage forms. Adv Drug Deliv Rev. 2004; 56: 371–90. https: //doi.org/10.1016/j.addr.2003.10.009.

[40] Nokhodchi A, Raja S, Patel P, Asare-Addo K. The role of oral controlled release matrix tablets in drug delivery systems. Bioimpacts. 2012; 2: 175–87. https: //doi.org/10.5681/bi.2012.027.

[41] Vivien-Castioni N, Gurny R, Baehni P, Kaltsatos V. Salivary fluoride concentrations following applications of bioadhesive tablets and mouthrinses. Eur J Pharm Biopharm. 2000; 49: 27–33. https: //doi.org/10.1016/s0939-6411(99)00041-7.

[42] Timur SS, Yüksel S, Akca G, Şenel S. Localized drug delivery with mono and bilayered mucoadhesive films and wafers for oral mucosal infections. Int J Pharm. 2019; 559: 102–12. https: //doi.org/10.1016/j.ijpharm.2019.01.029.

[43] Kockisch S, Rees GD, Young SA, Tsibouklis J, Smart JD. Polymeric microspheres for drug delivery to the oral cavity: an in vitro evaluation of mucoadhesive potential. J Pharm Sci. 2003; 92: 1614–23. https: //doi.org/10.1002/jps.10423.

[44] Boddupalli BM, Mohammed ZNK, Nath RA, Banji D. Mucoadhesive drug delivery system: an overview. J Adv Pharm Technol Res. 2010; 1: 381–7. https: //doi.org/10.4103/0110-5558.76436.

[45] Karki S, Kim H, Na S-J, Shin D, Jo K, Lee J. Thin films as an emerging platform for drug delivery. Asian J Pharm Sci. 2016; 11: 559–74. https: //doi.org/10.1016/j.ajps.2016.05.004.

[46] Aslani A, Rostami F. Medicated chewing gum, a novel drug delivery system. J Res Med Sci. 2015; 20: 403–11. http: //www.ncbi.nlm. nih.gov/pubmed/26109999.

[47] Fini A, Bergamante V, Ceschel GC. Mucoadhesive gels designed for the controlled release of chlorhexidine in the oral cavity. Pharmaceutics. 2011; 3: 665–79. https: //doi.org/10.3390/pharmaceutics3040665.

[48] ClinicalTrials.gov U.S. National Library of Medicine, dexamethasone to treat oral lichen planus, 2008. https: //clinicaltrials.gov/ct2/show/NCT00111072.

[49] ClinicalTrials.gov U.S. National Library of Medicine, study of the safety of BEMA™ fentanyl use for breakthrough pain in cancer subjects on chronic opioid therapy, 2012. https: //clinicaltrials. gov/ct2/show/NCT00293020.

[50] Giralt J, Tao Y, Kortmann R-D, Zasadny X, Contreras-Martinez J, Ceruse P, de la Vega FA, Lalla RV, Ozsahin EM, Pajkos G, Mazar A, Attali P, Bossi P, Vasseur B, Sonis S, Henke M, Bensadoun R-J. Randomized phase 2 trial of a novel clonidine mucoadhesive buccal tablet for the amelioration of oral mucositis in patients treated with concomitant chemoradiation therapy for head and neck cancer. Int J Radiat Oncol Biol Phys. 2020; 106: 320–8. https: //doi. org/10.1016/j.ijrobp.2019.10.023.

[51] ClinicalTrials.gov U.S. National Library of Medicine, efficacy and safety study of clonidine Lauriad® to treat oral mucositis, 2017. https: //clinicaltrials.gov/ct2/show/NCT01385748.

[52] ClinicalTrials.gov U.S. National Library of Medicine, a study to evaluate the efficacy of MuGard for the amelioration of oral mucositis in head and neck cancer patients (MuGard), 2013. https: //clinicaltrials.gov/ct2/show/NCT01283906.

[53] Allison RR, Ambrad AA, Arshoun Y, Carmel RJ, Ciuba DF, Feldman E, Finkelstein SE, Gandhavadi R, Heron DE, Lane SC, Longo JM, Meakin C, Papadopoulos D, Pruitt DE, Steinbrenner LM, Taylor MA, Wisbeck WM, Yuh GE, Nowotnik DP, Sonis ST. Multi-institutional, randomized, double-blind, placebo-controlled trial to assess the efficacy of a mucoadhesive hydrogel (MuGard) in mitigating

oral mucositis symptoms in patients being treated with chemoradiation therapy for cancers of the head and neck. Cancer. 2014; 120: 1433–40. https: //doi.org/10.1002/cncr.28553.
[54] ClinicalTrials.gov U.S. National Library of Medicine, clinical effect of phenytoin mucoadhesive paste on wound healing after oral biopsy, 2012. https: //clinicaltrials.gov/ct2/show/NCT01680042.
[55] Ghalayani P, Emami H, Pakravan F, Nasr Isfahani M. Comparison of triamcinolone acetonide mucoadhesive film with licorice mucoadhesive film on radiotherapy-induced oral mucositis: a randomized double-blinded clinical trial. Asia Pac J Clin Oncol. 2017; 13: e48–56. https: //doi. org/10.1111/ajco.12295.
[56] ClinicalTrials.gov U.S. National Library of Medicine, comparing triamcinolone acetonide mucoadhesive films with licorice mucoadhesive films, 2014. https: //clinicaltrials.gov/ct2/show/NCT02075749.
[57] ClinicalTrials.gov U.S. National Library of Medicine, comparison of triamcinolone acetonide mucoadhesive film and licorice mucoadhesive film effect on lichen planus, 2015. https: //www. clinicaltrials.gov/ct2/show/NCT02453503.
[58] ClinicalTrials.gov U.S. National Library of Medicine, efficacy and safety of forrad® for the management of radiation-induced mucositis in patients with nasopharyngeal carcinoma receiving IMRT, (2016). https: //clinicaltrials.gov/ct2/show/NCT02735317.
[59] ClinicalTrials.gov U.S. National Library of Medicine, efficacy of curcumin in oral submucous fibrosis (ECOSMF), 2018. https: //clinicaltrials.gov/ct2/show/NCT03511261.
[60] Hazarey VK, Sakrikar AR, Ganvir SM. Efficacy of curcumin in the treatment for oral submucous fibrosis – a randomized clinical trial. J Oral Maxillofac Pathol. 2015; 19: 145–52. https: //doi.org/10.4103/0973-029X. 164524.
[61] ClinicalTrials.gov U.S. National Library of Medicine, efficacy of a dietary supplement (Aqualief®) in xerostomic patients (Aqualief), 2018. https: //clinicaltrials.gov/ct2/show/NCT03612414.
[62] ClinicalTrials.gov U.S. National Library of Medicine, dexamethasone solution for the treatment of oral lichen planus, 2018. https: //clinicaltrials.gov/ct2/show/NCT02850601.
[63] ClinicalTrials.gov U.S. National Library of Medicine, Intra-oral treatment of OLP with Rivelin®-CLO patches, 2020. https: //clinicaltrials.gov/ct2/show/NCT03592342.
[64] ClinicalTrials.gov U.S. National Library of Medicine, effects of Aqualief® in patients with xerostomia as consequence of radiotherapy for head and neck cancer, 2020. https: //clinicaltrials. gov/ct2/show/NCT03601962.
[65] Braga FTMM, Santos ACF, Bueno PCP, Silveira RCCP, Santos CB, Bastos JK, Carvalho EC. Use of Chamomilla recutita in the prevention and treatment of oral mucositis in patients undergoing hematopoietic stem cell transplantation: a randomized, controlled, phase II clinical trial. Cancer Nurs. 2015; 38: 322–9. https: //doi.org/10.1097/NCC.0000000000000194.
[66] ClinicalTrials.gov U.S. National Library of Medicine, Topical chamomile in preventing chemotherapy-induced oral mucositis, 2020. https: //clinicaltrials.gov/ct2/show/NCT04317183.
[67] ClinicalTrials.gov U.S. National Library of Medicine, Carnosine supplementation on quantity/quality of oral salivae (PHoral), 2020. https: //www.clinicaltrials.gov/ct2/show/NCT04295525.
[68] Menon K, Mousa A, de Courten B. Effects of supplementation with carnosine and other histidine-containing dipeptides on chronic disease risk factors and outcomes: protocol for a systematic review of randomised controlled trials. BMJ Open. 2018; 8: e020623. https: //doi. org/10.1136/bmjopen-2017-020623.
[69] ClinicalTrials.gov U.S. National Library of Medicine, MucoLox formulation to mitigate mucositis symptoms in head/neck cancer, 2020. https: //clinicaltrials.gov/ct2/show/NCT03461354.
[70] Bhagavan HN, Chopra RK. Plasma coenzyme Q10 response to oral ingestion of coenzyme Q10 formulations. Mitochondrion. 2007; 7(Suppl): S78–88. https: //doi.org/10.1016/j. mito.2007.03.003.
[71] ClinicalTrials.gov U.S. National Library of Medicine, Clinical and biochemical assessment of the effect of topical use of coenzyme Q10 versus topical corticosteroid in management of symptomatic oral lichen planus: randomized controlled clinical trial, 2019. https: //clinicaltrials. gov/ct2/show/NCT04091698.
[72] Wen H, Jung H, Li X. Drug delivery approaches in addressing clinical pharmacology-related issues: opportunities and challenges. AAPS J. 2015; 17: 1327–40. https: //doi.org/10.1208/s12248-015-9814-9.
[73] Edsman K, Hägerström H. Pharmaceutical applications of mucoadhesion for the non-oral routes. J Pharm Pharmacol. 2005; 57: 3–22. https: //doi.org/10.1211/0022357055227.
[74] Sudhakar Y, Kuotsu K, Bandyopadhyay AK. Buccal bioadhesive drug delivery – a promising option for orally less efficient drugs. J Control Release. 2006; 114: 15–40. https: //doi. org/10.1016/j.jconrel.2006.04.012.
[75] Steward A, Bayley DL, Howes C. The effect of enhancers on the buccal absorption of hybrid (BDBB) α-interferon. Int J Pharm. 1994; 104: 145–9. https: //doi. org/10.1016/0378-5173(94)90189-9.
[76] Himanshi T, Sachdeva R. Transdermal drug delivery system: a review. Int J Pharm Sci Res. 2016; https: //doi.org/10.13040/IJPSR.0975-8232.7(6).2274-90.
[77] Das NG, Das SK. Development of mucoadhesive dosage forms of buprenorphine for sublingual drug delivery. Drug Deliv. 2004; 11: 89–95. https: //doi.org/10.1080/10717540490280688.
[78] Kováčik A, Kopečná M, Vávrová K. Permeation enhancers in transdermal drug delivery: benefits and limitations. Expert Opin Drug Deliv. 2020; 17: 145–55. https: //doi.org/10.1080/17425247.2020.1713087.
[79] Maher S, Brayden D, Casettari L, Illum L. Application of permeation enhancers in oral delivery of macromolecules: an update. Pharmaceutics. 2019; 11: 41. https: //doi.org/10.3390/pharmaceutics11010041.